rn c   ə las

(

Critical Pathways in Cardiology

Critical Pathways in Cardiology

Editors

Christopher P. Cannon, M.D.
Cardiovascular Division
Brigham and Women's Hospital
Assistant Professor of Medicine
Harvard Medical School
Boston, Massachusetts

Patrick T. O'Gara, M.D.
Director, Clinical Cardiology
Brigham and Women's Hospital
Associate Professor of Medicine
Harvard Medical School
Boston, Massachusetts

LIPPINCOTT WILLIAMS & WILKINS
A **Wolters Kluwer** Company

Philadelphia • Baltimore • New York • London
Buenos Aires • Hong Kong • Sydney • Tokyo

Acquisitions Editor: Ruth W. Weinberg
Developmental Editor: Stacey L. Baze
Production Editor: Emily Lerman
Manufacturing Manager: Colin J. Warnock
Cover Designer: Mark Lerner
Compositor: The PRD Group
Printer: R. R. Donnelley–Willard

© **2001 by LIPPINCOTT WILLIAMS & WILKINS**
530 Walnut Street
Philadelphia, PA 19106 USA
LWW.com

Printed in the USA

Library of Congress Cataloging-in-Publication Data

Critical pathways in cardiology / editors, Christopher P. Cannon, Patrick T. O'Gara.
    p. ; cm.
    Includes bibliographical references and index.
    ISBN 0-7817-2621-2 (alk. paper)
    1. Cardiology.   2. Critical path analysis.   3. Outcome assessment (Medical care).
  4. Medical protocols.   I. Cannon, Christopher P.   II. O'Gara, Patrick T.
    [DNLM: 1. Cardiovascular Diseases—diagnosis.   2. Cardiovascular Diseases—therapy.
  3. Critical Care—standards.   4. Critical Pathways. WG 141 C934 2001]
    RC669 .C755   2001
    616.1′2—dc21

                                                    00-067146

10 9 8 7 6 5 4 3 2 1

Contents

Part IV. Critical Pathways in the Outpatient Setting

Contributing Authors

Michelle A. Albert, M.D.,   *Research Fellow, Department of Medicine, Harvard Medical School, 116 Huntington Avenue; Research/Clinical Fellow, Department of Medicine, Cardiovascular Division, Brigham and Women's Hospital, 75 Francis Street, Boston, Massachusetts 02115*

Bruce Becker, M.D.,   *Associate Professor, Department of Community Health, Brown University School of Medicine; Department of Emergency Medicine, Rhode Island Hospital, 53 Eddy Street, Providence, Rhode Island 02903*

Richard C. Becker, M.D.,   *Professor, Department of Medicine, University of Massachusetts Medical School; Director, Coronary Care Unit, University of Massachusetts Memorial Medical Center, 55 Lake Avenue, Worcester, Massachusetts 01655*

Joshua A. Beckman, M.D.,   *Instructor, Cardiovascular Division, Department of Medicine, Harvard University; Cardiovascular Division, Department of Medicine, Brigham and Women's Hospital, 75 Francis Street, Boston, Massachusetts 02115*

Beth C. Bock, Ph.D.,   *Assistant Professor, Department of Psychiatry and Human Behavior, Brown University School of Medicine; Staff Psychologist, Center for Behavioral Medicine, The Miriam Hospital, 164 Summit Avenue, Providence, Rhode Island 02906*

J. Stephen Bohan, M.D., F.A.C.P., F.A.C.E.P.,   *Instructor, Harvard Medical School; Clinical Director, Department of Emergency Medicine, Brigham and Women's Hospital, 75 Francis Street, Boston, Massachusetts 02115*

John G. Byrne, M.D.,   *Associate Professor, Department of Surgery, Harvard Medical School; Associate Cardiac Surgeon, Department of Surgery, Brigham and Women's Hospital, 75 Francis Street, Boston, Massachusetts 02115*

Christopher P. Cannon, M.D.,   *Assistant Professor of Medicine, Harvard Medical School; Cardiovascular Division, Brigham and Women's Hospital, 75 Francis Street, Boston, Massachusetts 02115*

Shirley Chan, B.S.,   *Research Coordinator, Brigham and Women's Hospital, 75 Francis Street, Boston, Massachusetts 02115*

Paul R. Conlin, M.D.,   *Assistant Professor, Department of Medicine, Harvard Medical School; Director, Endocrinology Training Program, Endocrinology–Hypertension Division, Brigham and Women's Hospital, 221 Longwood Avenue, Boston, Massachusetts 02115*

Kirsten E. Fleischmann, M.D.,   *Assistant Professor of Medicine, Cardiology Division, University of California, San Francisco; Physician, Department of Cardiology, University of California San Francisco Medical Center, 505 Parnassus Avenue, San Francisco, California 94143*

Leonard I. Ganz, M.D.,   *Associate Professor, Department of Medicine, University of Pittsburgh School of Medicine; Director of Cardiac Electrophysiology, Cardiovascular Institute, University of Pittsburgh Medical Center, 200 Lothrop Street, Pittsburgh, Pennsylvania 15213*

Bernard J. Gersh, M.B., Ch.B., D.Phil.,   *Professor of Medicine, Department of Cardiovascular Diseases, Mayo Medical School; Consultant, Department of Cardiovascular Diseases, Mayo Clinic, 200 First Street SW, Rochester, Minnesota 55905*

Samuel Z. Goldhaber, M.D., *Associate Professor, Department of Medicine, Harvard Medical School; Director, Venous Thromboembolism Research Group and Director, Cardiac Center's Anticoagulation Service, Department of Medicine, Cardiovascular Division, Brigham and Women's Hospital, 75 Francis Street, Boston, Massachusetts 02115*

Cindy L. Grines, M.D., *Director, Cardiac Catheterization Laboratory and Director, Interventional Cardiology Fellowship, William Beaumont Hospital, 3601 West Thirteen Mile Road, Royal Oak, Michigan 48073*

L. Howard Hartley, M.D., *Associate Professor, Department of Medicine, Harvard Medical School, Shattuck Street; Director of Cardiac Rehabilitation, Division of Cardiology, Brigham and Women's Hospital, 75 Francis Street, Boston, Massachusetts 02115*

Thomas H. Lee., M.D., *Associate Professor, Department of Medicine, Harvard University, Cambridge, Massachusetts 02138; Physician, Department of Internal Medicine, Brigham and Women's Hospital, 75 Francis Street, Boston, Massachusetts 02115*

Norman W. Lindenmuth, M.D., *Clinical Faculty, Department of Medicine, University of Rochester, Elmwood Avenue, Rochester, New York 14627; Vice President of Medical Affairs, Finger Lakes Health System; Department of Medicine, Geneva General Hospital, 196 North Street, Geneva, New York 14456*

Nancy Sinclair McNamara, R.N., B.S.N., *Cardiology Resource/Research Nurse-Coordinator, Cardiovascular Specialties, Exeter Hospital, 10 Buzell Avenue, Exeter, New Hampshire 03833*

Patrick T. O'Gara, M.D., *Associate Professor of Medicine, Harvard Medical School; Director, Clinical Cardiology, Brigham and Women's Hospital, 75 Francis Street, Boston, Massachusetts 02115*

Joseph P. Ornato, M.D., F.A.C.C., F.A.C.E.P., *Professor and Chairman, Department of Emergency Medicine, Virginia Commonwealth University's Medical College of Virginia, 401 North 12th Street, Richmond, Virginia 23298*

Edward F. Philbin, III, M.D., F.A.C.C., *Associate Professor, Department of Medicine, Division of Cardiology, Albany Medical College; Division Head, Division of Cardiology, Albany Medical Center Hospital, 47 New Scotland Avenue, Albany, New York 12208*

Carísi A. Polanczyk, M.D., *Physician, Department of Cardiology, Hospital de Clinicas de Porto Alegre, Ramiro Barcelos 2350/2225, Porto Alegre, RS 9000, Brazil*

Jeffrey J. Popma, M.D., *Associate Professor, Department of Medicine, Harvard Medical School; Director, Interventional Cardiology, Brigham and Women's Hospital, 75 Francis Street, Boston, Massachusetts 02115*

Daniel J. Rader, M.D., *Director, Preventive Cardiovascular Medicine, University of Pennsylvania Health System, 4th Floor PHI Building, Presbyterian Medical Center, 39th and Market Streets; Associate Professor, Department of Medicine, University of Pennsylvania, 421 Curie Boulevard, Philadelphia, Pennsylvania 19104*

James D. Rawn, M.D., *Instructor and Associate Surgeon, Division of Cardiac Surgery, Brigham and Women's Hospital, 75 Francis Street, Boston, Massachusetts 02115*

Christopher F. Richards, M.D., *Assistant Professor and Assistant Director, Acute Care Services, Department of Emergency Medicine, Oregon Health Sciences University, 3181 SW Sam Jackson Park Road, Portland, Oregon 97201*

Donna M. Rosborough, M.S., R.N., *Care Coordinator, Cardiac Surgery Service, Brigham and Women's Hospital, 75 Francis Street, Boston, Massachusetts 02115*

Alan B. Storrow, M.D., *Assistant Professor, Department of Emergency Medicine, University of Cincinnati, 231 Albert B. Sabin Way; Faculty, Department of Emergency Medicine, University Hospital, 234 Goodman Street, Cincinnati, Ohio 45267*

Ron M. Walls, M.D., *Associate Professor, Department of Medicine, Division of Emergency Medicine, Harvard Medical School, 25 Shattuck Street; Chairman, Department of Emergency Medicine, Brigham and Women's Hospital, 75 Francis Street, Boston, Massachusetts 02115*

Thomas P. Wharton, Jr., M.D., F.A.C.C., *Medical Director, Cardiology Section and Cardiac Catheterization Laboratory, Exeter Hospital, The Perry Medical Services Building, 3 Alumni Drive, Exeter, New Hampshire 03833*

Robert Wolyn, M.D., *Interventional Cardiology Fellow, William Beaumont Hospital, 3601 West Thirteen Mile Road, Royal Oak, Michigan 48073*

R. Scott Wright, M.D., *Assistant Professor, Department of Medicine, Mayo Clinic and Foundation, 200 First Street SW, Rochester, Minnesota 55905*

Preface

The past 10 to 15 years have witnessed remarkable progress in the field of cardiology. The evidence that has emerged on effective new therapies for several important cardiovascular diseases is quite impressive. For example, the treatment of acute myocardial infarction 15 years ago consisted of nitroglycerin, beta-blockers, and morphine. Now patients also receive fibrinolytic therapy, aspirin, heparin, ACE inhibitors, statins, and, in some cases, glycoprotein IIb/IIIa inhibitors. Indeed, we are in an era when each year there are new therapies and approaches to the management of patients with every cardiac condition.

How do busy clinicians keep up with the latest advances and ensure that their patients receive current state-of-the-art therapy? One approach has been the development and use of critical pathways. These are standardized documents or computer order sets that incorporate new therapies and simultaneously attempt to streamline treatment in order to make it more cost-effective. Critical pathways have grown in use, initially as a means of reducing hospital length of stay. However, they offer a unique opportunity to raise the standard of care at institutions, while at the same time to include all the appropriate tests and treatments for patients. In this fashion, they serve as a readily available guide to the clinician when treating the patient. They also may serve as a means of improving compliance with current guidelines for treating patients.

We are delighted to present in this book a full array of critical pathways from leading institutions around the country. These pathways are the "best practices" for these hospitals, developed by leaders in their areas of expertise. The authors have done a superb job of integrating the key clinical data into brief summaries and then providing the critical pathways that they use at their hospitals. We have organized this book in a fashion to facilitate using the information. We begin with an overview of what critical pathways are and how to develop them. We then present several pathways for management of patients in the Emergency Department, focusing on patients with acute coronary syndromes. The next section covers the types of patients who are admitted to the hospital, and the final section includes several outpatient critical pathways, such as management of hypertension and lipid disorders. It is hoped that these pathways will allow clinicians around the world to adopt critical pathways more easily as a means of improving the care of their cardiac patients.

Christopher P. Cannon, M.D.
Patrick T. O'Gara, M.D.

PART I

General Principles

CHAPTER 1

Goals, Design, and Implementation of Critical Pathways in Cardiology

Christopher P. Cannon and Patrick T. O'Gara

"Critical pathways" are standardized protocols for the management of specific disorders aimed at optimizing and streamlining patient care. Numerous other names have been developed for such programs, including "clinical pathways" (so as not to suggest to patients that they are in a "critical" condition), or simply "protocols," such as acute myocardial infarction (MI) protocols used in emergency departments to reduce time to treatment with thrombolysis (1–3). A broader name—disease management—is currently used to denote that these pathways extend beyond the hospital phase of treatment, to optimize medical management over the long-term.

The complexity of the pathways has also been used to distinguish true critical pathways (e.g., coronary artery bypass surgery pathways; Chapter 14) as tools that detail the processes of care and potential inefficiencies, from "clinical protocols," which are algorithms and treatment recommendations focused on improving compliance with evidence-based medicine. Different disease states lend themselves to more complex pathways, such as those for coronary artery bypass surgery. In contrast, for medical conditions in which patients are treated in the ambulatory setting (e.g., hypertension or hyperlipidemia; Chapters 20 and 21), the critical pathways tend to be more algorithm-based documents. Notwithstanding these minor differences in terminology, a broader view of critical pathways is adopted in this book, where various types of pathways are presented by leading clinicians to summarize current, state-of-the art cardiology and cardiac surgical practice.

GOALS OF CRITICAL PATHWAYS

Critical pathway use initially emerged as a means to reduce length of hospitalization. However, clinicians have recognized many other goals for such pathways, the most important of which is the need to improve the quality of patient care (Table 1-1). Indeed, physicians involved in developing critical pathways should focus on the positive aspects of pathways and use them as a means to advance medical care. Other

specific goals focus on (a) improving the use of medications and treatments; (b) improving patient triage to the appropriate level of care; (c) increasing participation in research protocols; and (d) limiting the use of unnecessary tests to reduce costs and allow savings to be allocated to other treatments that have been shown to be beneficial (1,4). With involvement of physicians, nurses, and other clinicians in the development of these pathways, those responsible for patient care can control how the patients are managed. It should be noted that data are only now beginning to emerge regarding the success of various pathways. Indeed, we should remain critical of pathways, and monitor their performance to ensure that they meet the overall goal of reducing costs while improving (or at least maintaining) the quality of patient care.

NEED AND RATIONALE FOR CRITICAL PATHWAYS

Despite widespread dissemination of the clinical trial results, many patients with acute coronary syndromes do not receive evidence-based medical therapies. Such a glaring deficiency has been seen most dramatically for aspirin, but is also apparent with the use of thrombolytic therapy, beta-blockers, and many other classes of drugs (5–10).

Another need addressed by critical pathways is the marked variation in the use of cardiac procedures following admission for acute MI and unstable angina. In acute ST-segment elevation MI, numerous studies have found wide differences in the use of invasive cardiac procedures but no differences in mortality, suggesting that some of these procedures may be unnecessary or inappropriate (11–13).

Other areas of potential overutilization of testing also exist (e.g., laboratory tests and echocardiography) (14–16). Several studies have suggested that for patients with small non–Q-wave MIs, assessment of left ventricular function via echocardiography or ventriculography may not be necessary, a strategy which could have potential implications for more cost-effective care.

TABLE 1-1. *Goals of critical pathways*

Improve patient care
Increase use of recommended medical therapies (e.g., aspirin for all acute coronary syndromes, reperfusion therapy for ST-segment myocardial infarction elevation)
Decrease use of unnecessary tests
Decrease length of hospitalizations
Reduce costs
Increase participation in clinical research protocols

TABLE 1-2. *Steps in developing and implementing a critical pathway*

Identify problems in patient care. (e.g., underutilization of evidence-based therapies, excess resource use, long length of hospitalizations)
Identify committee to develop guidelines and critical pathway
Distribute a draft critical pathway to all departments involved
Revise pathway to reach a consensus
Implement the pathway
Collect and monitor data on critical pathway performance
Periodically modify or update the critical pathway as needed to further improve performance and keep current with new therapies and treatments

Reducing Hospital (and Intensive Care Unit) Length of Stay

Reduction in the length of hospitalization has been the driving force behind creation of critical pathways. As noted in the initial pathways for cardiac surgical patients, early discharge was the main outcome variable (17). In acute coronary syndromes, just 5 years ago hospitalization was very lengthy: in 1993, it was 9 days for patients with unstable angina in both the Thrombolysis in Myocardial Infarction (TIMI) IIIB trial and the parallel TIMI III registry. In the Global Utilization of Streptokinase and tPA for Occluded Coronary Arteries (GUSTO-I) trial, conducted in the early 1990s, the median length of stay was 9 days, and did not differ between patients with in-hospital complications versus those who had an uncomplicated course (18). In the TIMI-9 registry conducted in 1995 for uncomplicated patients with ST-segment elevation MI, the median length of stay was 8 days (9,19). Thus, it appears that hospitalizations have historically been lengthy for patients with acute coronary syndromes, and opportunities exist to safely reduce them, especially for patients at low risk.

Overutilization of Intensive Care

Overutilization of the intensive and coronary care units (CCU) is another area in which critical pathways can reduce costs. A decade ago, admission to the CCU was standard for all patients with unstable angina and MI (frequently to "rule out MI") (20,21). Even recently in the multicenter GUARANTEE registry conducted in the United States in 1996, 40% of patients with unstable angina and non–ST-segment elevation MI were admitted to the CCU (22). Because CCU admission is now generally recommended for patients at higher risk (i.e., those with ST-segment elevation MI, hemodynamic compromise, or other complications), such data suggest opportunities may exist for reducing the number of patients admitted to intensive care units.

METHODS FOR THE DEVELOPMENT OF CRITICAL PATHWAYS

The process of developing a critical pathway derives first from identifying the problem (Table 1-2). Beginning with a specific diagnosis, the obstacles to the appropriate care of patients are delineated (e.g., low use of aspirin, as noted above) in parallel with the prevailing issues at the institutional level. For example, the use of blood tests might be higher than necessary when left to an individual house officer or physician (e.g., multiple cholesterol measurements during a single hospital stay).

The next step is to establish a task force or committee (composed of clinicians recognized as local thought leaders) to create (or adapt) a critical pathway that would include recommended guidelines for the treatment of patients with specific diagnoses. The third step is to distribute the draft critical pathway(s) to all healthcare professionals and services involved in the management of patients with those diagnoses, to ensure adequate input from all parties involved. For example, an unstable angina pathway should include members of the cardiology, cardiac surgery, emergency medicine, nursing, noninvasive laboratory, cardiac rehabilitation, social service, case management, and dietary service. Comments from these parties are then included in the final pathway.

Implementation of the pathway can begin with a "pilot" and then be available for routine use. The fifth step in the process of establishing a critical pathway is to collect and monitor data regarding performance. This could include the number of patients for whom the pathway was used, use of recommended therapy and the hospital length of stay. The final step is to interpret the initial data and to modify the pathway as needed. These latter three steps collectively consist of the continuous quality improvement that must be ongoing during the implementation of any pathway. In addition, as new therapies become available, the data should be reviewed to determine which steps should be added or modified as part of optimal patient management.

Methods of Implementation

Several potential methods of implementation exist. First, voluntary participation in a pathway. Although this appears to be an inefficient means of ensuring participation with a critical pathway, it is frequently all that can be accomplished with limited resources at individual hospitals. The pathway could be sent to physicians and nurses and presented at appropriate staff meetings. Another means of triggering pathway use would be reminders via electronic mail messages triggered from the admission diagnosis, or monthly reminders to physicians and nurses. Another approach is to have independent screening of all admissions, with copies of the pathway placed in the chart. Use of the pathway would be expected to be low with such a voluntary approach. On the other hand, if a pathway becomes implemented in an initial group of patients, that treatment strategy may become the standard of care at a particular hospital. Later, it may no longer be necessary to actually involve additional personnel to implement the pathway.

An alternate approach that some hospitals have used is to have a designated case manager evaluate each patient and ensure that all steps in the pathway are carried out. Such an approach would be expected to improve the use of the pathway. However, this approach obviously requires additional resources from the hospital or healthcare system. The approach used by individual hospitals for specific diagnoses needs to be individualized. The ultimate goal is to improve the care of patients and make such care more cost-effective.

"Cardiac Checklist"

A very simplified version of a critical pathway is to use a "cardiac checklist." Although checklists exist for many purposes, including admission tests and procedures, this format can be extended to medical treatments. It is a simple method to ensure that each patient receives all the recommended therapies. Table 1-3 shows an example cardiac checklist for the patient with unstable angina or non–ST-segment elevation MI. This checklist could be used in two ways: physicians could keep a copy on a small index card in their pocket and scan down the list when writing admission orders, or the checklist could be used to develop standard orders for a patient with MI,

either printed or computerized, from which the physician can choose when admitting a patient (Chapters 4, 8–12). Such a system has worked well in ensuring extremely high compliance with evidence-based recommendations at Brigham and Women's Hospital (Cannon, unpublished data). In the era of "scorecard medicine," many outside observers (e.g., health maintenance organizations or insurers) tally up the use of recommended medications as quality of care measures (23,24). Use of a cardiac checklist should allow physicians (and patients) to "win" the game and improve the quality of care for patients.

CONCLUSIONS AND FUTURE DIRECTIONS

Use of critical pathways is increasing rapidly. They offer great potential for reducing both length of hospitalizations and costs, and for improving patient care. Standardized approaches with simple checklists to ensure the appropriate use of medications will be a significant improvement in patient care. Improving the administrative links between different departments to make these pathways work may also benefit patient care. After the development of pathways, their performance must be monitored to ensure that they meet the overall goal of reducing costs while improving the quality of patient care. It is our belief that this goal can be achieved.

The evolution of critical pathways is just beginning. Evidence is not yet available regarding the usefulness of these pathways, but research is ongoing to evaluate the patient outcomes. New ways of implementing the pathways need to be developed, the most promising of which appears to be use of computer technology.

TABLE 1-3. *"Cardiac checklist" for unstable angina and non–ST-segment elevation myocardial infarction*

Medications
1. Aspirin.. ☐
2. Heparin/LMWH .... ☐
3. IIb/IIIa inhibition .... ☐
4. Beta-blockers .... ☐
5. Nitrates... ☐
6. ACE inhibitors if low EF/CHF.................... ☐

Interventions
7. Catheterization and revascularization for recurrent ischemia or patients at medium to high risk.............. ☐

Secondary prevention
8. Cholesterol—check + Rx as needed......... ☐
9. Smoking cessation................................. ☐
10. Treat other risk factors (hypertension, diabetes)........ ☐

ACE, angiotensin converting enzyme; CHF, congestive heart failure; EF, ejection fraction; LMWH, low molecular weight heparin.
Adapted from Cannon CP. Optimizing the treatment of unstable angina. *J Thromb Thrombolysis* 1995;2:205–218; with permission.

REFERENCES

1. Cannon CP, Antman EM, Walls R, Braunwald E. Time as an adjunctive agent to thrombolytic therapy. *J Thromb Thrombolysis* 1994;1:27–34.
2. National Heart Attack Alert Program Coordinating Committee—60 Minutes to Treatment Working Group. Emergency department: rapid identification and treatment of patients with acute myocardial infarction. *Ann Emerg Med* 1994;23:311–329.
3. Every NR, Hochman J, Becker R, et al., for the Committee on Acute Cardiac Care, Council of Clinical Cardiology, American Heart Association. Critical pathways: a review. An AHA Scientific Statement. *Circulation* 2000;101:461–465.
4. Cannon CP. Optimizing the treatment of unstable angina. *J Thromb Thrombolysis* 1995;2:205–218.
5. Rogers WJ, Bowlby LJ, Chandra NC, et al. Treatment of myocardial infarction in the United States (1990 to 1993). Observations from the National Registry of Myocardial Infarction. *Circulation* 1994;90:2103–2114.
6. Ellerbeck EF, Jencks SF, Radford MJ, et al. Quality of care for Medicare patients with acute myocardial infarction. A four-state pilot study from the Cooperative Cardiovascular Project. *JAMA* 1995;273:1509–1514.
7. Scirica BM, Moliterno DJ, Every NR, et al. Differences between men and women in the management of unstable angina pectoris (The GUARANTEE Registry). *Am J Cardiol* 1999;84:1145–1150.
8. Barron HV, Bowlby LJ, Breen T, et al. Use of reperfusion therapy for acute myocardial infarction in the United States: data from the National Registry of Myocardial Infarction 2. *Circulation* 1998;97:1150–1156.
9. Cannon CP, Henry TD, Schweiger MJ, et al. Current management of ST elevation myocardial infarction and outcome of thrombolytic ineligible

patients: results of the multicenter TIMI 9 Registry. *J Am Coll Cardiol* 1995;(Special Issue):231A–232A.

10. Krumholz HM, Radford MJ, Wang Y, et al. Early beta-blocker therapy for acute myocardial infarction in elderly patients. *Ann Intern Med* 1999;131:648–654.

11. Every NR, Parson LS, Fihn SD, et al. Long-term outcome in acute myocardial infarction patients admitted to hospitals with and without on-site cardiac catheterization facilities. *Circulation* 1997;96:1770–1775.

12. Rouleau JL, Moye LA, Pfeffer MA, et al. A comparison of management patterns after acute myocardial infarction in Canada and the United States. *N Engl J Med* 1993;328:779–784.

13. Pilote L, Califf RM, Sapp S, et al. Regional variation across the United States in the management of acute myocardial infarction. *N Engl J Med* 1995;333:565–572.

14. Silver MT, Rose GA, Paul SD, et al. A clinical rule to predict preserved left ventricular ejection fraction in patients after myocardial infarction. *Ann Intern Med* 1994;121:750–756.

15. Tobin K, Stomel R, Harber D, et al. Validation of a clinical prediction rule for predicting left ventricular function post acute myocardial infarction in a community hospital setting. *J Am Coll Cardiol* 1996;27[Suppl A]:318A.

16. Krumholtz HM, Howes CJ, Murillo JE, et al. Validation of a clinical prediction rule for left ventricular ejection fraction after myocardial infarction in patients >65 years old. *Am J Cardiol* 1997;80:11–15.

17. Nickerson NJ, Murphy SF, Kouchoukos NT, et al. Predictors of early discharge after cardiac surgery and its cost-effectiveness. *J Am Coll Cardiol* 1996;27:264A.

18. Newby LK, Califf RM, for the GUSTO Investigators. Redefining uncomplicated myocardial infarction in the thrombolytic era. *Circulation* 1994;90(Pt. 2):I-110.

19. Cannon CP, Antman EM, Gibson CM, et al. Critical pathway for acute ST segment elevation myocardial infarction: evaluation of the potential impact in the TIMI 9 registry. *J Am Coll Cardiol* 1998;31[Suppl A]:192A.

20. Goldman L, Cook EF, Brand DA, et al. A computer protocol to predict myocardial infarction in emergency department patients with chest pain. *N Engl J Med* 1988;318:797–803.

21. Pozen MW, D'Agostino RB, Mitchell JB, et al. The usefulness of a predictive instrument to reduce inappropriate admissions to the coronary care unit. *Ann Intern Med* 1980;92:238–242.

22. Cannon CP, Moliterno DJ, Every N, et al. Implementation of AHCPR guidelines for unstable angina in 1996: unfortunate differences between men & women. Results from the multicenter GUARANTEE registry. *J Am Coll Cardiol* 1997;29[Suppl A]:217A.

23. Topol EJ, Califf RM. Scorecard cardiovascular medicine. Its impact and future directions. *Ann Intern Med* 1994;120:65–70.

24. Topol EJ, Block PC, Holmes DR, et al. Readiness for the scorecard era in cardiovascular medicine. *Am J Cardiol* 1995;75:1170–1173.

CHAPTER 2

Potential Pitfalls in the Development of Successful Critical Pathways

Carísi A. Polanczyk and Thomas H. Lee

In recent years, intense pressure to reduce costs of delivering healthcare has led many healthcare organizations to seek strategies that reduce resource utilization while maintaining or improving the quality of care. Among the most popular of the methods described are critical pathways (i.e., management plans that display goals for patients and provide the corresponding ideal sequence and timing of staff actions to achieve optimal efficiency under a specific medical condition) (1). They can be used both to describe a management plan for optimal care of the ideal uncomplicated patient and to collect information on the frequency and reasons for deviations from that plan.

Although conceptually pathways are attractive and have been rapidly disseminated in hospitals throughout the world, many uncertainties remain about their impact and use. Concerns have been raised about their effect on patient outcomes, physician autonomy, and malpractice liability. Beyond these issues is the paucity of evidence from controlled trials for the impact of critical pathways on quality or efficiency. Finally, even when data support the impact of a pathway, the findings may have limited generalizability, because (a) the effectiveness of pathways is likely to be strongly influenced by the local cultural and financial environment and (b) pathways should evolve over time to keep pace with medical progress.

DIFFICULTY IN ASSESSING EFFECTIVENESS OF CRITICAL PATHWAYS

Several institutions have described their experience with clinical pathways, but most "studies" have significant methodologic limitations and very few have been well-controlled trials. The limitations are not caused by a lack of sophistication by the investigators. It is difficult to perform a trial at a single institution in which patients are randomized because of the high probability of contamination: the care of patients randomly assigned to "usual care" is likely to be highly influenced by the caregiver's knowledge of the pathway's recommendations. A time-series study design is also difficult to perform, because management strategies recommended by the pathway are unlikely to "wash out" even after several weeks. In addition, most hospitals have had a secular trend toward reduction in length of hospitalizations in recent years; therefore, studies looking at resource use before and after the implementation of a trial are likely to find improvements that may have little to do with the pathway itself.

Most published studies of critical pathways have reported reductions in both length of hospitalizations and direct costs (2–6). These reports have generally found no adverse effects on quality of care, or some improvements (7–9). These findings must be interpreted with caution, however, because the possibility of "reporting bias" is likely to lead to overrepresentation of "positive" studies in the literature. Nevertheless, reason exists to encourage the experience described in some studies.

In one study, for example, a critical pathway for elective coronary artery bypass grafting was implemented by a multidisciplinary team. Introduction of the critical pathway was associated with a reduction in total length of hospitalization (11.1 $\pm$ 6.6 days versus 7.7 $\pm$ 2.3 days, $p < 0.001$). Mean hospital costs were $1,181 lower in the critical pathway group when compared with the control group. Postoperative mortality and readmission rates were similar for the two groups (10).

One of the most rigorous studies of pathway use was a recent multicenter, controlled clinical trial of a critical pathway for community-acquired pneumonia, performed at 19 hospitals in Canada. Hospitals were assigned to conventional management or critical pathway implementation. The investigators found that pathway use was associated with a 1.7-day reduction in bed days per patient managed and an 18% decrease in the admission of patients at low risk. No differences were seen on quality of life, occurrence of complications, readmission, and mortality rate between the two strategies (9).

Nevertheless, reports also suggest little or no impact from critical pathways (11). In an observational study, Holmboe et al. (12) compared hospitals with and without specific critical pathways for myocardial infarction. Of 32 nonfederal hospitals evaluated, 10 developed critical pathways and 18 of 22 nonpathway hospitals employed some combination of standard orders, multidisciplinary teams, or physician champions. The study used outcomes, including the proportion of patients who received evidence-based medical therapies, length of stay, and 30-day mortality rate. Hospitals that instituted critical pathways did *not* have increased use of proved medical therapies (e.g., aspirin, beta-blockers, and reperfusion therapy), shorter length of stay, or reductions in mortality compared with other hospitals (12).

The physicians and others who develop pathways are often surprised that it is difficult to derive a major impact from these initiatives. One possible explanation is the difficulty of isolating the impact of pathways from that of other continuous quality improvement strategies being implemented concurrently. Pathways might be only one piece of the puzzle involved in improving the quality and efficiency of care. Hence, improvements in performance through implementation of a pathway should never be accepted as certain.

PRIORITIZATION

Some institutions mistakenly try to implement many (even dozens) critical pathways at once. Overly ambitious efforts keep the institution from focusing attention on the most important areas and committing itself to achieving success in them. A more appropriate strategy is for institutions to identify a small number of protocols (e.g., 3–4) on which to concentrate these efforts. Data should be analyzed to assess objectively which areas offer the most opportunity. The criteria by which projects are chosen should generally include the following:

- Patient volume: Staff will not find it worthwhile to invest the time to standardize care for low volume procedures or diagnoses.
- Perceived opportunity: Data should be analyzed to determine whether the local institution or provider group lags behind quality or efficiency in benchmarks or "best practices" from elsewhere. Examples might be longer hospitalizations than a competitor or a longer period before administration of thrombolytic therapy for patients with acute myocardial infarction.
- Economic and strategic importance: Because the time and attention of healthcare providers is currently under such pressure, efforts generally should be focused on developing pathways that are likely to be rewarded economically, either through greater efficiency or improved marketability because of better quality. If a certain procedure (e.g., coronary artery bypass graft surgery) is of particular interest to a payer or the business community, that interest should be considered in choosing topics for pathway implementation.
- Availability of a local champion: Although pathways from other institutions are almost invariably sound, success is often dependent on the availability of a local physician opinion leader who can articulate the case for using a pathway and can help make the pathway something locally "owned."

TEAM DEVELOPMENT

Pathway development can stall if the team is inappropriately organized or does not understand its goal. The involvement of true local opinion leaders is advisable, as is the invitation of opinion leaders who are most likely to be critics at the end of the process. The team should be multidisciplinary and include nonclinicians (e.g., hospital administrators and office staff). An ideal size for a team is 7 to 10 members.

In organizing the team, it is useful to establish explicit goals, including a time by which key milestones will be achieved. Weekly or biweekly meetings (often at an early hour) are useful to clarify that the team is engaged in a time-limited process. Meetings should include a clear agenda, and tasks for the next meeting should be established.

The team should also understand that the goal of the pathway is not just to codify current practices. Establish target changes in length of hospitalization or other measures so that the team can ultimately decide whether the project succeeded or failed. Otherwise, a real danger exists that the targets of the pathway will not be sufficiently ambitious to change practice patterns. Some data suggest that the major impact of a pathway can be accomplished simply by organizing the teams and reaching consensus on the need to achieve the goals. For example, one institution reported that a protocol for renal transplantation was associated with declines in length of stay, complications, and infection, but much of the effect was seen during development rather than during implementation (13). Such findings do not imply a failure of the pathway, because the development of a pathway is part of the overall process.

ACCEPTANCE

Physicians and others who do not participate in the development of a pathway are often resistant to its use. They may assert that it is not appropriate for their patients because of illness severity or other reasons. (One common reaction of physicians to pathways is: "Very nice—but not for me or my patients.") In some institutions, strong leadership can achieve a consensus that a pathway will be the standard management protocol for patients with a given diagnosis. At most hospitals, however, physicians must be convinced individually to allow their patients to participate. For this reason, it is important to have true opinion leaders (not just junior physicians who are available) lead these initiatives.

Participation can often be enhanced by profiling length of hospitalization or other measures for those physicians who use the pathway and for those who do not. Another strategy is to make care simpler for physicians who use the pathway by establishing order sets that reduce writing and other burdens.

Acceptance can also be facilitated by keeping pathways simple. They should really just include the absolutely key steps that must be performed to accomplish the goal. They need not include every step in the care process. Focusing attention on a small number of steps decreases the opportunity for criticizing pathways over issues for which no controlled data exist (e.g., nasal oxygen use for patients suspected of having myocardial ischemia).

SUSTAINABILITY

Pathway implementation is often accompanied by a decline in length of hospitalization or other form of improvement. However, some hospitals note difficulty sustaining these effects over time. The most effective strategy to counter this problem is to build collection and feedback of data on pathway performance into routine care. When physicians understand that they are going to see data on their success or failure in performing certain processes on an ongoing basis, they tend to maintain high levels of performance.

The effectiveness of changing behavior can also be enhanced by reporting data as failure rates. For example, it is more compelling to physicians to hear that they failed to administer thrombolytic therapy within 30 minutes in 25% of cases than to hear that their average time to thrombolysis was 35 minutes. In fact, their average performance may be within a target period, whereas they are still failing to achieve the goal for an unacceptable percentage of cases.

Many institutions find it useful to update periodically the pathways and then reintroduce the protocol to renew interest and focus. One study evaluated a pathway for abdominal aortic aneurysm surgery in three different periods: prepathway, first year of the pathway, and later when data from the pathway were analyzed after some modifications. Although positive results were seen in the first year, practice modifications based on interim data analysis yielded further reductions in charges and length of hospitalizations and no change in mortality rate (14).

RELEVANCE

Pathways are developed to be the ideal plan of care for patients with uncomplicated specific conditions. However, these plans may be unachievable for patients with comorbid medical conditions (15). Similarly, some conditions and procedures have more variable outcomes than others. For example, compliance with length of stay goals with carotid endarterectomy pathways tends to be greater than with aortic surgery pathways (16).

Although the heterogeneity of patients and procedures is an important factor in considering the potential impact of pathways, physicians should not be too quick to give up on individual patients or diagnoses as candidates for pathways. Very elderly patients, for example, may "fall behind" the pathway a day or so early in their course, but the availability of a plan can promote quality and efficiency later in the hospitalization. In addition, high rates of "success" as expressed as the percentage of patients who meet length of stay goals for a pathway do not actually mean the pathway is "good." They may mean that the length of stay goal is not sufficiently ambitious.

OTHER CULTURAL FACTORS

As noted, critical factors for success with pathways seem to include involvement of local clinicians, a unified or closed medical staff, as well as non-physician clinicians (nurses, pharmacists, nurse practitioners, and physician assistants), who may be more likely than physicians to comply with the protocol (17). "Real time" feedback of information on deviation from the pathway has been shown to reduce resource use in a variety of syndromes including chest pain, pulmonary edema, and syncope (18–20). Finally, pathways that exert their influence by making recommendations to act (rather than withhold) appear to be more likely to be implemented, especially when doing less involves abandoning established practices (21).

CONCERNS ABOUT CRITICAL PATHWAYS

Autonomy versus Standardization

A common response of physicians to critical pathways is to view them as just one more threat to their autonomy (22–24). An appropriate counter to the charge of "cookbook medicine" is that pathways have the potential to codify the practices that the physicians deem important: they do not even have to be present to ensure that their patients are managed as they wish. In short, physicians can gain even greater control over the care of their patients by helping define these standards. However, achieving this control requires that physicians participate in the development of the standards with their peers. (One "management pearl" now widely quoted is: "The world is run by people who show up.")

It is also useful to emphasize that physicians must remain in control of patients' care at all times and that they can and must order deviations from the pathway when appropriate. Physicians at our institution can and do write orders that change pathways for a patient or they can remove a patient from a pathway completely. Indeed, it is important to remind physicians that they do not surrender their responsibilities to follow patients carefully when they are on a pathway.

Malpractice Risk

Physicians are often concerned about whether a pathway will increase their risk for a malpractice suit by pushing too hard for efficiency. Although some theoretic hazard is seen, the opposite is more likely to be true. Malpractice involves a deviation from the local standard of care that leads to harm to a patient. In many law suits, no clearly defined local standard of care is found, so that plaintiffs can easily find an "expert witness" who will charge that he or she would have handled the case differently. However, some evidence indicates that the availability of pathways does inhibit suits by discouraging plaintiff attorneys (25).

A clinical pathway represents a local standard of care and, therefore, can potentially protect physicians in malpractice litigation, assuming that the pathway has been executed and the patient met appropriateness criteria for the pathway. On the other hand, physicians may be more liable to suits if the care of a patient deviates from the pathway without a documented reason. Deviations from the standard of care that injure a patient may not increase liability if the deviation is caused by an error in judgment, as opposed to negligence. Therefore, critical pathway implementation should include a method for capturing the reason for any deviations.

Overall, data available suggest that the impact of pathways and guidelines on malpractice litigation is complex (26). Guidelines have been used by both plaintiffs and defendants to implicate and to exonerate physicians and hospitals and thus far have been used more often against the defendant (27). Attorneys surveyed in one study reported that the existence of guidelines in certain cases had induced them not to bring suit in the first place (28); other attorneys have described several ways in which pathways can decrease overall malpractice risk (25).

In the United Kingdom and other countries, guidelines and protocols can be introduced into court by an expert witness as evidence of accepted and customary standards of care, but they cannot be introduced as a substitute for expert testimony. Courts are unlikely to adopt guidelines as "gold standards of care" because the simple fact that the a guideline exists does not of itself establish that compliance with it is reasonable, or that the noncompliance is negligent (26).

The extent to which this legal experience with guidelines is generalizable to critical pathways is unclear. Disagreement over the standard of care is less likely to occur with critical pathways than with other types of guidelines, which are often quite vague. Perhaps the most important impact of pathways on malpractice is prevention of errors. By establishing a management protocol that has been reviewed by local opinion leaders, a critical pathway identifies the appropriate standard of care and helps keep the caregiver's attention focused on the most vital steps (1).

Research and Education

The research and educational missions of teaching hospitals are already in jeopardy, and critical pathways are sometimes perceived as potentially further undermining training by discouraging experimentation and independent thinking by trainees. Those responsible for housestaff education may feel that critical pathways establish processes of care that stifle the questioning through which residents learn.

On the other hand, medical training may be well served by incorporating methods such as critical pathways to teach students about cost-effective practice. At our institution, we have incorporated critical pathways into our teaching programs by involving housestaff in all phases of pathway development and implementation. We have also used the pathways themselves as teaching instruments in lectures that explore the clinical controversies of pathways. These activities have helped many members of the housestaff overcome the natural resistance they have for clinical protocols and have smoothed the integration of pathways into our teaching hospital.

Physicians involved in clinical research may be concerned that strong institution support will create an atmosphere in which patients will be steered away from clinical research studies into treatment according to critical pathways. Critical pathways, however, are not meant to supplant clinical research but rather to improve the "usual care" that is delivered. For example, one critical pathway at our institution includes explicit instructions to consider patients for a clinical research protocol and to contact the research team when appropriate. We have also encouraged the pathway development teams to think of research questions that can be embedded within their pathways, the answers for which may be discovered during the implementation of the pathway (e.g., during variance analysis) (1).

CONCLUSIONS

Critical pathways have attracted considerable attention as important methods for improving quality and efficiency in recent years. The effectiveness of pathways, however, is not clearly supported by rigorously collected data, for a variety of methodologic reasons. Nevertheless, some data support pathways as a useful strategy for improving care, even if they were to act mainly by focusing the attention of caregivers on a topic and key issues. The most appropriate interpretation of currently available information is that the potential impact of pathways on efficiency and quality is real, but far from guaranteed.

Even with the best of intentions, many potential pitfalls can undermine the effectiveness of a pathway. Efforts to address cultural issues, appropriate development of the pathway, and the collection and feedback of data can increase the chances that a pathway will lead to improvements in care.

REFERENCES

1. Pearson SD, Goulart-Fisher D, Lee TH. Critical pathways as a strategy for improving care: problems and potential. *Ann Intern Med* 1995;123:941–948.
2. Goldberg R, Chan L, Haley P, et al. Critical pathway for the emergency department management of acute asthma: effect on resource utilization. *Ann Emerg Med* 1998;31:562–567.
3. Pritts TA, Nussbaum MS, Flesh LV, et al. Implementation of a clinical pathway decreases length of stay and cost for bowel resection. *Ann Surg* 1999;230:728–733.
4. Leibman BD, Dillioglugil O, Abbas F, et al. Impact of a clinical pathway for radical retropubic prostatectomy. *Urology* 1998;52:94–99.
5. Bailey R, Weingarten S, Lewis M, et al. Impact of clinical pathways and practice guidelines on the management of acute exacerbations of bronchial asthma. *Chest* 1998;113:28–33.

6. Back MR, Harward TR, Huber TS, et al. Improving cost-effectiveness of carotid endarterectomy. *J Vasc Surg* 1997;26:463–464.

7. Chang L, Wang TM, Huang ST, et al. Effects of implementation of 18 clinical pathways on costs and quality of care among patients undergoing urological surgery. *J Urol* 1999;161:1858–1862.

8. Hay JA, Maldonado L, Wiengarten SR, et al. Prospective evaluation of a clinical guideline recommending hospital length of stay in upper gastrointestinal tract hemorrhage. *JAMA* 1997;278:2151–2156.

9. Marrie TJ, Lau CY, Wheeler SL, et al. A controlled trial of a critical pathway for treatment of community-acquired pneumonia. CAPITAL Study Investigators. Community-acquired pneumonia intervention trial assessing levofloxican. *JAMA* 2000;283(6):749–755.

10. Velasco FT, Ko W, Rosengart T, et al. Cost containment in cardiac surgery: results with a critical pathway for coronary bypass surgery at the New York Hospital–Cornell Medical Center. *Best Pract Benchmarking Healthhc* 1996;1:21–28.

11. Stanley AC, Barry M, Scott TE, et al. Impact of critical pathway on postoperative length of stay and outcomes after infrainguinal bypass. *J Vasc Surg* 1998;27:1056–1064.

12. Holmboe ES, Meehan TP, Radford MJ, et al. Use of critical pathways to improve the care of patients with acute myocardial infarction. *Am J Med* 1999;197:324–331.

13. Holtzman J, Bjerke T, Kane R. The effects of clinical pathways for renal transplant on patient outcomes and length of stay. *Med Care* 1998;36:826–834.

14. Muluk SC, Painter L, Sile S, et al. Utility of clinical pathway and prospective management to achieve cost and hospital stay reduction for aortic aneurysm surgery at a tertiary care hospital. *J Vasc Surg* 1997;25:84–93.

15. Paone G, Higgins RS, Havstad SL, et al. Does age limit the effectiveness of clinical pathway after coronary artery bypass graft surgery? *Circulation* 1998;98:1141–1145.

16. Schneider JR, Droste JS, Colan JF. Impact of critical pathways on surgical outcome and hospital stay. In: Yao JST, Pearce WH, eds. *Practical vascular surgery*, 1st ed. New York: McGraw-Hill, 1999:18–25.

17. Changing from top to bottom [Editorial]. *Lancet* 1998;351:997–998.

18. Weingarten SR, Agoes L, Tankel N, et al. Reducing length of stay for patients hospitalized with chest pain using medical practice guidelines and opinion leaders. *Am J Cardiol* 1993;71:259–262.

19. Weingarten SR, Riendinger MS, Conner L, et al. Practice guidelines and reminders to reduce duration of hospital stay for patients with chest pain. *Ann Intern Med* 1994;120:257–263.

20. Eagle KA, Mulley AG, Skates SJ, et al. Length of stay in the intensive care unit. Effects of practice guidelines and feedback. *JAMA* 1990;264:992–997.

21. Larson EB. Evidence-based medicine: is translating evidence into practice a solution to the cost-quality challenges facing medicine? *Jt Comm J Qual Improv* 1999;25:480–485.

22. Audet AM, Greenfield S, Field M. Medical practice guidelines: current activities and future directions. *Ann Intern Med* 1990;113:709–714.

23. Brook RH. Practice guideline and practicing medicine: are they compatible? *JAMA* 1989;262:3027–3030.

24. Holoweiko M. What cookbook medicine will mean for you. *Med Econ* 1989;66:118–133.

25. Garnick DW, Hendricks AM, Brennan TA. Can practice guidelines reduce the number and costs of malpractice claims? *JAMA* 1991;266:1856–1860.

26. Hurwitz B. Legal and political considerations of clinical practice guidelines. *BMJ* 1999;318:661–664.

27. Eagle KA, Lee TH, Brennan CA, et al. Task Force 2: guideline implementation. *J Am Coll Cardiol* 1997;29:1141–1148.

28. Nolin CE. Malpractice claims, patient communications, and critical paths: a lawyer's perspective. *Qual Manag Health Care* 1995;3:65–70.

PART II

Critical Pathways in the Emergency Department

CHAPTER 3

Emergency Department Critical Pathways for Acute Coronary Syndromes

Christopher P. Cannon and Christopher F. Richards

In the United States, approximately 6 to 7 million patients annually present to emergency departments (EDs) with a complaint of chest pain or other symptoms suggestive of possible acute coronary syndrome. Of these, only 20% to 25% have a final diagnosis of unstable angina or myocardial infarction (MI) for whom rapid treatment is necessary (1–3). For the remainder, the diagnostic evaluation to exclude acute coronary syndromes is the key step. Critical pathways can be particularly useful in providing standardization and guidance in these cases.

At Brigham and Women's Hospital, five pathways were established for the evaluation of chest pain. An overview of these critical pathways is shown in Fig. 3-1. Five pathways are set up for the different types of syndromes: two for patients with acute ST-segment elevation MI (one for thrombolysis, and one for primary angioplasty; Chapters 4 and 10); one for unstable angina and non–ST-segment elevation MI (Chapter 12); and two for patients with chest pain of unclear etiology (one 6-hour ED-based "rule out MI" pathway for patients with low likelihood of acute coronary syndrome and one pathway that involved direct exercise stress testing for patients with very low likelihood of acute coronary syndrome based on clinical evaluation). In addition, beyond the ED is extended the ED-based 6-hour rule-out MI pathway for patients with chest pain and a low likelihood of coronary artery disease, but who have other comorbid conditions requiring acute care (e.g., pneumonia, atrial fibrillation) or have conditions that preclude standard exercise testing who are admitted to the short stay unit and have their care carried out in 24 to 48 hours.

GOALS

The overall goals of these ED pathways are similar to all pathways. In the ED, however, the focus is on (a) rapid diagnosis and treatment with fibrinolytic therapy or primary percutaneous intervention (PCI); (b) standardizing and improving the use of appropriate medications (e.g., aspirin, beta-blockers,

heparin, IIb/IIIa inhibitors); and (c) improving triage of the patient to the appropriate level of care (4,5).

FORMAT

The format of the pathways has evolved from a pathway of several pages listing all the indications, contraindications, and dosages for each medicine (e.g., fibrinolytic therapy, heparin, beta-blockers), to a one-page document with all five pathways in a simple "checklist" format (4–7). This checklist format was developed to simplify the pathway and increase both its usability and use. The design is such that is serves as a quick reminder of the key goals, tests to perform, and medications to consider using. In this way, a busy ED physician could use the pathway rapidly to improve care, but the pathway would not burden the physician with a lot of paperwork.

Recently, moves have been made to make these checklists standardized order sets for the ED physician and nurse to use (Fig. 3-2). Because all medications and other orders are now entered electronically, having a computerized order template associated with the critical pathway ensures that the physician sees the checklist of orders (Fig. 3-3). The physician simply chooses a pathway based on the clinical diagnosis and clicks on the medications desired. Verbal orders still can be taken, as in the case for administering fibrinolytic therapy, to speed delivery of the drug. It is hoped that this system, which guarantees that physicians will see the critical pathway for every patient, will further increase the use of evidence-based medications.

ST-SEGMENT ELEVATION MYOCARDIAL INFARCTION CRITICAL PATHWAYS

The critical pathway for all acute coronary syndromes begins immediately with the triage nurse who brings patients with chest pain into an "acute" room of the ED. A brief history is obtained and an electrocardiogram (ECG) performed. If

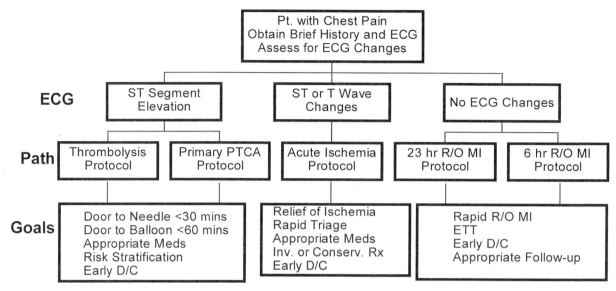

FIG. 3-1. Overview of the critical pathways for acute coronary syndromes at Brigham and Women's Hospital. (Adapted from Cannon CP. Optimizing the treatment of unstable angina. *J Thromb Thrombolysis* 1995;2:205–218; with permission.)

Brigham and Women's Hospital Chest Pain Pathway Summary (9/1999)

Description	ST ↑ MI-Angioplasty	ST ↑ MI-Thrombolysis	Unstable Angina/ Non-ST↑ MI	Possibly Angina	Probably not Angina
Category	1	2	3	4	5
Clinical	Acute MI	Acute MI	Good Story and/or	Fair story	Atypical story
EKG	ST elevation/New LBBB	ST elevation/New LBBB	(+)EKG	(-)EKG[1]	(-)EKG[1]
			(+)enzymes	(-)enzymes	(-)CAD risk factors
			(+)Hx MI, PCI, CABG	(+)CAD risk factors	
Goals	☐ Call Cath lab <20 min[2]	☐ Door to Needle <30 min	☐ Weight = _ _ _ _ kg		
	☐ Leave ED <45 min	(Actual_ _ _)			
	(Actual_ _ _)	☐ Weight = _ _ _ kg			
	☐ Door to Balloon <90 min				
	(Actual_ _ _)				
Tests	☐ CBC, CMP[3], PT/PTT	☐ CBC, CMP[3], PT/PTT	☐CBC, CMP[3], PT/PTT	☐ CBC, BMP[3]	☐ ETT
	☐ CPK/MB	☐ CPK/MB	☐ CPK/MB, TNI	☐ CPK/MB, TNI (0 hrs)	☐ Consider CPK 6 hrs
	☐ Lipid profile	☐ Lipid profile	☐ Lipid profile	☐ CPK/MB, TNI (6 hrs)	after pain then ETT
	☐ Clot to BB	☐ Clot to BB		☐ ETT if enzymes normal	
Medications	☐ ASA 325mg chew	☐ ASA 325mg chew	☐ ASA 325mg chew	☐ ASA 325mg chew	☐ ASA 325mg chew
	☐ Heparin IV[4]	☐ r-PA 10U & 10U in 30 min	☐ Metoprolol IV/PO	☐ Consider Metoprolol PO	☐ NTG PRN
	☐ Metoprolol IV	☐ Heparin IV[5]	☐ discuss with Cards B	☐ NTG PRN	
	☐ Consider IIb/IIIa	☐ Metoprolol IV/PO	☐Heparin IV + IIb/IIIa		
	☐ Clopidogrel 300 mg PO	☐ Consider ACE inhibitor	☐Enoxaparin SQ		
	☐ Consider ACE inhibitor	☐ NTG PRN	☐Cath Lab		
	☐ NTG PRN		☐NTG PRN		
Disposition	Cath Lab/CCU	CCU	Monitored Bed	ED Observation Unit (OBS)	ETT/OBS[6]
	☐ Arrange admission	☐ Arrange admission	☐ Arrange admission	☐ OBS Packet[7]	☐ OBS Packet[7]
			(Cardiology B Team)	☐ PCP consult @ D/C[8]	☐ PCP consult @ D/C

[1] (-)EKG means normal or unchanged from previous
[2] Cath lab coordinator B13612, call cath attending >6pm
[3] CMP: Comprehensive Metabolic Panel BMP: Basic Metabolic Panel
[4] Heparin IV dose: 60U/kg bolus, 12U/kg/hr infusion
[5] Maximum Heparin bolus 4000U and infusion 1000 U/hr with thrombolysis
[6] Very Low risk patients may undergo ETT directly from ED without enzyme testing
[7] OBS and RACE forms
[8] Consider Cardiology consult if ETT positive or indeterminate

FIG. 3-2. Emergency department critical pathways for acute coronary syndromes at Brigham and Women's Hospital.

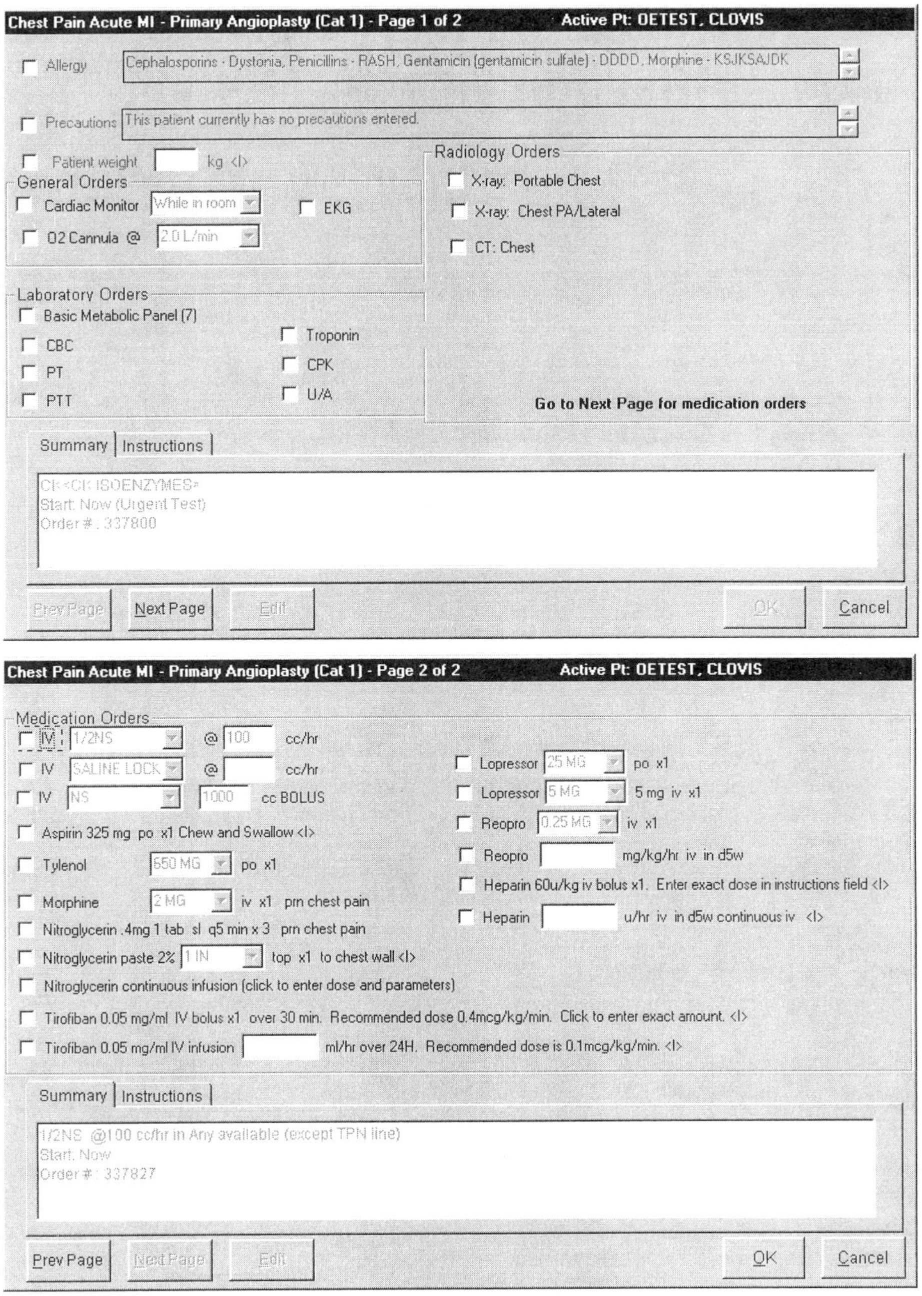

FIG. 3-3. Emergency department critical pathway order template for patients with acute myocardial infarction undergoing percutaneous coronary intervention at Brigham and Women's Hospital.

ST-segment elevation is present, the patient is immediately evaluated for thrombolysis or primary angioplasty. One critical guideline (based on the importance of time to reperfusion with either thrombolysis or primary percutaneous transluminal coronary angioplasty) is to triage patients to that strategy which will achieve infarct-related artery patency most quickly (4,8,9). During the day, primary angioplasty is the preferred strategy, whereas on nights and weekends thrombolysis is considered (and might be preferred), in recognition of the time necessary to mobilize the cardiac catheterization laboratory (CL) team.

After initial diagnosis, if the patient is eligible, thrombolytic therapy is administered in the ED with the goal of starting drug in <30 minutes from arrival in the ED (4). As described in Chapter 4 a significant reduction in door-to-needle time occurred when a fibrinolysis critical pathway was instituted (7). In recognition of the benefits of bolus thrombolysis in reducing door-to-needle time, and in simplifying treatment, we use a bolus thrombolytic, currently reteplase (10–12).

For the primary PCI patients, rapid door-to-balloon time is equally important. In a recent study, it was observed that

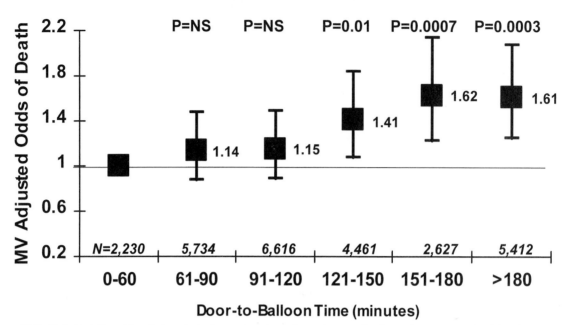

FIG. 3-4. Relationship of door-to-balloon time to adjusted mortality in patients treated with primary angioplasty for acute myocardial infarction. (Adapted from Cannon CP, Gibson CM, Lambrew CT, et al. Relationship of symptom-onset-to-balloon time and door-to-balloon time with mortality in patients undergoing angioplasty for acute myocardial infarction. *JAMA* 2000;283:2941–2947; with permission.)

if door-to-balloon times were >2 hours, adjusted mortality was 40% to 60% higher than in patients with optimal door-to-balloon times of <60 minutes (Fig. 3-4). To achieve a target door-to-balloon time of 90 ± 30 minutes, as recommended by the American College of Cardiology/American Heart Association (ACC/AHA) *Guidelines for the Management of Acute MI,* the process has been simplified to a single telephone call to the CL coordinator (13). This person simultaneously arranges for an open room, and asks the CL attending to contact the ED for clinical details. The goal is for this step to occur within 20 minutes of the patient's arrival in the ED. The patient's care continues and a nurse or fellow from the CL is dispatched to assist in transferring the patient to the CL, with the time of leaving the ED targeted to be <45 minutes after hospital arrival. The exact times are recorded on the pathway (Fig. 3-2).

For both thrombolysis and primary PCI, the second goal of the pathways is to treat the patient with all other appropriate medications (e.g., aspirin, intravenous heparin, beta-blockers, angiotensin converting enzyme inhibitors, nitrates, and antiischemic drugs). We have specified the weight-based dose of heparin, because it is the new, lower dose recommended in the 1999 update of the ACC/AHA MI guidelines (13). This dose is a bolus of 60 U/kg, with a maximum of 4,000 U, and 12 U/kg/h initial infusion with a maximum of 1,000 U/h. Clopidogrel (300 mg) is frequently

administered in patients going directly for primary PCI. Glycoprotein IIb/IIIa inhibition is generally administered in the CL, but consideration can be given to starting these agents in the ED, because this appears to "facilitate" early reperfusion (14,15). The third goal is to ensure that patients are considered for ongoing clinical research trials, and reminders are listed in the "Goals" section.

UNSTABLE ANGINA AND NON–ST-SEGMENT ELEVATION MYOCARDIAL INFARCTION PATHWAY

The pathway for unstable angina and non–ST-segment elevation MI at Brigham and Women's Hospital emphasizes (a) early relief of ischemic pain, a symptom found to be a determinant of development of MI; (b) administration of antithrombotic and antiischemic therapy; (c) reminders of eligibility criteria for ongoing clinical research trials (e.g., trials of new IIb/IIIa inhibitors or treatment strategy trials); (d) a detailed list of suggested blood tests in an effort to reduce unnecessary tests; and (e) choice of either an early conservative strategy or an early invasive strategy (5,16).

Inclusion criterion for the pathway is essentially true unstable angina. This is defined as ischemic pain occurring either at rest or with minimal exertion and with an accelerating

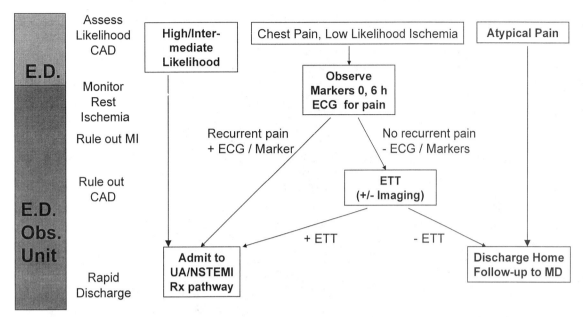

FIG. 3-5. Brigham and Women's Hospital Emergency Department "Chest Pain/Rule Out MI" critical pathway. (From Cannon CP, Braunwald E. Unstable angina. In: Braunwald E, Zipes DP, Libby P, eds. *Heart disease: a textbook of cardiovascular medicine.* Philadelphia: WB Saunders, 2000; with permission.)

pattern (i.e., Braunwald class 1–3 unstable angina) (17). Corroborative information that supports the clinical history is helpful in establishing the diagnosis and identifying patients at higher risk: prior history of MI or documented coronary disease by catheterization, or ST–segment- or T-wave changes with the presenting syndrome (18). ST-segment deviation of ≥0.5 mm is used because it appears to have equal prognostic significance as ≥1 mm ST-segment depression (16). Because only a third of patients presenting with unstable angina have ECG changes, much of the admission diagnosis relies on the history (16).

The treatment involves aspirin, nitrates, and beta-blockers. If the latter is contraindicated, heart rate lowering calcium antagonists can be used. Then, a decision is needed regarding the use of glycoprotein IIb/IIIa inhibition, which has clear benefits in this patient population, especially for those at high risk for positive troponin, ST-segment changes, diabetes, prior aspirin use, or recurrent episodes of rest pain (19–22). Similar benefits have been shown for the low-molecular weight heparin (LMWH) enoxaparin as compared with unfractionated heparin (23–25). Initially, trials used IIb/IIIa inhibition with unfractionated heparin and, thus, a decision had to be made regarding the use of either unfractionated heparin plus IIb/IIIa inhibitors versus LMWH. As data emerge, it is believed that the combination of enoxaparin and IIb/IIIa inhibitors will be safe, as shown to date in one small pilot study, and this combination may be more effective (26). Thus, the pathway will likely move to start enoxaparin in all patients in the ED, and IIb/IIIa inhibition in patients with high-risk features.

Tests on Admissions

In addition to ECG, the pathway recommends serial creatine kinase MB (CK-MB) determinations for diagnosis of non–ST-segment elevation MI. In addition, a troponin I at entry is measured, as well as serial measurements every 8 hours over the first 24 hours, because these tend to increase sensitivity of identifying a positive test (27,28). The Treat Angina with Aggrastat and determine Cost of Therapy with an Invasive or Conservative Strategy (TACTICS)–Thrombolysis in Myocardial Infarction (TIMI) 18 trial should help determine whether the treatment strategy should be different as a function of the troponin value (29). The acute cardiac ischemia time-insensitive predictive instrument (ACI-TIPI) ECG analysis tool has recently been added to the protocol and is being assessed in our patient population (30).

Treatment Strategy

Patients are managed by either an early invasive or early conservative strategy. Because TIMI IIIB showed equivalent outcomes through one year, the choice of which strategy is left to the discretion of the treating cardiologist. Thus, in the ED pathway, early contact is made to decide on the treatment strategy.

"RULE-OUT MYOCARDIAL INFARCTION PATHWAYS"

The large population of patients without ECG changes are risk stratified. Patients, with clearly atypical pain, not suggestive of ischemia, are discharged home with follow-up to their primary physicians. The remaining patients with pain possibly suggestive of ischemia are observed in the ED observation unit. These patients are monitored for recurrent rest pain, and have a panel of markers (CK-MB, troponin I, and myoglobin) at arrival and 6 hours later. If the onset of pain was >6 hours before arrival, the baseline sample is frequently considered sufficient to "rule out" a MI. If cardiac markers are positive or if the patient develops recurrent pain with ECG changes, the patient is admitted to the hospital and treated for unstable angina (Fig. 3-5).

If the patient remains pain free and the markers are negative, the patient goes on to exercise stress testing (31). For most patients, ECG stress testing is used; however, for patients with fixed abnormalities (e.g., left bundle branch block), perfusion imaging is used, and for those who cannot walk, pharmacologic stress is used. In some patients, if the clinical history suggests an extremely low likelihood of acute infarction, but some possibility of unstable angina exists, the cardiac marker testing is omitted and the patient is sent directly for stress testing (last column, Fig. 3-2). If the stress test is positive, the patients are admitted to the cardiology service for further evaluation and treatment. If negative, they are discharged home with follow-up from their physicians (31). The goal is to carry out the testing and discharge (or admit) of patients within 6 to 12 hours from ED arrival, with follow-up from their primary physicians.

In addition, we have also established a "23-hour" rule out MI pathway that essentially extends the extension of the ED-based, 6-hour rule out MI pathway. It is for patients with chest pain and a low likelihood of coronary artery disease, but who have other comorbid conditions requiring acute care (e.g., pneumonia, atrial fibrillation) or have conditions that preclude standard exercise testing. They are admitted to the short stay unit and have their care carried out within 24 to 48 hours.

CONCLUSIONS

For the full spectrum—from atypical chest pain to acute MI—we have moved to a quick "checklist" format with computerized "template" prompts for our ED critical pathways. The focus is on reminding physicians of the key steps in treating the patients—the tests to do and medication to administer. For ST-segment elevation MI, rapid treatment with reperfusion therapy is an additional goal. These checklists have also be used to create standardized order sets in the ED—to facilitate rapid and appropriate care for our patients.

REFERENCES

1. Pope JH, Ruthazer R, Beshansky JR, et al. Clinical features of emergency department patients presenting with symptoms suggestive of acute cardia ischemia: a multicenter study. *J Thromb Thrombolysis* 1998;6:63–74.
2. Kontos MC, Ornato JP, Tatum JL, et al. How many patients are eligible for treatment with GP IIb/IIIa inhibitors? Results from a clinical database. *Circulation* 1999;100 [Suppl I]:I-775.
3. Pope JH, Aufderheide TP, Ruthazer R, et al. Missed diagnoses of acute cardiac ischemia in the emergency department [see comments]. *N Engl J Med* 2000;342:1163–1170.
4. Cannon CP, Antman EM, Walls R, et al. Time as an adjunctive agent to thrombolytic therapy. *J Thromb Thrombolysis* 1994;1:27–34.
5. Cannon CP. Optimizing the treatment of unstable angina. *J Thromb Thrombolysis* 1995;2:205–218.
6. Sagarin MJ, Cannon CP, Cermignani MS, et al. Delay in thrombolysis administration: causes of extended door-to-drug times and the asymptote effect. *J Emerg Med* 1998;16:557–565.
7. Cannon CP, Johnson EB, Cermignani M, et al. Emergency department thrombolysis critical pathway reduces door-to-drug times in acute myocardial infarction. *Clin Cardiol* 1999;22:17–22.
8. Cannon CP, Braunwald E. Time to reperfusion: the critical modulator in thrombolysis and primary angioplasty. *J Thromb Thrombolysis* 1996;3:117–125.
9. Cannon CP, Gibson CM, Lambrew CT, et al. Relationship of symptom-onset-to-balloon time and door-to-balloon time with mortality in patients undergoing angioplasty for acute myocardial infarction. *JAMA* 2000;283:2941–2947.
10. Seyedroudbari A, Kessler ER, Mooss AN, et al. Time to treatment and cost of thrombolysis: a multicenter comparison of tPA and rPA. *J Thromb Thrombolysis* 2000;9:303–308.
11. Cannon CP. Bridging the gap with new strategies in acute ST elevation myocardial infarction: bolus thrombolysis, glycoprotein IIb/IIIa inhibitors, combination therapy, percutaneous coronary intervention, and "facilitated PCI." *J Thromb Thrombolysis* 2000;9:235–241.
12. Cannon CP. Thrombolysis medication errors: benefits of bolus thrombolytic agents. *Am J Cardiol* 2000;85:17C–22C.
13. Ryan KA, Rizzo M, Kelley MB, et al. Relationship between the presence and duration of chest pain and blood flow at 90 minutes following thrombolytic administration. *J Am Coll Cardiol* 1999;33[Suppl A]:375A.
14. Antman EM, Giugliano RP, Gibson CM, et al. Abciximab facilitates the rate and extent of thrombolysis: results of TIMI 14 trial. *Circulation* 1999;99:2720–2732.
15. van den Merkhof LF, Zijlstra F, Olsson H, et al. Abciximab in the treatment of acute myocardial infarction eligible for primary percutaneous transluminal coronary angioplasty. Results of the Glycoprotein Receptor Antagonist Patency Evaluation (GRAPE) pilot study. *J Am Coll Cardiol* 1999;33:1528–1532.
16. Cannon CP, McCabe CH, Stone PH, et al. The electrocardiogram predicts one-year outcome of patients with unstable angina and non-Q wave myocardial infarction: results of the TIMI III Registry ECG Ancillary study. *J Am Coll Cardiol* 1997;30:133–140.
17. Braunwald E. Unstable angina: a classification. *Circulation* 1989;80:410–414.
18. Braunwald E, Mark DB, Jones RH, et al. Unstable angina: diagnosis and management. *Clinical practice guideline number 10.* Rockville, MD: Agency for Health Care Policy and Research and the National Heart, Lung, and Blood Institute, Public Health Service, US Department of Health and Human Services, 1994:154.
19. A comparison of aspirin plus tirofiban with aspirin plus heparin for unstable angina. The Platelet Receptor Inhibition for Ischemic Syndrome Management (PRISM) Study Investigators. *N Engl J Med* 1998;338:1498–1505.
20. Inhibition of the platelet glycoprotein IIb/IIIa receptor with tirofiban in unstable angina and non–Q-wave myocardial infarction. The Platelet Receptor Inhibition for Ischemic Syndrome Management in Patients Limited by Unstable Signs and Symptoms (PRISM-PLUS) Trial Investigators. *N Engl J Med* 1998;338:1488–1497.
21. Inhibition of platelet glycoprotein IIb/IIIa with eptifibatide in patients with acute coronary syndromes. The PURSUIT Trial Investigators. Platelet Glycoprotein IIb/IIIa in Unstable Angina: Receptor Suppression Using Integrilin Therapy. *N Engl J Med* 1998;339:436–443.
22. Cannon CP. Targeting high-risk patient subsets in acute coronary syndromes: greater benefit from antithrombotic and interventional therapies. *Acute Coronary Syndromes (in press).*
23. Cohen M, Demers C, Gurfinkel EP, et al. A comparison of low-molecular-weight heparin with unfractionated heparin for unstable coronary artery disease. *N Engl J Med* 1997;337:447–452.
24. Antman EM, McCabe CH, Gurfinkel EP, et al. Enoxaparin prevents death and cardiac ischemic events in unstable angina/non-Q-wave myocardial infarction: results of the Thrombolysis in Myocardial Infarction (TIMI) 11B trial. *Circulation* 1999;100:1593–1601.

25. Antman EM, McCabe CH, Gurfinkel EP, et al. Treatment benefit of enoxaparin in unstable angina/non-Q wave myocardial infarction is maintained at one year in TIMI 11B. *Circulation* 1999;100[Suppl I]: I-497.

26. Cohen M, Theroux P, Weber S, et al. Combination therapy with tirofiban and enoxaparin in acute coronary syndromes. *Int J Cardiol* 1999;71:273–281.

27. Antman EM, Tanasijevic MJ, Thompson B, et al. Cardiac-specific troponin I levels to predict the risk of mortality in patients with acute coronary syndromes. *N Engl J Med* 1996;335:1342–1349.

28. Newby LK, Christenson RH, Ohman EM, et al. Value of serial troponin T measures for early and late risk stratification in patients with acute coronary syndromes. The GUSTO-IIa investigators. *Circulation* 1998;98:1853–1859.

29. Cannon CP, Weintraub WS, Demopoulos LA, et al. Invasive versus conservative strategies in unstable angina and non–Q wave myocardial infarction following treatment with tirofiban: rationale and study design of the international TACTICS-TIMI 18 trial. *Am J Cardiol* 1998;82:731–736.

30. Selker HP, Beshansky JR, Griffith JL, et al. Use of the acute cardiac ischemia time-insensitive predictive instrument (ACI-TIPI) to assist with triage of patients with chest pain or other symptoms suggestive of acute cardiac ischemia. A multicenter, controlled clinical trial. *Ann Intern Med* 1998;129:845–855.

31. Nichol G, Walls R, Goldman L, et al. A critical pathway for management of patient with acute chest pain at low risk for myocardial ischemia: recommendations and potential impact. *Ann Intern Med* 1997;127:996–1005.

CHAPTER 4

Thrombolysis for Acute Myocardial Infarction

Christopher F. Richards, J. Stephen Bohan, and Ron M. Walls

OVERVIEW

Patients with acute ST-segment elevation myocardial infarction (MI) comprise the population of patients with chest pain at highest risk seen in the emergency department (ED). These patients require rapid diagnosis, early stabilization, and rapid reperfusion. Whether reperfusion involves administration of thrombolytic agents or primary percutaneous coronary intervention (PCI), delays in intervention increase morbidity and mortality (1,2). Typically, thrombolytic therapy is delivered in the ED, where the conflicting demands of multiple high acuity patients can increase the potential for delay or error. Thus, although time to administration is critical, errors in administration can have disastrous consequences and must be avoided. The combination of time-critical interventions and high morbidity and mortality make the application of critical pathways to this population especially appropriate. Recently, the issue of medication errors has received substantial attention (3–5). The specific issue of medication errors during the administration of thrombolytic therapy has also been addressed, with patients who have been subjected to drug error having an increase in morbidity and mortality (4). Frequent comparison is made with the airline industry, which has reduced error to an astoundingly low rate. Activities involving a series of complex tasks are particularly susceptible to error and, therefore, are especially amenable to adaptation of critical pathways such as those discussed below. These pathways help to simplify the tasks and are analogous to the checklists that pilots have been using for decades (6). Computer-assisted decision-making may also be helpful in this context (7).

Thrombolysis may be the only available method for reperfusion in many community hospitals, whereas larger centers can use combination approaches, involving PCI and thrombolysis. Critical pathways can draw on national consensus, but must be customized for the local environment in which they are to be applied. As such, critical pathways should be developed by collaboration between the departments of emergency medicine and cardiology, specifying, for example, when primary angioplasty should be performed and when thrombolytic administration is appropriate. Although such pathways must always allow some latitude for clinical judgment in unique circumstances, clear and unambiguous understanding of the pathway must be had by all parties, and improvisation and case-by-case negotiation must be minimized.

RATIONALE

The three crucial, interrelated determinations for the patient with chest pain patient presenting to the ED are:

1. Does this pain represent an acute coronary syndrome?
2. Does the acute coronary syndrome require reperfusion?
3. Could the pain could be caused by aortic dissection?

The most simple, direct, and efficient way to answer these questions is still a matter of some debate. Extensive literature, however, can aid in the decision-making for both diagnosis and therapy. This evidence can be condensed and arranged in a pathway that can both structure the patient's care and act as an "aide de memoire." A condensed version of our pathway is shown in Fig. 4-1.

Pathway

The key determinant and entry point for the pathway is suspected acute coronary syndrome. Two essential elements guide all further actions: the electrocardiogram (ECG) and the character of the patient's chest pain. ST-segment elevation of at least 1 ml in at least two "geographically contiguous" leads or the presence of a new, or presumed new, left bundle branch block in the context of an acute coronary syndrome indicates active MI and mandates immediate steps to reopen the occluded infarct-related artery.

Because time is of the essence, the ED must be structured to allow a prompt ECG, immediate interpretation of the ECG, and prompt therapeutic intervention if indicated. Even before the thrombolytic decision is made, empiric therapy (aspirin, nitroglycerin, etc.) can be initiated, often in the ED triage area.

The pathway in Fig. 4-1 is designed both to act as a schematic representation of the critical steps in diagnosis and

Summary of the BWH Thrombolytic Pathway

THROMBOLYTIC PATHWAY

GOALS
- ◆ Rapid decision on need for reperfusion
- ◆ Rapid decision on optimum method of reperfusion
- ◆ Safe administration of thrombolytic agent
- ◆ Prompt completion of adjunctive therapies

I.   Determine Need for Reperfusion Therapy:

<u>TIME</u>

_____   Patient arrives—obtain immediate ECG

_____   ECG done—shown to physician—request old ECG

_____   Place patient on oxygen, establish IV, administer 160-325 mg of non-enteric
          coated ASA (chewed) and perform other nursing interventions

_____   Patient assessed by physician

    1. Suspicion of ischemia > 30 min duration
    2. Onset of pain < 12 hours
    3. ST segment elevation >0.1 mV in at least 2 contiguous leads or LBBB not
       known to be old
    NOTE: Consider possibility of Aortic Dissection

    If yes to 1,2,3 proceed to Step II (below). If no to any of 1,2,3 proceed according
    to Ischemic Chest Pain Pathway

II.   Determine Optimum Method of Reperfusion:

    <u>Assess for Contraindications:</u>
        Intracerebral Neoplasm, AVM, or aneurysm
        Active Internal Bleeding
        Suspected Aortic Dissection
        Previous Hemorrhagic stroke, anytime;
        Any Stroke within 1 year
        Known bleeding diathesis

FIG. 4-1A.

treatment of acute MI, and to provide a record of the critical time elements. It states the general goals of the pathway and constructs an orderly set of intermediate goals in determining a patient's need.

Goal 1: Determine the Need for Thrombolytic Therapy

All patients more than 30 years of age with active chest pain suspected of acute coronary syndrome should have an ECG within 10 minutes of presenting to the ED. This ECG should be promptly (within 1 to 2 minutes) shown to the emergency physician who should assess it for ST-segment elevation (>0.1 mV in at least two contiguous leads) or new, or presumed new, left bundle branch block. If either is present, the patient should be examined and interviewed before 10 more minutes have elapsed. Careful confirmation of the patient's presenting symptoms and history, and evaluation for possible aortic dissection will guide the decision whether reperfusion therapy is indicated.

Goal 2: Determine the Optimal Method of Reperfusion

The patient should now be assessed for any contraindication to thrombolysis. If any of these are present, PCI is necessary.

When reperfusion is indicated and no contraindication is seen to thrombolysis, a prompt decision is required to which method should be used to open the infarct-related artery. The role of PCI should be established by policy. As such, implementation of the angioplasty branch of the pathway should be protocol driven and should not be determined on a case-by-case basis, as such determinations will unnecessarily delay reperfusion by confounding the decision-making process.

Use of primary PCI requires operational "door-to-balloon" times of 90 minutes or less (1,8). With cooperation between

Assess for Cautions (Relative Contraindications):
Severe uncontrolled BP (>180/110 mm Hg)
Active anticoagulation (INR > 2-3): known bleeding diathesis
Recent trauma (2-4 weeks) especially head trauma or spinal trauma
Traumatic or prolonged (>10 min) CPR
History of prior CVA or other intracranial pathology not covered in contraindications
Non-compressible vascular punctures
Pregnancy
Recent (2-4 weeks) internal bleeding or surgery
History of chronic severe hypertension
Streptokinase/APSAC prior exposure (especially 5d-2wks)/prior allergy

Assess for PCI availability.
If contraindications (or significant cautions) present, or <90 minutes to balloon inflation, send patient to PCI.
If no contraindications or balloon inflation >90 minutes, continue.
NOTE: See text for assessing PCI availability.

_____ **Administer thrombolytic agent (See Figure 4-2)**

_____ Heparin
Give **IV heparin** 4000 unit bolus
Start continuous infusion of 1000 U/hr
(if patient weighs <65kg, start infusion 800 U/hour)

_____ Metoprolol: evaluate for any contraindications, including:
a. Heart rate <60/min, or SBP < 90 mmHg
b. History of asthma or COPD requiring chronic medications
c. History of LV ejection fraction <30%
d. Clinical evidence of CHF
e. PR $\geq$ 0.24
If no contraindication, administer **intravenous metoprolol** 5 mg bolus q2 minutes x3,
Or until HR <55. Check BP between boluses. Administer oral metoprolol 50 mg, 15 minutes after last dose of IV metoprolol.

_____ Captopril (optional): consider captopril if BP >110/80, especially for anterior MIs and for hypertensive patients. Dosage: **Captopril PO** 6.25 mg x 1.

FIG. 4-1B.

referring and receiving hospitals, this standard can be achieved even in facilities without a cardiac catheterization laboratory, by using "direct to catheterization laboratory" transfer agreements with invasive cardiology centers. Hospitals with a cardiac catheterization laboratory must establish whether PCI is to be used in all cases, regardless of time of day, or as a hybrid approach using PCI or thrombolytic therapy, depending on time of day. Operation of a rapidly mobilized cardiac catheterization team around the clock may be cost-prohibitive, and hours must be clearly defined for PCI versus thrombolytic therapy. If a contraindication to thrombolytic therapy is present, then PCI is indicated regardless of time of day, which may require transfer to another facility.

Goal 3: Accurate and Safe Administration of the Thrombolytic Agent

The choice of agent (see text below) should be established by policy and guidelines for administration should be part of the pathway. The standard administration regimens of the four most commonly used agents are shown in Fig. 4-2.

Goal 4: Adjunctive Therapy

Adjunctive therapies (aspirin, heparin, beta-blockade, angiotensin converting enzyme inhibitors) have been shown to improve outcome, and should be integrated into the pathway. Indications, contraindications, and doses and routes of administration should be clearly stated.

SELECTION OF THROMBOLYTIC AGENTS

The timely administration of thrombolytic therapy can reduce mortality by 25% when compared with placebo (9–12). Accelerated dose tissue plasminogen activator (tPA) became the favored agent after publication of the Global Utilization of Streptokinase and tPA for Occluded Arteries (GUSTO-I) trial results. Bolus therapy may prove safer and equally effective.

Administration of Thrombolytic agents

<u>t-PA: Alteplase® (Genentech):</u>
Accelerated dose (90 minutes total)
15 mg IV bolus, then
0.75 mg/kg (up to 50mg) IV over 30 minutes, then
0.50 mg/kg (up to 35mg) IV over 60 minutes.
Plus IV heparin and aspirin
NOTE: Administer via dedicated IV line

<u>r-PA: Retavase® (Centocor):</u>
10U IV bolus over 2 minutes, then
10U IV bolus over 2 minutes 30 minutes later
Plus IV heparin and aspirin
Note: Incompatible with heparin, stop heparin during bolus or use alternative IV site.

<u>TNK-tPA: Tenecteplase® (Genentech):</u>
Weight based, administer by IV bolus over 5 seconds.
Plus IV heparin and aspirin

Weight	Dose	Volume
< 60 kg	30 mg	6 cc
60-70 kg	35 mg	7 cc
70-80 kg	40 mg	8 cc
80-90 kg	45 mg	9 cc
> 90 kg	50 mg	10 cc

Note: Incompatible with Dextrose solutions.

<u>Streptokinase: Streptase® (Hoechst Marion Roussel):</u>
1.5 million units (45 cc) over 60 minutes.
Plus Aspirin
Begin Heparin after Streptokinase infusion
Note: Administer via dedicated IV line

Note all agents are supplied in a kit as lyophilized powder and solutions appropriate for reconstitution. Avoid shaking any of them to facilitate reconstitution.

FIG. 4-2.

When selecting an agent for use as part of a thrombolytic pathway, it is important to consider cost, availability, ease of administration, and the complexity of calculating the dose and of administering the drug.

Thrombolytic agents are more precisely called "fibrinolytic" agents, because they function as plasminogen activators that initiate the blood fibrinolytic system by converting the proenzyme plasminogen to the active enzyme plasmin. Plasmin, in turn, digests fibrin into soluble byproducts. The seven agents currently available for clinical use can be divided into three "generations" based on their origin and pharmacokinetics. The first generation agents are naturally occurring and include streptokinase and urokinase, as well as anisoylated plasminogen streptokinase activator complex (APSAC). The second generation agent is the genetically engineered version of human tPA. The third generation agents are versions of human tPA that have been modified in various ways to have greater fibrin specificity or a longer plasma half life in order to accommodate bolus administration. The three agents in this class are: rPA (Retavase, Centocor), TNK-tPA (Tenecteplase, Genentech), and nPA (Lanoteplase, Bristol-Myers Squibb, New York, NY). nPA is not yet approved by the US Food & Drug Administration (FDA). All agents are given by bolus administration. tPA and nPA require weight-based dosing. rPA is administered as a fixed-dose double bolus and, thus, does not require weight estimation or dose calculation.

Agents can also be classified on the basis of "fibrin specificity." The plasminogen occurring naturally in the bloodstream is inhibited by two plasminogen activator inhibitors and plasmin is inhibited by α_2-antiplasmin. At the level of the clot, a key lysine-binding site on plasmin is protected from α_2-antiplasmin. Non–fibrin-specific agents (e.g., streptokinase, APSAC, and urokinase) produce large amounts of circulating plasmin, which also degrades other clotting factors such as von Willebrand factor and factors V, VIII, and XII. This activation overwhelms the circulating α_2-antiplasmin and produces a state of systemic thrombolysis. The more clot-specific plasminogen activators—tPA, rPA, and TNK-PA—are said to be fibrin specific because they activate plasminogen preferentially at the fibrin surface and less so in the circulation (13).

Comparing the first and second generation agents, no difference was seen with the 3-hour regimen of tPA with no heparin or subcutaneous heparin as compared with streptokinase in the GISSI-2 (Gruppo Italiano per lo Studio Della Strep-tochinasi Nell' Infarcto Miocardico) and ISIS-3 (International Study of Infarct Survival) trials (11,14,15). However, an absolute 1% reduction in 30-day mortality was observed in GUSTO-I, and an absolute 1% reduction in 30-day mortality was observed with front-loaded tPA and intravenous (i.v.) heparin versus streptokinase and heparin (2).

Recombinant tPA has three separate dosing regimens: for (a) acute MI, (b) acute stroke, and (c) acute pulmonary embolism. The dose for an acute MI is 15 mg i.v. bolus; then 0.75 mg/kg (up to 50 mg) i.v. over 30 minutes; then 0.5 mg/kg (up to 35 mg) i.v. over 60 minutes given with aspirin and i.v. heparin. In the GUSTO-I trial, 13.5% of patients had a medication error (incorrect dose or infusion length) and a higher (7.7%) mortality when compared with those who received the correct (5.5%) dose of tPA (16,17). Similar results were found for streptokinase. The weight-based dosing of tPA adds the challenge of measuring or accurately estimating a patient's weight. Patients frequently over- or underestimate their weight for a variety of reasons, and healthcare professionals have been shown to have limited ability to estimate a supine patient's weight (18,19). Total drug dose is important. In the dose-ranging studies with rPA, doses lower than the approved dose (10 U plus 10 U 30 minutes apart) yielded lower infarct-related artery patency rates (20). With tPA, an infusion rate that results in infusion over a period longer than 90 minutes also has a lower rate of infarct-related artery patency and thrombolysis in myocardial infarction (TIMI) grade 3 flow (21–23). Data from the National Registry of Myocardial Infarction (NRMI-2) examined doses of tPA. Patients who received an excessive dose of tPA (>1.5 mg/kg), had a 2.3 times increase in intracranial hemorrhage rate. After adjusting for differences in baseline characteristics, a 49% increase in intracranial hemorrhage was attributable to the higher dose (24).

Bolus thrombolytics are easier to administer and should limit the number of medication errors (16). The two bolus thrombolytics currently available are rPA and TNK-tPA. Both have been shown to have clinical efficacy similar to tPA (25–28). rPA is administered as two boluses (10 U each) 30 minutes apart. Initially some concern was seen that the second bolus would be overlooked, leading to medication errors and inadequate coronary reperfusion. This appears to be unfounded, with fewer than 1% of patients failing to receive the full dose, whereas 4% of tPA patients fail to receive the full dose for one reason or another (29). TNK-tPA is a single bolus injection that requires weight-based dosing. Serious and intracranial bleeding were significantly higher (5.6% and 12%, respectively) in those who received too high a dose (>0.53 mg/kg) versus those who received the correct dose (0% and 4.5%, respectively). Thus, the trade-off becomes one of weight-based dosing and the errors associated with improper weight estimates versus the extra steps involved in double bolus therapy. We have chosen double bolus therapy at our institution but will review this approach at regular intervals as more data become available.

EXPANDING THE HORIZON

As the therapy of acute coronary syndrome becomes more complex, standardization becomes more imperative. State-of-the-art care now includes multiple medications, including aspirin (both oral and i.v.), beta-blockers, nitrates, heparin, and frequent or even continuous ECG monitoring. Prehospital thrombolyis has been proposed for more than a decade but was impractical before the advent of bolus thrombolytics (30). The ongoing TIMI-19 trial will help delineate where prehospital use might be most appropriate. Recent literature has pointed to the importance of appropriate weight-based doses of heparin (31,32), and heparin doses must be adjusted with the glycoprotein IIb/IIIa inhibitor agents (33,34). The GUSTO-IV trial using lower doses of thrombolytic agents combined with the glycoprotein IIb/IIIa agents is soon to be released and may add to the complexity of the decision-making in the therapy of acute coronary syndromes, including acute MI.

A similar checklist to the one used for thrombolytic administration can be adapted to the care of all ED patients with chest pain suspected of having an acute coronary syndrome. Such a system should be simple, and should include only the critical information necessary to guide the physician. Such a system works best in conjunction with a "Chest Pain Center" pathway, as described elsewhere in this text. Such a checklist guides the patient from admission through disposition, providing critical reminders along the way. It is clear, however, that the increasing complexity described above may present opportunity for error in the busy ED setting. Computerized physician order entry, which has been shown to standardize care and reduce errors, clearly will play a central role in managing the complex interactions and calculations necessary for safe and effective treatment.

CONCLUSIONS

Few areas in medicine have evolved as dramatically over the past 20 years as the approach to acute coronary ischemia. Myocardial infarction used to be considered an "untreatable" event, and physicians stood by (with often ineffective therapies) to treat only the complications of the MI. Death of heart tissue, once expected, is now considered a measure of individual and system failure. Well-conducted, randomized clinical trials have proved the effectiveness of aspirin, beta-blockers, nitroglycerin, platelet IIb/IIIa inhibitors, lytic therapy, and PCI in reducing infarct size, ejection fraction compromise, recurrent events, and mortality. Although providing astonishing improvement in outcome for patients, these interventions have greatly increased the complexity of emergency treatment of acute coronary syndromes and the time pressures on the emergency physicians caring for these patients. A well-defined critical pathway, using principles supported by the literature and agreed on by both cardiologists and emergency physicians, represents the best approach to incorporating these crucial interventions safely into daily clinical use. Although interpretation of the literature allows for some discretion with respect to choice or sequencing of the individual agents, it is clear that rapid, decisive, comprehensive therapy is now the standard of care in acute coronary syndrome.

REFERENCES

1. Cannon CP. Relationship of symptom-onset-to-balloon time and door-to-balloon time with mortality of patients undergoing angioplasty for acute myocardial infarction. *JAMA* 2000;283:2941–2947.
2. Boersma E, Maas AC, Deckers JW, et al. Early thrombolytic treatment in acute myocardial infarction: reappraisal of the golden hour. *Lancet* 1996;348:771–775.
3. Leape LL, Woods DD, Hatlie MJ, et al. Promoting patient safety by preventing medical error. *JAMA* 1998;280:1444–1447.
4. Wears R, Leape LL. Human error in emergency medicine. *Ann Emerg Med* 1999;34:370–372.
5. Bates DW, Miller EB, Cullen DJ, et al. Patient risk factors for adverse drug events in hospitalized patients. ADE Prevention Study Group. *Arch Intern Med* 1999;159:2553–2560.
6. Pearson SD, Goulart-Fisher D, Lee TH. Critical pathways as a strategy for improving care: problems and potential. *Ann Intern Med* 1995;123:941–948.
7. Bates DW, Leape LL, Cullen DJ, et al. Effect of computerized physician order entry and a team intervention on prevention of serious medication errors. *JAMA* 1998;280:1311–1316.
8. Ryan TJ, Antman EM, Brooks NH, et al. 1999 Update: ACC/AHA Guidelines for management of patients with acute myocardial infarction. *Circulation* 1999;100:1016–1030.
9. GISSI (Gruppo Italiano per lo Studio Della Streptochinasi Nell'Infarto Miocardico). Effectiveness of intravenous thrombolytic treatment in acute myocardial infarction. *Lancet* 1986;1(8478):397–401.
10. ISIS-2 (Second International Study of Infarct Survival) Collaborative Group. Randomized trial of intravenous streptokinase, oral aspirin, both, or neither among 17,187 cases of suspected acute myocardial infarction: ISIS-2. *Lancet* 1998;2:349–360.
11. ISIS-3. A randomized trial of streptokinase versus tissue plasminogen activator versus anistreplase and of aspirin plus heparin versus aspirin alone among 41,299 cases of suspected acute myocardial infarction. ISIS-3 (Third International Study of Infarct Survival) Collaborative Group. *Lancet* 1992;339:753–770.
12. A prospective trial of intravenous streptokinase in acute myocardial infarction (ISAM): mortality, morbidity and infarct size at 21 days. The ISAM Study Group. *N Engl J Med* 1986;314:1465–1471.
13. Collen D, Lijnen HR. Basic and clinical aspects of fibrinolysis and thrombolysis. *Blood* 1991;78:3114–3124.
14. An international randomized trial comparing four thrombolytic strategies for acute myocardial infarction. The GUSTO Investigators. *N Engl J Med* 1993;329:673–682.
15. GISSI-2. A factorial randomized trial of alteplase versus streptokinase and heparin versus no heparin among 12,490 patients with acute myocardial infarction. *Lancet* 1990;336:65–71.
16. Cannon CP. Thrombolysis medication errors: benefits of bolus thrombolytic agents. *Am J Cardiol* 2000;85(8A):17C–22C.
17. Vorchheimer DA, Baruch L, Thompson TD, et al. North American vs non–North American streptokinase use in GUSTO-I: impact of protocol deviation on mortality benefit of TPA. *Circulation* 1997;96[Suppl 1]:I-535(abst).
18. Fernandes CM, Clark S, Price A, et al. How accurately do we estimate patient's weight in emergency departments? *Can Fam Physician* 1999;45:2373–2376.
19. Harris M, Patterson J, Morse J, et al. Doctors, nurses, and parents are equally poor at estimating pediatric weights. *Pediatr Emerg Care* 1999;15:17–18.
20. Smelling RW, Bode C, Kalbfleisch J, et al. More rapid, complete and stable coronary thrombolysis with bolus administration of reteplase compared with alteplase infusion in acute myocardial infarction. *Circulation* 1995;91:2725–2732.
21. Neuhaus KL, Feuerer W, Jeep-Teebe S, et al. Improved thrombolysis with a modified dose regimen of recombinant tissue-type plasminogen activator. *J Am Coll Cardiol* 1989;14:1566–1569.
22. Carney RJ, Murphy GA, Brandt TR, et al. Randomized angiographic trial of recombinant tissue-type plasminogen activator (alteplase) in myocardial infarction. *J Am Coll Cardiol* 1992;20:17–23.
23. Granger CB, Califf RM, Topol EJ. Thrombolytic therapy for acute myocardial infarction. *Drugs* 1992;44:293–325.
24. Gurwitz JH, Gore JM, Goldberg RJ, et al. Risk for intracranial hemorrhage after tissue plasminogen activator treatment for acute myocardial infarction. Participants in the National Registry of Myocardial Infarction 2. *Ann Intern Med* 1998;129:597–604.
25. The Global Use Strategies to Open Occluded Coronary Arteries (GUSTO-III) Investigators. A comparison of reteplase with alteplase for acute myocardial infarction. *N Engl J Med* 1997;337:1118–1123.
26. Cannon CP, Gibson CM, McCabe CH, et al. TNK–tissue plasminogen activator compared with front-loaded alteplase in acute myocardial infarction: results of the TIMI 10B trial. *Circulation* 1998;98:2805–2814.
27. Gibson CM, Cannon CP, Murphy SA, et al. Weight adjusted dosing of TNK–tissue plasminogen activator and its relation to angiographic outcomes in the thrombolysis in myocardial infarction 10B trial. *Am J Cardiol* 1999;84:976–980.
28. Assessment of the Safety and Efficacy of a New Thrombolytic Investigators. Single-bolus tenecteplase compared with front-loaded alteplase in acute myocardial infarction: the ASSENT-2 double-blind randomized trial. *Lancet* 1999;354:716–722.
29. Hilleman DE, Seyedroudbari A, Tejani A, et al. Cost-minimization analysis of direct injection and infusion thrombolytic therapy in acute myocardial infarction: a multi-center study. *Circulation* 1998;98:I-381(abst).
30. Cannon CP, Sayah AJ, Walls RM. Prehospital thrombolysis: an idea whose time has come. *Clin Cardiol* 1999;22[Suppl IV]:IV-9–IV-10.
31. Antman EM, for the TIMI 9A Investigators. Hirudin in acute myocardial infarction: safety report from the thrombolysis and thrombin inhibition in myocardial infarction (TIMI) 9A trial. *Circulation* 1994;90:1624–1630.
32. The Global Use of Strategies to Open Occluded Coronary Arteries (GUSTO) IIA Investigators. A randomized trial of intravenous heparin versus recombinant hirudin for acute coronary syndromes. *Circulation* 1994;90:1631–1637.
33. The Epic Investigators. Use of a monoclonal antibody directed against platelet glycoprotein IIb/IIIa receptor in high-risk coronary angioplasty. *N Engl J Med* 1994;330:956–961.
34. The Epilog Investigators. Platelet glycoprotein IIb/IIIa receptor blockade and low-dose heparin during percutaneous coronary revascularization. *N Engl J Med* 1997;336:1689–1696.

CHAPTER 5

Critical Pathways for Evaluating the Chest Pain Patient at Low Risk

Kirsten E. Fleischmann and Thomas H. Lee

Critical pathways for the management of patients with acute chest pain, who are at low risk, have been developed and implemented at many institutions, reflecting the importance and the potential opportunity for improvement in the care of patients with this syndrome. It is estimated that more than 5 million people present annually with acute chest pain to emergency departments (EDs) in the United States alone (1). Most of these patients are admitted for further evaluation and to exclude myocardial infarction (MI). However, a much smaller percentage actually develops MI, or even leaves the hospital with a defined cardiac cause of their chest pain. Conversely, approximately 2% to 4% of patients with MI are discharged directly from the ED, often with worse outcomes (2,3).

Thus, identifying the patient likely to suffer from ischemic disease who can benefit from the aggressive treatments developed over the past 10 to 15 years, while avoiding large numbers of admissions for noncardiac or benign conditions, has become a major focus of research and quality improvement efforts. This problem is particularly acute for patients without clear-cut evidence of an acute coronary syndrome (e.g., MI or unstable angina). Typically, these patients present without signs and symptoms of congestive heart failure (CHF) on examination; their electrocardiograms (ECG) are normal or unremarkable; and the initial enzyme determinations may be negative.

A variety of different approaches has been taken to help triage this "low risk" patient population, including the development of rapid testing for cardiac enzyme markers such as troponin, creatine kinase (CK)-isoforms, or myoglobin (4–6). Rest imaging, either with scintigraphy or echocardiography, has also been investigated (7–11). Stress testing, either alone or in conjunction with cardiac enzyme testing, to assess for provocable ischemia has been widely studied (12–21). More recently, stress scintigraphy and stress echocardiography have been used (22,23). Concurrently, a shift has occurred toward lower intensity care settings for the evaluation of these patients, including step-down units, observation units, or "chest pain ERs," units adjacent to or within the ED where patients can receive expedited evaluation (15,24,25).

Critical pathways for patients with chest pain at low risk incorporate many of these approaches with the goal of maintaining or improving outcomes, while increasing efficiency (26). The pathways in use at various institutions around the country share many common features, including:

- Rapid risk stratification through the history, examination, and ECG.
- Expedited interventions for patients at high risk with probable acute ischemic heart disease.
- Short observation periods for patients at low risk, followed by further risk stratification through exercise testing or other noninvasive strategies.
- Arrangement of follow-up in ambulatory settings for patients who are candidates for early discharge.

To provide insight into the development, implementation, and potential impact of such pathways, this chapter describes in detail one such critical pathway, developed at Brigham and Women's Hospital, Boston, Massachusetts, and validated prospectively with regard to safety.

DEVELOPMENT OF THE CRITICAL PATHWAY

The process of developing a critical pathway requires support or "buy-in" from the many disciplines involved in the care of these patients. We convened a group consisting of ED physicians, cardiology experts in noninvasive testing and acute care, and personnel in laboratory medicine, nursing, and quality improvement, as well as representatives from a large health maintenance organization that accounts for about 20% of admissions for acute chest pain at our hospital.

We initially conducted a comprehensive literature search, as the critical pathway was designed to be evidence-based to the extent possible (26). For many issues (e.g., the safety of early exercise testing, or the optimal use of cardiac markers

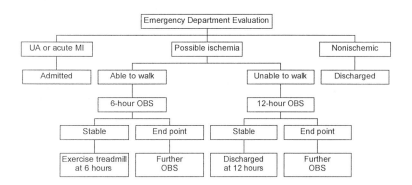

FIG. 5-1. Critical pathway for patients with acute chest pain at low risk. Adapted from Nichol G, Walls R, Goldman L, et al. A critical pathway for management of patients with acute chest pain who are at low risk for myocardial ischemia: recommendations and potential impact. *Ann Intern Med* 1997; 127(11):996–1005.

for injury), no controlled trial data were available, or no data focused on the low risk population eligible for the pathway. Using a combination of published literature and expert opinion, and building on experience from other institutions, an initial draft of the pathway was created.

The pathway then underwent several cycles of commentary and revision, until consensus was achieved over a period of about 4 months. By involving all of the clinical and administrative groups who were "stakeholders" in the process, we hoped to encourage utilization of the pathway, foster a proprietary attitude toward its development (i.e., "ownership"), and ensure that the practical expertise of clinical leaders involved in the day-to-day care of these patients was incorporated.

CRITICAL PATHWAY FOR PATIENTS AT LOW RISK

An overview of the critical pathway developed and its place in the overall triage of patients with chest pain is given in Fig. 5-1. Patients older than 30 years of age who presented with a chief complaint of chest pain, not explained by trauma or chest x-ray abnormality, were urgently assessed. On the basis of the initial history and physical examination as well as an ECG, the patient was triaged into one of three groups. The first group, which contained those with clear-cut evidence of an acute coronary syndrome, was treated aggressively, with reperfusion as appropriate, and admitted. Critical pathways developed for patients with acute ischemic heart disease were implemented for the care of these patients. Conversely, those patients for whom the attending physician felt the pain was clearly noncardiac were evaluated and treated further according to the cause of their chest pain, and discharged directly from the ED, as appropriate.

However, an intermediate group whose pain was felt probably not to be ischemic remained. These patients typically had no signs of CHF on examination, and their initial ECGs were normal or showed only nonspecific changes. Patients meeting these criteria and able to exercise underwent a period of observation of 6 hours from their last episode of chest pain. During this time, they received at least one set of cardiac enzymes (CK-MB) drawn at least 4 hours after pain. If they remained stable, without recurrent symptoms or other worrisome signs or symptoms, and if their initial

enzyme determination was normal, they underwent standard treadmill exercise testing. Final triage was at the discretion of the treating attending physician, although guidelines based on the results of exercise testing were provided (Table 5-1).

Patients unable to exercise were typically observed for a longer period of time, as previous work by our group has shown that serial enzyme determinations over 12 hours is sufficient to exclude MI in patients at low risk (2). Alternately, they could undergo pharmacologic stress testing. Imaging in conjunction with standard exercise testing was performed at the discretion of the treating physician. Standard exercise testing was made available for 13 hours each weekday (8 a.m. to 9 p.m.) and for 4 hours on each weekend day (10 a.m. to 2 p.m.).

RETROSPECTIVE APPLICATION

As a first step in determining the safety of such a pathway, we applied the pathway retrospectively to a cohort of 4,585 patients evaluated in the ED at Brigham and Women's Hospital for acute chest pain from July, 1990 to February 24, 1994 (26). Of these patients, 1,687 were discharged directly from the ED, and 2,898 were admitted for further evaluation. Of patients admitted to the hospital, 1,152 (40%) were eligible for the pathway according to the entry criteria described above. Over a 6-hour observation period, 67 (2.3%) developed an endpoint requiring further observation; 1,085 remained on the pathway. Outcomes for these patients included 163 (15%) who left the hospital with a diagnosis of unstable angina, and 13 cases (1.2%) of MI, as determined by the criteria of the Chest Pain Study—Multiphase Study of ED patients with chest pain conducted at Brigham and women's Hospital over many years (26–35). Serious complications developed in 5/1085 (0.5%). Length of stay in these patients averaged 2.8 ± 4.8 days.

Retrospectively, it was estimated that application of the pathway in this cohort of patients could have saved substantial days of hospitalization without compromising patient outcomes. Lengthening the observation period to 12 hours would have decreased the number of patients remaining on the pathway to 1,068, of which 163 (15%) developed unstable angina, 4 (0.4%) developed MI, and 5 (0.5%) developed life-threatening complications. Thus, a 6-hour observation

TABLE 5-1. *Recommendations for the triage of patients undergoing ETT after 6 hours of observation*

ETT interpretation	Test criterion	Suggested triage
Negative	No ST-segment changes or symptoms at ≥85% MPHR	Discharge with follow-up within 7 days
Consistent with ischemia (but not diagnostic)	Symptoms typical of angina *or* 1 millimeter ST-segment depression at >85% MPHR	Discharge with follow-up in 1–2 days
Highly predictive	≥2 mm ST-segment depression *or* 1 mm ST-segment depression *and* typical symptoms	Admit
Strongly positive	Fall of blood pressure with exercise Marked ST-segment changes in multiple leads Prolonged, persistent ST-segment changes in recovery	Admit
Indeterminate/ inadequate	Failure to achieve 85% of MPHR with absence of above criteria	Review with physician performing stress test

ETT, exercise treadmill testing; MPHR, maximum age-predicted heart rate. Adapted from Nichol G, Walls R, Goldman L, et al. A critical pathway for management of patients with acute chest pain who are at low risk for myocardial ischemia: recommendations and potential impact. *Ann Intern Med* 1997;127(11):996–1005.

period was felt to represent a reasonable compromise between published experiences with a 9-hour observation period (15) and immediate exercise testing in the absence of prior cardiac enzyme determination (12,17).

It is important to note that a single enzyme determination 4 hours after pain is not sufficient to fully rule out MI. We estimated that a single enzyme determination 3 hours after pain has a sensitivity of 76% for MI (26). However, in a population with low *a priori* risk of infarction (<5%), a negative enzyme determination at this time reduces the risk of MI to 1.9% (95% confidence interval, 0.9% to 3.0%), which was felt low enough to proceed with provocative testing. Thus, after retrospective evaluation, we felt the pathway for patients at low risk would help achieve the goals of our chest pain protocol (Table 5-2) while preserving safety and potentially improving efficiency.

IMPLEMENTATION AND VALIDATION

Our critical pathway was introduced as a quality improvement initiative. To facilitate assessment of the pathway, two to three research assistants from the Department of Quality Improvement were charged with collecting clinical and outcomes data for patients in the pathway. These data included a detailed history and physical examination; findings from ECG, laboratory tests, and exercise testing; and other information concerning survival, MI, and cardiac procedures at discharge, 1 week, and 6 months after discharge. Data were also collected on health status and patient satisfaction at 1 week and 6 months after discharge, and also on follow-up visits, both to the ED and to patients' physicians.

TABLE 5-2. *Goals of chest pain protocol*

Rapid diagnosis of ischemia
Rapid reperfusion of acute myocardial infarction as indicated
Resolution of ischemic pain
Triage to the appropriate level of care

Protocol implementation of the pathway was aided by "in-services" with both ED physicians and nursing staff, to facilitate their familiarity with the protocol. Exercise testing laboratory personnel were also familiarized with the protocol and with the need for prompt testing of these patients.

OUTCOMES

During the first 6 months of implementation, 1,363 visits of 1,207 patients met the entry criteria described above. Of these, 145 visits (10.6%) were deemed eligible for the pathway by the treating physician—a proportion considerably lower than that predicted from the retrospective analysis. We believe that this lower percentage reflects the challenge of getting physician acceptance, even after considerable efforts to do so. However, an additional factor is the logistical difficulty of making the pathway easily accessible and implemented in a busy, often chaotic ED.

Clinical characteristics for the patients are given in Table 5-3. Generally, risk factor profiles for patients triaged to the clinical pathway were intermediate in risk between those who were discharged directly from the ED and those admitted directly without pathway evaluation. By definition, none had ECG changes suggestive of ischemia. All patients were at low or very low risk for major events as defined by the Goldman algorithm for major complications (1). Initial CK levels averaged 157 ± 124 U/L, ranging from 29 to 904 U/L. The initial CK-MB exceeded 5 ng/ml in one case, but the percentage of MB was only 1.7% of the total CK value.

Hospital Outcomes

Of the 145 patients felt eligible for the low risk critical pathway, most (90.3%) were discharged from the ED or the adjacent observation unit. The remainder (14 patients, 9.7%) were admitted, either on the basis of an event during observation or the results of their exercise test. No MIs were diagnosed in the critical pathway group and all patients survived to hospital discharge.

TABLE 5-3. *Characteristics of the critical pathway patient visits in comparison with those admitted or discharged directly from the emergency department*

	Directly admitted (n = 805)	Critical pathway (n = 145)	Directly discharged (n = 413)	P value
Age (yr)	63 ± 14	51 ± 12	51 ± 16	
Male gender	416 (52%)	67 (46%)	169 (41%)	0.001
Race				0.001
–White	481 (61%)	63 (46%)	177 (43%)	
–Black	190 (24%)	40 (29%)	145 (36%)	
–Hispanic	98 (12%)	32 (23%)	78 (19%)	
–Asian/other	20 (3%)	3 (2%)	7 (2%)	
Family history	200 (25%)	31 (21%)	54 (13%)	0.001
Hypercholesterolemia	401 (50%)	42 (29%)	98 (24%)	0.001
Hypertension	514 (64%)	47 (32%)	139 (34%)	0.001
Diabetes	254 (32%)	19 (13%)	41 (10%)	0.001
Current or past smoker	393 (49%)	61 (42%)	134 (32%)	0.001
Previous MI	275 (34%)	7 (5%)	48 (12%)	0.001
Previous PTCA	94 (12%)	4 (3%)	9 (2%)	0.001
Previous CABG	128 (16%)	5 (3%)	20 (5%)	0.001
Ischemic changes on electrocardiogram	194 (24%)	0 (0%)	10 (2%)	0.001
Risk of MI >7%	222 (32%)	1 (1%)	14 (4%)	0.001

CABG, coronary artery bypass graft; MI, myocardial infarction; PTCA, percutaneous transluminal coronary angioplasty.

Seven-Day Outcomes

Survival status was directly determined in 141 of 145 patient visits (97.2%). Data on the remaining four patient visits were checked against death records of the Massachusetts Bureau of Vital Statistics. No deaths were recorded in the cohort. Of patients completing the 7-day questionnaire, only two reported presenting to an ED since their evaluation (1.7%). No deaths or MIs were recorded. Patients' satisfaction with the pathway was good, with 83.1% of respondents rating the care they received as very good or excellent; 93% stated they would return to the same ED if they had another problem requiring emergency care. Approximately 90% recalled receiving their discharge instructions. However, despite the availability of the special follow-up described, 55% were unaware of any follow-up appointment made before discharge from the ED.

Six-Month Outcomes

At 6 months, survival status was directly available in 90% of patients, all of whom survived. A check of the remaining names against the Massachusetts Bureau of Vital Statistics revealed no additional deaths. In the interim, 19% had visited an ED at least once, but only seven patients reported a visit for the same or similar symptoms. In addition, 13 respondents (12%) reported hospital admission, 6 reported an exercise test, and 2 reported cardiac catheterization. Both cardiac catheterizations occurred in patients with initially nondiagnostic exercise tests. These 6-month outcome statistics were similar to those in a previous cohort of patients at low or very low risk of major complications who were admitted and underwent expedited exercise testing within 48 hours of admission. Patients with negative exercise tests had a very low event rate over the next 6 months and only four patients (2%) had a cardiac event (MI, percutaneous transluminal coronary angioplasty, or coronary artery bypass graft).

LENGTH OF STAY AND DISCHARGE RATES

Median time to exercise testing for patients triaged by means of the pathway was 5.5 hours and the median length of stay was 7.7 hours—representing an approximate 74% decrease from the average length of stay for rule-out MI (DRG 143) in our hospital during the same period. The overall admission rate was 60%, a decrease from 63% in the earlier cohort in which retrospective validation of the pathway had been performed ($p < 0.05$). It is estimated that the average cost of a day of hospitalization for a patient with chest pain at low risk exceeds $1,000 (24). Therefore, a reduction of 3% in the admission rate was consistent with substantial reduction in inpatient costs.

LIMITATIONS

Our critical pathway was implemented as a quality improvement initiative, rather than as a randomized, controlled trial. Therefore, we cannot fully distinguish the effect of the pathway from secular temporal trends. Our follow-up relied on self-report, and some adverse outcomes may have been missed. However, the follow-up rate in the 7 days after presentation was excellent and suggested very low rates of representation to acute care or complications in this low risk population. Rates of follow-up after ED evaluation were disappointing, and suggest that new strategies are needed to ensure patient follow-up in the ambulatory setting.

FUTURE DIRECTIONS

Our critical pathway addressed patients clearly defined as low risk by the absence of persistent chest pain, CHF, and significant ECG changes. Future work will focus on expanding the population of patients at low risk eligible for the pathway; for example, to patients with nonspecific ECG changes in addition to normal tracings or to patients with ongoing, but clearly atypical chest pain. Experience with immediate exercise testing for patients at low risk is being extended at many medical centers, and can be expected to become routine for carefully defined patient subsets. The role of markers for myocardial injury is uncertain in this low risk population, and is being explored in ongoing investigations.

In summary, critical pathways for patients at low risk with acute chest pain can be expected to be revised and improved as economic pressures increase and hospitals redesign care to improve quality and efficiency. During this evolution, the importance of continual monitoring of the safety and efficacy of the pathway in new iterations is critical.

REFERENCES

1. deFilippi CR, Runge MS. Evaluating the chest pain patient: scope of the problem. *Cardiol Clin* 1999;17(2):307–326.
2. Lee TH, Rouan GW, Weisberg MC, et al. Clinical characteristics and natural history of patients with acute myocardial infarction sent home from the emergency room. *Am J Cardiol* 1987;60(4):219–224.
3. McCarthy BD, Beshansky JR, D'Angostino RB, et al. Missed diagnoses of acute myocardial infarction in the emergency department: results from a multicenter study. *Ann Emerg Med* 1993;22(3):579–582.
4. Hamm CW, Goldman BU, Heeschen C, et al. Emergency room triage of patients with acute chest pain by means of rapid testing for cardiac troponin T or troponin I. *N Engl J Med* 1997;337(23):1648–1653.
5. DeWinter RJ, Koster RW, Sturk A, et al. Value of myoglobin, troponin T, and CK-MB in ruling out an acute myocardial infarction in the emergency room. *Circulation* 1995;92(12):3401–3407.
6. Puleo PR, Meyer D, Wathen C, et al. Use of a rapid assay of subforms of creatinine kinase MB to diagnose or rule out acute myocardial infarction. *N Engl J Med* 1994;331(9):561–566.
7. Sabia P, Abbot RD, Afrookteh A, et al. Importance of two-dimensional echocardiographic assessment of left ventricular systolic function in patients presenting to the emergency room with cardiac-related symptoms. *Circulation* 1991;84(4):1615–1624.
8. Sabia P, Afrookteh A, Touchstone DA, et al. Value of regional wall motion abnormality in the emergency room diagnosis of acute myocardial infarction. *Circulation* 1991;84[Suppl 3]:I-85–I-92.
9. Kontos MC, Jesse RL, Schmidt KL, et al. Value of acute rest sestamibi perfusion imaging for evaluation of patients admitted to the emergency department with chest pain. *J Am Coll Cardiol* 1997;30(3):976–982.
10. Varetto T, Cantalupi D, Altieri A, et al. Emergency room technetium-99m sestamibi imaging to rule out acute myocardial ischemic events in patients with nondiagnostic electrocardiograms. *J Am Coll Cardiol* 1993;22(7):1804–1808.
11. Hilton TC, Thompson RC, Williams HJ, et al. Technetium-99m sestamibi myocardial perfusion imaging in the emergency room evaluation of chest pain. *J Am Coll Cardiol* 1994;23(5):1016–1022.
12. Kirk JD, Turnipseed S, Lewis WR, et al. Evaluation of chest pain in low-risk patients presenting to the emergency department: the role of immediate exercise testing. *Ann Emerg Med* 1998;32(1):1–7.
13. Gomez MA, Anderson JL, Karagounis LA, et al. An emergency department based protocol for rapidly ruling out myocardial ischemia reduces hospital time and expense: results of a randomized trial (ROMIO). *J Am Coll Cardiol* 1996;28(1):25–33.
14. Zalenski RJ, McCarren M, Roberts R, et al. An evaluation of a chest pain diagnostic protocol to exclude acute cardiac ischemia in the emergency department. *Arch Intern Med* 1997;157(10):1085–1091.
15. Gibler W, Runyon JP, Levy RC, et al. A rapid diagnostic and treatment center for patients with chest pain in the emergency department. *Ann Emerg Med* 1995;25(1):1–8.
16. Kerns JR, Shaub TF, Fontanarosa PB. Emergency cardiac stress testing in the evaluation of emergency department patients with atypical chest pain. *Ann Emerg Med* 1993;22(5):794–798.
17. Lewis WR, Amsterdam EA. Utility and safety of immediate exercise testing of low-risk patients admitted to the hospital for suspected acute myocardial infarction. *Am J Cardiol* 1994;74(10):987–990.
18. Mikhail MG, Smith FA, Gray M, Britton C, Frederiksen SM. Cost-effectiveness of mandatory stress testing in chest pain center patients. *Ann Emerg Med* 1997;29(1):88–98.
19. Roberts RR, Zalenski RJ, Mensah EK, et al. Costs of an emergency department–based accelerated diagnostic protocol vs hospitalization in patients with chest pain. *JAMA* 1997;278(20):1670–1676.
20. Tsakonis JS, Shesser R, Rosenthal R, et al. Safety of immediate treadmill testing in selected emergency department patients with chest pain: a preliminary report. *Am J Emerg Med* 1991;9(6):557–559.
21. Uretsky BF, Farquhar DS, Berezin AF, et al. Symptomatic myocardial infarction without chest pain: prevalence and clinical course. *Am J Cardiol* 1977;40(4):498–503.
22. Trippi JA, Lee KS, Kopp G, et al. Dobutamine stress tele-echocardiography for evaluation of emergency department patients with chest pain. *J Am Coll Cardiol* 1997;30(3):627–632.
23. Ritchie JL, Bateman TM, Bonow RO, et al. Guidelines for Clinical Use of Cardiac Radionuclide Imaging. Report of the American College of Cardiology/American Heart Association Task Force on Assessment of Diagnostic and Therapeutic Cardiovascular Procedures (Committee on Radionuclide Imaging), developed in collaboration with the American Society of Nuclear Cardiology. *J Am Coll Cardiol* 1995;25:521–547.
24. Gaspoz JM, Lee TH, Weinstein MC, et al. Cost-effectiveness of a new short-stay unit to rule out acute myocardial infarction in low risk patients. *Am J Cardiol* 1994;24(5):1249–1259.
25. Graff L, Joseph T, Andelman R, et al. American College of Emergency Physicians Information Paper: chest pain units in emergency departments—a report from the Short-Term Observation Services section. *Am J Cardiol* 1995;76(14):1036–1039.
26. Nichol G, Walls R, Goldman L, et al. A critical pathway for management of patients with acute chest pain who are at low risk for myocardial ischemia: recommendations and potential impact. *Ann Intern Med* 1997;127(11):996–1005.
27. Goldman L, Cook EF, Brand DA, et al. A computer protocol to predict myocardial infarction in emergency department patients with chest pain. *N Engl J Med* 1988;318(13):797–803.
28. Goldman L, Weinberg M, Weisberg M, et al. A computer-derived protocol to aid in the diagnosis of emergency room patients with acute chest pain. *N Engl J Med* 1982;307(10):588–596.
29. Lee TH, Cook EF, Weisberg M, et al. Acute chest pain in the emergency room: identification and examination of low-risk patients. *Arch Intern Med* 1985;145(1):65–69.
30. Lee TH, Cook EF, Weisberg MC, et al. Impact of the availability of a prior electrocardiogram on the triage of the patient with acute chest pain. *J Gen Intern Med* 1990;5(5):381–388.
31. Lee TH, Goldman L. The coronary care unit turns 25: historical trends and future directions. *Ann Intern Med* 1988;108(6):887–894.
32. Lee TH, Pearson SD, Johnson PA, et al. Failure of information as an intervention to modify clinical management: a time-series trial in patients with acute chest pain. *Ann Intern Med* 1995;122(6):434–437.
33. Lee TH, Rouan GW, Weisberg MC, et al. Clinical characteristics and natural history of patients with acute myocardial infarction sent home from the emergency room. *Am J Cardiol* 1987;60(4):219–224.
34. Lee TH, Rouan GW, Weisberg MC, et al. Sensitivity of routine clinical criteria for diagnosing myocardial infarction within 24 hours of hospitalization. *Ann Intern Med* 1987;106(2):181–186.
35. Lee TH, Weisberg MC, Cook EF, et al. Evaluation of creatine kinase and creatine kinase–MB for diagnosing myocardial infarction: clinical impact in the emergency room. *Arch Intern Med* 1987;147(1):115–121.

CHAPTER 6

Critical Pathways Approach Using Nuclear Cardiac Imaging in the Emergency Department

Joseph P. Ornato

OVERVIEW

Precise and cost-effective assessment of chest pain in the emergency department (ED) is a well-recognized problem. Despite the high rate of false-positive admissions, the traditional diagnostic paradigm fails to detect 1% to 8% of patients with acute myocardial infarction (MI), resulting in an inappropriate discharge home (1–8). Such false-negative cases ("missed" acute MIs) are associated with a relatively high short-term morbidity, mortality, and medicolegal burden for emergency physicians. Although the actual number of missed unstable angina or acute coronary syndrome (ACS) cases is not known precisely, it is also of concern because these patients are at significant risk.

The advent of highly effective, time-dependent treatment for acute MI and ACS, coupled with the need to reduce healthcare costs, adds further incentive for clinicians to get the "right answer" quickly and to reduce unnecessary admissions and lengthy hospitalizations. Investigators have tried various diagnostic tools (e.g., clinical decision algorithms, cardiac markers, echocardiography, and myocardial perfusion imaging) in an attempt to avoid missing patients with acute MI (and, to a lesser extent, ACS). The most successful strategies to emerge thus far tend to use a combination of myocardial markers, short-term observation, diagnostic imaging, and provocative stress testing.

This chapter describes a specific strategy that has evolved at the Medical College of Virginia (MCV) in Richmond, Virginia, which incorporates several different complementary technologies, with a special reliance on the use of single photon emission computed tomography (SPECT)-gated nuclear myocardial perfusion imaging

RATIONALE FOR THE STRATEGY

An 890-bed tertiary care academic medical center, MCV has a 65-bed ED complex that treats more than 82,000 patients per year, approximately 3,000 of whom present with symptoms suggesting the possibility of acute MI, ACS, or both. Given this high volume and potential for diagnostic error, in January 1994 MCV implemented a sophisticated critical pathway approach to the triage and treatment of patients with suspected acute cardiac ischemia. The strategy has four basic goals: (a) to rule out acute MI; (b) to rule out an ACS other than acute MI; (c) to screen for the presence of clinically significant coronary artery disease in patients who were felt to be at risk; and (d) to identify nonischemic and noncardiovascular causes for a patient's symptoms if acute MI and ACS were not present.

This strategy relies heavily on the use of both rest and stress SPECT-gated nuclear perfusion imaging. Myocardial perfusion imaging using radionuclides is a valuable tool proved for the detection of ischemic and infarcted myocardium. A variety of radiopharmaceuticals are available that can be used clinically to define gross cardiac anatomy, myocardial perfusion, and global and regional ventricular function. Radioisotope myocardial perfusion imaging is virtually noninvasive (except for a low risk injection of radionuclide through a peripheral vein) and imposes little if any risk to patients.

Myocardial perfusion imaging is widely available in most hospitals and provides adequate images in most adult patients. Most major medical centers and community hospitals have had considerable experience in the use of thallium-201 (^{201}Tl). Myocardial perfusion abnormalities can be detected in cases of acute ischemia or scarring from prior MI. If a perfusion abnormality is detected when ^{201}Tl is injected following exercise, it is beneficial to reimage the patient several hours later after the thallium has had time to "redistribute" in the myocardium. If the defect disappears on the rest study ("reversible defect"), likely, the patient had reversible ischemia (angina). If the defect persists, an MI or scar from a prior MI is likely present.

Technetium 99m-sestamibi (^{99m}Tc sestamibi) offers an important advantage over ^{201}Tl for decision-making in the acute clinical setting. Because ^{99m}Tc sestamibi does not redistribute in the myocardium significantly after intravenous injection,

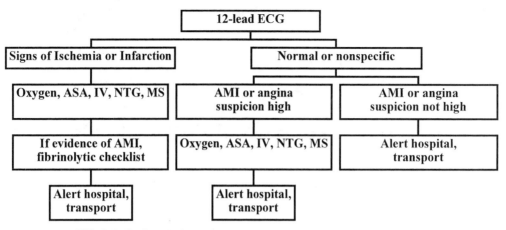

FIG. 6-1. Prehospital protocol used by paramedics in Richmond, VA.

it "freezes time" and captures a "snapshot" of the state of myocardial perfusion at the time of injection (9). The patient does not need to be placed under a scanner immediately after the injection, but can be stabilized clinically and imaged 1 to 4 hours after the injection. This makes it particularly useful and practical for detecting myocardial ischemia in patients with spontaneous chest pain. In fact, perfusion abnormalities can often be detected by either ^{201}Tl or ^{99m}Tc sestamibi for up to several hours after the last episode of chest pain in patients with cardiac ischemia (10,11).

Gated SPECT imaging can be performed with ^{99m}Tc sestamibi to study myocardial perfusion better and to look for segmental abnormalities of left ventricular wall motion (hypokinesis, dyskinesis, or akinesis), or failure of a portion of the left ventricle to thicken during systole (12,13).

In experienced hands, ^{99m}Tc sestamibi scintigraphy can provide valuable, accurate diagnostic and prognostic information in patients presenting to the ED with symptoms of acute cardiac ischemia (11,14–22). If the rest study is negative, a provocative stress study (exercise or pharmacologic) can be performed with ^{99m}Tc sestamibi the following day on adult patients with atypical symptoms, nondiagnostic electrocardiograms (ECG), and no clinical or laboratory evidence (e.g., serial ECG and enzymes) of acute MI to screen for the presence of hemodynamically significant coronary artery disease.

VERTICALLY INTEGRATED CRITICAL PATHWAY STRATEGY

The MCV strategy is built on a vertically integrated approach to comprehensively serve the needs of the patient with chest pain. Vertical integration refers to the fact that the program begins in the community with our highly advanced prehospital care system and flows seamlessly through care in the ED and on to the various diagnostic and therapeutic inpatient and outpatient services at MCV.

The multidisciplinary acute coronary treatment ("ACT") team at MCV is actively involved in the design and operation

of Richmond's high-performance emergency medical services (EMS) system. All ambulances (including emergency and nonemergency vehicles) in the city are staffed continuously with advanced life support paramedics who are trained and equipped to perform prehospital 12-lead ECGs on patients with chest pain. Therapy in the field is driven by the results of the prehospital ECG using a formal protocol (Fig. 6-1). Because MCV strategy relies heavily on the use of cardiac nuclear imaging, the use of nitroglycerin is restricted to those patients who manifest objective electrocardiographic evidence of myocardial ischemia, because this coronary vasodilator can decrease the sensitivity of myocardial perfusion imaging.

Prehospital ECG tracings are sent by cell phone to the ED, allowing paramedics to sound an alert early when a patient need lifesaving reperfusion therapy. Paramedics are also trained to complete a "fibrinolytic checklist" in the field when the ECG indicates an ST-segment elevation infarction.

All patients with chest pain or other symptoms suggestive of myocardial ischemia are brought directly into the treatment unit where an immediate ECG is performed by nurses or specially trained emergency care technicians. Based on the baseline ECG, presenting character of the chest pain, the patient's past medical history, and risk factor profile, the ED attending physician assigns patients to one of five pathways or "levels" that are based on the probability of acute MI or ACS (Fig. 6-2) (21). A detailed definition of each chest pain level is discussed below.

Level 1

Patients are assigned to level 1 (Fig. 6-3) if the ECG shows evidence of an acute MI with ST elevation (or signs of acute true posterior infarction). Therapy includes early fibrinolysis or acute percutaneous coronary intervention. All level 1 patients are admitted to the CCU as soon as possible. Serial ECG and myocardial markers [creatine kinase (CK)-MB, myoglobin, troponin] are performed over a 24-hour interval, primarily to quantitate the extent of the infarction.

Level	AMI risk	ACS risk	Strategy	Disposition
1	Very High	Very High	Fibrinolysis &/or PCI	CCU
2	High	High	Heparin, ASA, NTG, IIb/IIIa inhibitors	CCU
3	Moderate	Moderate	Markers + nuclear imaging	Observation (ED or CCU)
4	Low	Moderate or Low	Nuclear imaging	Home + outpatient stress test
5	Very Low	Very Low	As needed	Home

FIG. 6-2. The five track critical pathways at the Medical College of Virginia in Richmond, VA.

Level 2

Patients are assigned to level 2 (Fig. 6-4) in cases of a high clinical suspicion of non–ST-elevation acute MI, ACS based on prolonged (typically >20–30 minutes) symptoms accompanied by ischemic ST-T changes on ECG (horizontal or downsloping ST depression >1 mm 80 msec after the J-point and/or T wave inversion). Therapy includes nitroglycerin, heparin (unfractionated or low molecular weight), aspirin, beta-blockers, or glycoprotein IIb/IIIa inhibitors unless contraindicated. All level 2 patients are admitted to the CCU as soon as possible and receive serial ECG and markers as for level 1 patients.

Level 3

Patients are assigned to level 3 (Fig. 6-5) when a moderate suspicion of ACS or a low suspicion of acute MI exists. Typical patients in this category have prolonged symptoms (typically >20–30 minutes) unaccompanied by ischemic changes (either a normal ECG, nonspecific ST-T abnormality, or a complex ECG because of ventricular hypertrophy, intraventricular conduction disturbance, or bundle branch block). Level 3 patients are injected with ^{99m}Tc sestamibi (MIBI) as soon as possible (usually within 10 minutes after the ECG is taken).

A SPECT-gated myocardial perfusion imaging study is performed 60 to 90 minutes later. The scan itself takes approximately 10 to 15 minutes. Patients are transported to and from the nuclear medicine department with continuous cardiac monitoring by either a nurse or advanced life support paramedic technician. Level 3 patients are observed in the ED or CCU with cardiac monitoring, serial ECG, and myocardial markers drawn on ED arrival and at hours 3, 6, and 8 after ED arrival. If any of these tests confirm the presence of acute MI or ACS, the patient is treated appropriately and, in many cases, will undergo further invasive or noninvasive diagnostic testing before hospital discharge. If all of these tests are negative, a provocative stress test (either a treadmill or dipyridamole study with SPECT-gated myocardial perfusion imaging using MIBI or a stress echocardiogram) is performed. If the stress test is also negative, the patient is discharged home directly from the ED or CCU.

Level 4

Patients assigned to level 4 (Fig. 6-6) are considered to have an extremely low probability of either acute MI or ACS based on the initial clinical evaluation. They all have a normal or nondiagnostic ECG by definition, and the episodes of chest pain are typically brief (usually <20 minutes) in duration.

All level 4 patients are injected with ^{99m}Tc sestamibi (MIBI) as soon as possible (usually within 10 minutes after the ECG is taken) in the ED. A SPECT-gated myocardial perfusion imaging study is performed 60 to 90 minutes later, just as for level 3 patients, by a cardiac nuclear technician. Images are processed immediately and read by a nuclear imaging resident, attending physician, or both. Results are transmitted immediately to the ED by fax machine.

Level 1: Pt. Weight: _____
THROMBOLYTIC THERAPY PROTOCOL

Initial Assessment
1. *Confirm acute MI by ECG. Must have ST elevation infarct &/or evidence of true posterior MI or LBBB with ischemic symptoms.*

2. Allergy to aspirin: [ ] No   [ ] Yes
3. Check initial blood pressures (both arms)
   Initial BP: R arm ____/____mm Hg
                      L arm ____/____mm Hg
   Gradient between R & L arm SBP:
                      _____mm Hg

****
If SBP > 180 or DBP >110 mm Hg, urgently consider NTG (SL until the initiation of IV) and/or Metoprol IV . Titrate NTG drip every 5 min. to control BP.
****

4. Check stool for blood [ ] negative
                          [ ] positive
5. Notify CICU team ASAP   [ ] done

General Orders
1. Bedrest
2. Nasal oxygen at _____L/min by cannula PRN.
3. Check VS q5min (by monitor if necessary for patient safety) until 15 min after tPA infusion completed. Then, q15 min x 1h; q30 min x 1h; and q1 - 2 h x 24h per nursing standards.
4. Neurochecks q1h x 12h.
5. Adjust heparin using CICU/CMICU Heparin Management Nomogram and aPTT results.

Labs
1. Start 2-3 venous access lines (avoid central access unless absolutely necessary).
2. STAT Heme 18, Chem 7, U/A, PT, APTT, Magnesium.
3. CK Mass/Relative Index, Troponin I, Hepatic Panel, Lipid profile,STBB.
4. CK Mass/Relative Index, Troponin I at 6, 12, 18, and 24 hrs.
5. APTT drawn 3 and 6 hrs after starting heparin.

Medication preparation
1. Reconstitute tPA (100 mg) with 100 ml of STERILE WATER for Injection (no other diluent is acceptable) and administer by buretrol without inline filter. Do not shake.
2. When the tPA infusion is completed, flush IV line with 25cc of D5W at the same rate of infusion to clear tPA from the line.

Baby aspirin 2 tabs (162 mg) PO chewed stat if not allergic.

If ASA allergic: Plavix 300 mg po stat.

If no contraindications exist:
tPA 15 mg IV bolus STAT.
Do not delay tPA for 3rd IV line placement.

Start tPA _____mg (0.75 mg/kg DO NOT EXCEED 50 mg) infuse over next 30 min.,
And then follow with tPA _____mg (0.50 mg/kg, DO NOT EXCEED 35 mg) over the next 60 min.

Heparin 60u/kg IV bolus (max dose = 4000u) followed by Heparin 20,000u in 500 ml D5W maintenance infusion at 12u/kg/hr (max dose = 1000u/hr).

IV NTG (100mg/ 250 D5W). Initiate at 3cc/hr; titrate up to relieve chest pain while keeping SBP >90 mm Hg.

Metoprolol 5 mg IV over 5 min if no evidence of CHF, bronchospasm, hypotension, or heart rate < 60 bpm. Repeat x 2 additional doses 5 mins apart (total of 15 mg over 15 min)

Metoprolol 25 mg PO 30-60 min. after IV metoprolol given.

Morphine Sulfate _____ mg IV x 1.

FIG. 6-3. The level 1 pathway.

If the study results are normal, the patient is sent home directly from the ED with a scheduled appointment for a provocative stress test (either a treadmill or dipyridamole study with SPECT-gated myocardial perfusion imaging using MIBI or a stress echocardiogram) on the next working day. If the stress test is abnormal, the patient is admitted to the hospital for further evaluation. If the stress test is negative, a cardiologist conducts an exit evaluation of the patient. The test results are discussed with the patient and, when appropriate, the patient is referred for further evaluation (e.g., a gastrointestinal endoscopy), consultation, medical treatment, or risk factor modification. Special emphasis is placed on

referring patients back to their primary care physicians as soon as possible. A program support nurse practitioner has responsibility for communicating all test results back to the patient's primary care physician promptly and helping to schedule the patient's follow-up appointment.

Level 5

Patients in level 5 (Fig. 6-7) are typically young (<30 years of age), without significant coronary risk factors or cocaine use, and have clinically obvious noncardiac chest pain (e.g., a 20-year-old basketball player with a bruised rib, no risk

text continues on page 43

Medical College of Virginia Hospitals
Virginia Commonwealth University
Richmond, Virginia 23298

PHYSICIAN'S ORDERS

All orders must include date, time, and physician's signature. Do not abbreviate drug names. Circle route of administration or indicate other.*

MEDICATION ORDERS (ONLY ONE DRUG EACH ℞)

Patient Identification (Patient Plate)

DATE & TIME	ORDERS (OTHER THAN MEDICATION)

Level 2:

PROBABLE UNSTABLE ANGINA

Initial Assessment

1. *Typical anginal symptoms with evidence of ST segment depression, ischemic T wave inversion, new onset CHF, and/or significant cardiac history.*

2. Allergy to aspirin: ☐ No   ☐ Yes

3. Check initial blood pressures (*both arms*)
   Initial BP: R arm _____ / _____ mm Hg
                      L arm _____ / _____ mm Hg
   Gradient between R & L arm SBP
                      _____ mm Hg

4. Check stool for blood   ☐ negative   ☐ positive
   Consult CICU Fellow if positive.

5. Notify CICU Team ASAP   ☐ done

General Orders

1. Bedrest until painfree.

2. Nasal oxygen at _____ L/min by cannula PRN.

3. Check VS q5min (*by monitor if necessary for patient safety*) until painfree and then per nursing care standards.

4. ECG on admit, repeat for persistent pain or change in status or symptoms (*i.e. pain free*).

5. Consider IV NTG/Beta blockers for persistent pain.

6. Consider ST Segment monitoring in patients with nondiagnostic ECG's.

7. Adjust heparin using CICU/CMICU Heparin Management Nomogram and aPTT results.

8. ACS pts refractory to conventional Rx are candidates for IIb/IIIa inhibitors. Eligibility criteria attached. Notify the CCU team prior to administration.

Labs

1. Start 1-2 venous access lines (*avoid central access unless absolutely necessary*).

2. STAT Heme 18, Chem 7, CK Mass/Relative Index, Myoglobin, Troponin I, U/A, PT, APTT, Magnesium.

3. Chem 12, Lipid profile.

4. Serial Cardiac Markers:
   3 hr. _____ (*time*): CK Mass/Relative Index, Myoglobin
   8 hr. _____ (*time*): CK Mass/Relative Index
   8 hr. _____ (*time*): CK Mass/Relative Index, Troponin I

5. If pt. rules in, repeat CK Mass/Relative Index, Troponin I at 12, 18 & 24 hrs.

6. APTT drawn 6 hrs after starting heparin.

A   DATE | TIME | AM PM   PATIENT

℞
Baby aspirin 2 tabs (160 mg) PO chewed stat if not allergic.

PO IM IV RECTAL*   M.D.

B   DATE | TIME | AM PM   PATIENT

℞
Heparin 5,000 u IV bolus followed by Heparin 20,000 u in 500 ml D5W at 1,000 u/hr.

PO IM IV RECTAL*   M.D.

C   DATE | TIME | AM PM   PATIENT

℞   NTG oint _____" apply topically.
    or
    IV NTG (100mg / 250 D5W). Initiate at 3cc / hr; titrate up to relieve chest pain while keeping SBP > 90 mm Hg.

PO IM IV RECTAL*   M.D.

D   DATE | TIME | AM PM   PATIENT

℞   Metoprolol, 5 mg IV over 5 min if no evidence of CHF, bronchospasm, hypotension, or profound bradycardia. Repeat x 2 additional doses 5 mins apart (total of 15 mg over 15 min)

PO IM IV RECTAL*   M.D.

E   DATE | TIME | AM PM   PATIENT

℞
Metoprolol, 25 mg 30-60 min. after IV metoprolol given.

PO IM IV RECTAL*   M.D.

F   DATE | TIME | AM PM   PATIENT

℞
Morphine Sulfate _____ mg IV x 1.

PO IM IV RECTAL*   M.D.

G   DATE | TIME | AM PM   PATIENT

℞

PO IM IV RECTAL*   M.D.

H   DATE | TIME | AM PM   PATIENT

℞

PO IM IV RECTAL*   M.D.

FIG. 6-4. The level 2 pathway.

Medical College of Virginia Hospitals
Virginia Commonwealth University
Richmond, Virginia 23298

PHYSICIAN'S ORDERS

All orders must include date, time, and physician's signature. Do not abbreviate drug names. Circle route of administration or indicate other.*

Patient Identification (Patient Plate) LEVEL 3 – PAGE 1 OF 2

MEDICATION ORDERS (ONLY ONE DRUG EACH ℞)

DATE & TIME	ORDERS (OTHER THAN MEDICATION)

Level 3:

FAST TRACK

Initial Assessment

1. *Typical anginal pain >30 min with normal ECG. Atypical symptoms with nondiagnostic ECG.*
2. Allergy to aspirin: ☐ No ☐ Yes
3. Check initial blood pressures (both arms)

   Initial BP: R arm _____ / _____ mm Hg

   L arm _____ / _____ mm Hg

   Gradient between R & L arm SBP

   _____ mm Hg
4. Notify CICU team ASAP. ☐ done
5. Admit to CICU/CMICU for observation.

General Orders

1. ECG on admission.
2. Cardiolite baseline study. (*Nuclear Medicine 8-6828*)

   NOTE: Injection should precede any antianginal therapy whenever possible.

   If baseline study is at rest and negative, schedule for follow-up stress study and make pt. NPO at 3 hrs.
3. Nasal oxygen at _____ L/min by cannula PRN.
4. Check VS q5min (*by monitor if necessary for patient safety*) until painfree and then per nursing care standards.
5. Repeat ECG for persistent pain or change in status or symptoms (*i.e. painfree*)
6. Bedrest x3 hours, advance activity if painfree.
7. *If baseline study is positive and consistent with ischemia, advance pt. to Level 2 care: IV heparin +/- NTG and repeat ECG.*

Labs

1. Start 1-2 venous access lines (*avoid central access unless absolutely necessary*).
2. STAT CK Mass/Relative Index, Myoglobin, Troponin I, Heme 18, Basic Metabolic.
3. Lipid profile.
4. Serial Cardiac Markers:

   3 hr. _____ (*time*): CK Mass/Relative Index, Myoglobin

   6 hr. _____ (*time*): CK Mass/Relative Index

   8 hr. _____ (*time*): CK Mass/Relative Index, Troponin I
5. If pt. rules in, repeat CK Mass/Relative Index, Troponin I at 12, 18 & 24 hrs.

A DATE | TIME | AM PM | PATIENT

℞

Baby aspirin 2 tabs (160 mg) PO chewed stat if not allergic.

PO IM IV RECTAL* | _____ M.D.

B DATE | TIME | AM PM | PATIENT

℞

0.9 Normal Saline at KVO.

PO IM IV RECTAL* | _____ M.D.

C DATE | TIME | AM PM | PATIENT

℞

Nitroglycerin tab 0.4 mg 1 SL prn chest pain or anginal equivalent. May repeat x2.

PO IM IV RECTAL* | _____ M.D.

D DATE | TIME | AM PM | PATIENT

℞

Morphine Sulfate _____ mg IV x 1

PO IM IV RECTAL* | _____ M.D.

E DATE | TIME | AM PM | PATIENT

℞

PO IM IV RECTAL* | _____ M.D.

F DATE | TIME | AM PM | PATIENT

℞

PO IM IV RECTAL* | _____ M.D.

G DATE | TIME | AM PM | PATIENT

℞

PO IM IV RECTAL* | _____ M.D.

H DATE | TIME | AM PM | PATIENT

℞

PO IM IV RECTAL* | _____ M.D.

FIG. 6-5. The level 3 pathway.

Medical College of Virginia Hospitals
Virginia Commonwealth University
Richmond, Virginia 23298

PHYSICIAN'S ORDERS

All orders must include date, time, and physician's signature. Do not abbreviate drug names. Circle route of administration or indicate other. *
MEDICATION ORDERS (ONLY ONE DRUG EACH ℞)

Patient Identification (Patient Plate)

DATE & TIME	ORDERS (OTHER THAN MEDICATION)

Level 4:

ED EVALUATION OF POSSIBLE UNSTABLE ANGINA

Initial Assessment

1. *Typical anginal pain < 30 min with normal ECG.*
   Atypical symptoms normal ECG.
   History of cocaine use with normal or nondiagnostic ECG.

2. Check initial blood pressures (*both arms*)
   Initial BP:　　　　R arm _____ / _____ mm Hg
   　　　　　　　　　L arm _____ / _____ mm Hg
   　　Gradient between R & L arm SBP
   　　　　　　　　　_____ mm Hg

General Orders

1. ECG on admission.

2. Cardiolite baseline study. (*Nuclear Medicine 8-6828*)
   Note: Injection should precede any antianginal therapy
   　　　　whenever possible.

3. If baseline study is at rest and negative:

   A. Schedule outpatient follow-up stress Cardiolite.
   B. Give D/C instructions including prep for stress testing.

4. If rest cardiolite study is abnormal (suggestive of ischemia)
   pt. should be advanced to Level 2 care:

   A. Repeat ECG.
   B. Initiate IV Heparin +/- NTG, Metoprolol as ordered.
   C. Send original FAST TRACK cardiac markers.
   D. Draw 3 hr. labs including PT & aPTT and continue as
   　　indicated by Level 2 order set.

5. Check VS per ED nursing standard.

6. CXR.

7. Bedrest.

8. Clear liquid diet.

A　DATE _____　TIME _____　AM/PM　PATIENT _____
℞
　　0.9 Normal Saline at KVO or Saline Lock IV
PO IM IV RECTAL* _____　M.D. _____

B　DATE _____　TIME _____　AM/PM　PATIENT _____
℞
PO IM IV RECTAL* _____　M.D. _____

C　DATE _____　TIME _____　AM/PM　PATIENT _____
℞
PO IM IV RECTAL* _____　M.D. _____

D　DATE _____　TIME _____　AM/PM　PATIENT _____
℞
PO IM IV RECTAL* _____　M.D. _____

E　DATE _____　TIME _____　AM/PM　PATIENT _____
℞
PO IM IV RECTAL* _____　M.D. _____

F　DATE _____　TIME _____　AM/PM　PATIENT _____
℞
PO IM IV RECTAL* _____　M.D. _____

G　DATE _____　TIME _____　AM/PM　PATIENT _____
℞
PO IM IV RECTAL* _____　M.D. _____

H　DATE _____　TIME _____　AM/PM　PATIENT _____
℞
PO IM IV RECTAL* _____　M.D. _____

FIG. 6-6. The level 4 pathway.

Medical College of Virginia Hospitals
Virginia Commonwealth University
Richmond, Virginia 23298

PHYSICIAN'S ORDERS

All orders must include date, time, and physician's signature. Do not abbreviate drug names. Circle route of administration or indicate other.*
MEDICATION ORDERS (ONLY ONE DRUG EACH ℞)

Patient Identification (Patient Plate)

DATE & TIME	ORDERS (*OTHER THAN MEDICATION*)

Level 5:

ED EVALUATION OF NON-CARDIAC CHEST PAIN

Initial Assessment
1. A*typical chest pain of non-cardiac origin.*

General Orders
1. Check VS per ED nursing standard.
2. Arrange evaluation as appropriate to history and physical.

Discharge Diagnosis

_____

Physician Signature

_____

A	DATE		TIME	AM PM	PATIENT

℞

PO IM IV RECTAL* — M.D.

B	DATE		TIME	AM PM	PATIENT

℞

PO IM IV RECTAL* — M.D.

C	DATE		TIME	AM PM	PATIENT

℞

PO IM IV RECTAL* — M.D.

D	DATE		TIME	AM PM	PATIENT

℞

PO IM IV RECTAL* — M.D.

E	DATE		TIME	AM PM	PATIENT

℞

PO IM IV RECTAL* — M.D.

F	DATE		TIME	AM PM	PATIENT

℞

PO IM IV RECTAL* — M.D.

G	DATE		TIME	AM PM	PATIENT

℞

PO IM IV RECTAL* — M.D.

H	DATE		TIME	AM PM	PATIENT

℞

PO IM IV RECTAL* — M.D.

FIG. 6-7. The level 5 pathway.

factors or cocaine use, and a normal ECG). Patients in this category usually require little or no additional testing and are treated and discharged promptly from the ED.

If it is not clear to the ED attending physician what level the patient should be assigned, an ACT team cardiologist is usually consulted. At MCV, three attending cardiologists take call for the ACT team. One is on call at all times. A printed ACT team schedule is always posted in the ED and is available to the hospital page operators. The advantage of limiting the number of cardiologists who are available for this duty is that it has allowed the individuals on call to get to know the ED attending physicians well (>30 ED attending physicians and >30 cardiologists are at MCV). Each of the ACT team cardiologists have a fax machine at home to receive an ECG transmitted from the ED when any question arises regarding its interpretation. The ACT team cardiologists are also available for physicians from the community to refer patients for immediate evaluation in the system.

Not all patients fit clearly into each of these five categories, which is handled by a simple rule: if the category assignment is unclear between two adjacent levels, the patient should be assigned to the higher of the two levels (e.g., if it is not clear whether a patient should be evaluated on level 3 or 4, the patient should be treated as a level 3). In addition, if a level 3 or 4 patient has an abnormal cardiac perfusion scan, the patient is reassigned immediately to a higher level (usually at least a level 2).

The ACT team meets for 1 hour on a weekly basis to go over cases and to further improve the process. Cardiac nuclear perfusion scans, which are brought to the CCU every morning, are available for attending cardiologists to view during patient care rounds. At a monthly quality improvement meeting with all attending emergency physicians, individual cases are reviewed and various topics are discussed that relate to the care of the patients. Also, an extensive community outreach program is in place to make the system available to as many of our referring Richmond area physicians as possible.

PROTOCOL EXPERIENCE AT MCV

Experience with these critical pathways at MCV has been extensive. To date more than 10,000 cardiac nuclear imaging studies have been performed on patients presenting to the ED with chest pain or other symptoms suggestive of cardiac ischemia. Rest myocardial perfusion imaging is abnormal suggesting ischemia, infarction, or both in 30% of level 3 patients and 11% of level 4 patients at MCV. An abnormal rest myocardial perfusion imaging study identifies a subset of patients who are at high risk of acute MI, cardiac death, or the need for coronary artery revascularization over the next 12 months (15,18,21). Most importantly, a normal rest myocardial perfusion imaging study identifies a subset of patients who are at very low risk of subsequent adverse coronary events (15,18,21).

In our experience, rest myocardial perfusion imaging and serial troponin determinations have comparable sensitivities for identifying acute MI (15). Myocardial perfusion imaging identifies more patients who subsequently require coronary revascularization or have significant coronary artery disease than serial troponin determinations, but it has lower specificity than serial markers. Both tests provide complementary information for identifying patients at risk for ACS.

Rest nuclear imaging has been highly effective in detecting acute MI in patients with atypical symptoms and a normal or nondiagnostic ECG. Most (approximately two thirds) of such patients have acute MI involving the posterior, lateral left ventricle, or both. These locations are relatively "silent" electrocardiographically and the use of rest perfusion nuclear imaging appears to be a highly effective method for detecting such infarctions.

This protocol has also been highly useful for evaluating patients with cocaine-associated chest pain. In a recent study, we found that acute MI is infrequent in patients presenting with cocaine-associated chest pain (23). An abnormal myocardial rest perfusion scan was uncommon, suggesting that myocardial ischemia rather than frank infarction is infrequently the cause of cocaine-associated chest pain. At MCV, myocardial rest perfusion imaging provides an effective alternative to routine ED admission of patients with cocaine-related cardiac symptoms.

Finally, the use of this protocol at MCV has been highly cost-effective. A significant decrease in unnecessary hospital admissions has resulted from our being able to send level 4 patients who have a negative cardiac scan home directly from the ED. This has resulted in a 17% net decrease in our institutional costs for managing patients who present to the ED with chest pain. The effectiveness and cost-savings resulting from this approach has been confirmed by experience at other institutions (19,24).

REFERENCES

1. Jesse RL, Kontos MC. Evaluation of chest pain in the emergency department. *Curr Probl Cardiol* 1997;22:149–236.
2. Karcz A, Korn R, Burke MC, et al. Malpractice claims against emergency physicians in Massachusetts: 1975–1993. *Am J Emerg Med* 1996;14(4):341–345.
3. Karcz A, Holbrook J, Burke MC, et al. Massachusetts emergency medicine closed malpractice claims: 1988–1990. *Ann Emerg Med* 1993;22:553–559.
4. McCarthy BD, Beshansky JR, D'Agostino RB, et al. Missed diagnoses of acute myocardial infarction in the emergency department: results from a multicenter study. *Ann Emerg Med* 1993;22:579–582.
5. McCarthy BD, Beshansky JR, D'Agostino RB, et al. Missed diagnoses of acute myocardial infarction in the emergency department: results from a multicenter study. *Ann Emerg Med* 1993;22(3):579–582.
6. Quattrone MS. Missed myocardial infarction: violation of federal law? *J Emerg Nurs* 1991;17:40–42.
7. Pelberg AL. Missed myocardial infarction in the emergency room. *Qual Assur Util Rev* 1989;4(2):39–42.
8. Rusnak RA, Stair TO, Hansen K, et al. Litigation against the emergency physician: common features in cases of missed myocardial infarction. *Ann Emerg Med* 1989;18(10):1029–1034.
9. Okada R, Glover D, Gafney T, et al. Myocardial kinetics of technetium-99m-hexakis-2-methoxy-2-methylpropyl isonitrile. *Circulation* 1988;77:491–498.
10. Wackers F, Lie K, Liem K, et al. Potential value of thallium-201

scintigraphy as a means of selecting patients for the coronary care unit. *Br Heart J* 1979;41:111–117.

11. Varetto T, Cantalupi D, Altieri A, et al. Emergency room technetium 99m sestamibi imaging to rule out acute myocardial ischemic events in patients with nondiagnostic electrocardiograms. *J Am Coll Cardiol* 1993;22:1804–1808.

12. Gregoire J, Theroux P. Detection and assessment of unstable angina using myocardial perfusion imaging: comparison between technetium-99m sestamibi SPECT and 12-lead electrocardiogram. *Am J Cardiol* 1990;66:42–46.

13. Bilodeau L, Theroux P, Gregoire J, et al. Technetium-99m sestamibi tomography in patients with spontaneous chest pain: correlations with clinical, electrocardiographic and angiographic findings. *J Am Coll Cardiol* 1991;1:1684–1691.

14. Kosnik JW, Zalenski RJ, Shamsa F, et al. Resting sestamibi imaging for the prognosis of low-risk chest pain. *Acad Emerg Med* 1999;6:998–1004.

15. Kontos MC, Jesse RL, Anderson FP, et al. Comparison of myocardial perfusion imaging and cardiac troponin I in patients admitted to the emergency department with chest pain. *Circulation* 1999;99:2073–2078.

16. Kontos MC, Arrowood JA, Jesse RL, et al. Comparison between 2-dimensional echocardiography and myocardial perfusion imaging in the emergency department in patients with possible myocardial ischemia. *Am Heart J* 1998;136:724–733.

17. Summers RL, Tisdale B, Kolb JC, et al. Role of technetium-99m sestamibi myocardial imaging in the emergency department evaluation of chest pain. *J Miss State Med Assoc* 1998;39:176–179.

18. Kontos MC, Jesse RL, Schmidt KL, et al. Value of acute rest sestamibi perfusion imaging for evaluation of patients admitted to the emergency department with chest pain. *J Am Coll Cardiol* 1997;30:976–982.

19. Weissman IA, Dickinson CZ, Dworkin HJ, et al. Cost-effectiveness of myocardial perfusion imaging with SPECT in the emergency department evaluation of patients with unexplained chest pain. *Radiology* 1996;199:353–357.

20. Tatum JL, Ornato JP, Jesse RL, et al. A diagnostic strategy using Tc-99m sestamibi for evaluation of patients with chest pain in the emergency department. *Circulation* 1994;90:I-367.

21. Tatum JL, Jesse RL, Kontos MC, et al. Comprehensive strategy for the evaluation and triage of the chest pain patient. *Ann Emerg Med* 1997;29:116–125.

22. Hilton TC, Thompson RC, Williams HJ, et al. Technetium-99m sestamibi myocardial perfusion imaging in the emergency room evaluation of chest pain. *J Am Coll Cardiol* 1994;23(5):1016–1022.

23. Kontos MC, Schmidt KL, Nicholson CS, et al. Myocardial perfusion imaging with technetium-99m sestamibi in patients with cocaine-associated chest pain. *Ann Emerg Med* 1999;33:639–645.

24. Farkouh ME, Smars PA, Reeder GS, et al. A clinical trial of a chest-pain observation unit for patients with unstable angina. Chest Pain Evaluation in the Emergency Room (CHEER) Investigators. *N Engl J Med* 1998;339:1882–1888.

CHAPTER 7

Chest Pain Centers

Alan B. Storrow

OVERVIEW

Chest pain center (CPC) protocols have proved to be cost-effective and safe for the emergency department (ED) management of patients with chest pain. Cost management of patients with chest pain, including the half of inpatients eventually discharged with a noncardiac diagnosis, is estimated at $6 billion annually.

Emergency department diagnosis of acute coronary syndrome (ACS) is often challenging and limited by traditional diagnostic tools. Most patients with chest pain will present with a nondiagnostic initial electrocardiogram (ECG) and, if obtained, a negative first set of cardiac markers. Of patients, 2% to 8% will be discharged from the ED and subsequently have a cardiac event (1–3). Such inadvertent discharges represent the group with the highest total amount of malpractice awards in emergency medicine. Many will be considered candidates for further serial diagnostic testing over time, often termed a "rule-out MI" protocol.

The CPC protocols expand this approach to "rule-in ACS." ACS describes a spectrum of conditions that include unstable angina (UA), non–Q-wave myocardial infarction (MI), and Q-wave MI (4). The CPC provides a framework within the ED to evaluate for (a) myocardial necrosis, (b) rest ischemia, and (c) exercise-induced ischemia. This three-item strategy is the foundation for a safe evaluation and appropriate disposition decisions. It addresses the observation that the prevalence of ACS without acute MI is two- to threefold greater than acute MI itself, and that patients with suspected acute MI who are diagnosed without infarction have similar long-term prognosis to those with acute MI (5). The strategy (a) provides rapid identification and treatment of those patients eligible for reperfusion therapy; (b) safely identifies those patients with ACS who require inpatient admission; and (c) reduces inadvertent release home of patients who will subsequently have a cardiac event.

RATIONALE

The first CPC was designed to reduce the incidence of cardiac arrest by educating the public regarding chest pain and the importance of seeking care early (6). The American College of Emergency Physicians Short Term Observation Services Section (7) has further defined three distinct programs of a CPC:

1. Program for rapid treatment of ST-segment elevation acute MI
2. Observation program to exclude ACS in patients at low to moderate risk
3. Outreach program for education

The Society of Chest Pain Centers and Providers has further resolved that the CPC strategy represents a public initiative calling on all hospitals to focus on the heart attack program through a comprehensive triage evaluation using protocol-driven algorithms.

A national survey in the United States reported 520 designated CPCs existed in 1995, most located within an ED (8). The most common goals of these CPCs were to (a) reduce inappropriate release of patients with acute MI or UA, (b) promote cardiac care team work, and (c) reduce hospital admissions. These centers were more likely to utilize extended diagnostic protocols and perform advanced testing (e.g., echocardiography, exercise stress test, or radionuclide imaging).

The observation, or diagnostic, CPC program is particularly well suited for a protocol-driven approach to exclude or confirm ACS in patients with initially nondiagnostic findings. A growing body of evidence suggests that CPC protocols within EDs are diagnostically accurate and cost-effective. It is estimated that 80% of CPC patients without evidence of ACS can be released safely from the ED (9–17).

Although CPCs were not originally developed for cost-effectiveness, but rather to improve care, the financial impact of these centers is undergoing critical appraisal. For individual patients, CPCs have provided equivalent outcomes at a reduced cost compared with inpatient hospitalization. However, their impact on total healthcare expenditure is yet to be determined (11–16).

PATHWAY

Identification of patients with ACS on initial ED presentation is frequently difficult, given the variable presentation of symptoms and the lack of highly specific tests. A CPC is ideally suited for patients at low to moderate risk of ACS, a low likelihood of complications, no contraindication to the protocol's tests, and no comorbid conditions that could interfere with assessment or ED release at the conclusion of the evaluation (18,19). Classic presentations of ACS, by history and initial ECG, do not represent a diagnostic problem and should be addressed with protocol-driven care, stressing reperfusion, when appropriate, and critical care unit admission. Such patients are not candidates for a CPC. However, they represent only a small percentage of total emergency presentations for chest pain.

Most CPC protocols broadly define their candidates as hemodynamically stable patients with symptoms suggestive of ACS and a nondiagnostic initial ECG. Tools to aid in this process include the *Goldman Chest Pain Protocol* (20), and the Pozen/Selker *Acute Cardiac Ischemia—Time Insensitive Predictive Instrument* (ACI/TIPI) (21). However, neither has received widespread use. Published CPC protocols frequently cite following or modifying the UA guidelines from the Agency for Healthcare Policy Research/National Heart, Lung, and Blood Institute (AHCPR/NHLBI) (22). CPC protocols generally address the low-risk population and exclude most patients with intravenous vasoactive medication requirements or those receiving antiplatelet therapy beyond aspirin administration. Such patients at higher risk may be more frequently considered for CPC management in the future.

Sample inclusion and exclusion criteria from the University of Cincinnati "Heart ER" are found in Table 7-1. They broadly define a population at lower risk, but thought to be at risk for an ACS and with a negative initial ED evaluation. Added to the inclusion criteria were patients with recent sympathomimetic drug use (e.g., cocaine) (23). Before the addition of rest nuclear imaging as a test option, the inability to exercise, in order to complete a stress test, was an exclusion criterion for this protocol. Other institutions have been more detailed in further dividing the group eligible for CPC

evaluation into low- or moderate-risk, depending on history, risk factors, and initial ECG.

Once a candidate is identified for a CPC, several reported protocols are suggested to be effective and safe. Most are broadly based on a shortened version of a typical inpatient "rule-out MI" protocol, followed by provocative testing (Fig. 7-1). This pathway—serial serum makers, serial ECGs, and stress testing—addresses the diagnosis of the three components: necrosis, rest ischemia, and exercise-induced ischemia.

Electrocardiography

The initial ECG in most patients with ACS is nondiagnostic (24), providing a specific ED diagnosis in only 5% of patients with chest pain (25). However, the ECG remains a convenient, fast, noninvasive, inexpensive, and widely available test for risk stratification of patients with chest pain. Findings consistent with, and highly reliable for, transmural acute MI (ST-segment elevation or new bundle branch block) must indicate expedient reperfusion and exclude a patient from further ED-based CPC evaluation. ST-segment elevation remains the principal criterion for consideration of fibrinolytic therapy. Nonspecific findings (e.g., ST-segment depression or T-wave inversion) evolve into non–Q-wave MI in approximately 15% of cases, and represent UA in 20% (26).

Serial ECGs detect evolving changes of ischemia at rest and are an important component of a CPC protocol. Patients also undergo continuous cardiac monitoring for the detection of dysrhythmias. ST-segment trend monitoring may detect ischemic changes before symptom onset (27–30), identify revascularization candidates earlier (31), and detect changes suggestive of UA earlier. However, randomized studies need to be performed to confirm ST-segment trend monitoring utility and cost-effectiveness in the CPC population.

Cardiac Markers

Serial biochemical marker testing addresses the time-dependent process of myocardial necrosis, provides a degree

TABLE 7-1. *Inclusion and exclusion criteria for the "Heart ER"*[a]

Inclusion	Exclusion
Either sex	Acute myocardial infarction (ST-segment elevation >1 mm in two contiguous leads)
Age >25 yr, or any age with recent sympathomimetic drug ingestion	Acute unstable angina; uncontrolled pain; trauma
Chest pain or other signs and symptoms suggestive of acute coronary syndrome	Hemodynamic instability
Nondiagnostic ECG	Inability to complete, or contraindications to, exercise ECG testing (if planned)
Patient likely able to complete GXT (if planned)	History of known significant coronary artery disease

ECG, electrocardiogram; GXT, graded exercise testing.
[a]A chest pain center at the University of Cincinnati, Cincinnati, Ohio.

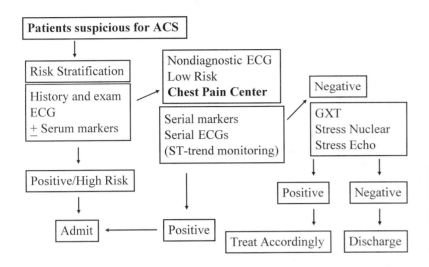

FIG. 7-1. Simplified schema of a typical chest pain center (CPC) protocol. ST-segment–trend monitoring is used at some centers. Stress testing is frequently an exercise electrocardiogram, stress echocardiography, or stress nuclear imaging. This approach addresses necrosis, rest ischemia, and exercise-induced ischemia in a step-wise fashion. GXT, graded exercise test.

of risk stratification, and has received increased attention as a criterion for the use of newer antiplatelet agents. Although the optimal combination and timing are debatable, attention to serum marker kinetics allows an institution to develop a protocol-driven approach.

Serial marker testing, a mainstay for ACS evaluation, has high sensitivity for the diagnosis of acute MI. A single negative determination of a marker, or set of markers, at initial presentation has a low sensitivity for acute MI diagnosis (32) and should not be relied on for disposition decisions. Some have suggested, however, that a single negative creatine kinase (CK)-MB level obtained in a patient at low risk at least 4-hours after pain onset, complemented by a benign 6-hour observation period, can identify those who can safely exercise (33).

Myoglobin's early release after myocardial necrosis (34,35) and high negative predictive value makes it a useful marker to consider. However, it is not cardiac specific, a universally accepted reference standard is lacking, and standardization between different assays is problematic. Myoglobin's rapid rise (compared with that of CK-MB) makes it particularly well suited for identification of myocardial necrosis in the first 3 to 4 hours after patient presentation (36,37). The likelihood of myocardial necrosis is low if myoglobin levels are not elevated within 4 hours in a patient with acute symptoms.

Creatine kinase isoenzyme MB mass assays, which have been the "gold standard" for acute MI diagnosis, become abnormal 4 to 8 hours after myocardial necrosis. CK-MB can be an important tool for detecting necrosis during the typical 6 to 12 hours of a CPC evaluation. A 90% sensitivity has been reported for serial measurements over 3 hours in patients with nondiagnostic ECGs (24). Early CK-MB testing has prognostic value in admitted patients (38).

The cardiac troponins I and T (cTnI and cTnT) are highly sensitive and moderately specific markers for myocardial cell damage (39–41); they have similar kinetics to CK-MB and are useful for prognosis and risk stratification (39,42–48). Their increased sensitivity for minor myocardial damage has

likely resulted in reports of lower specificity when CK-MB has been used as the standard. Elevated troponins, with a normal CK-MB, may indicate damage not detected conventionally (49) or, perhaps, represent UA (40,43,46). Two negative troponin values, one obtained at least 6 hours after symptom onset, have been suggested to allow safe ED discharge (40). However, the unclear natural history of UA should limit such ED triage decisions to the lowest risk subgroup (50).

The National Association of Clinical Biochemistry has recommended a division of the serum markers into early (myoglobin, CK-MB isoforms) and later or definitive (CK-MB, cTnI, cTnT) (49). It further recommends a timing protocol for patients with a nondiagnostic ECG (Table 7-2) and suggests the definitive marker of choice is a cardiac troponin. Whereas the high sensitivity and risk stratification properties of the cardiac troponins are attractive, it remains to be seen if they will replace the more familiar CK-MB.

Point-of-care cardiac marker testing, which is widely available and, reportedly, effective (40,51–54) may shorten the time to diagnosis and treatment. The clinical impact of such tests depends on the timing of traditional laboratory assays, volume of testing, and decrease in need for inpatient hospitalization. Further investigation is needed before point-of-care testing becomes commonplace.

Stress Testing

For patients with negative serial ECG and marker results, provocative testing, with or without imaging, is the final diagnostic test used to identify clinically significant coronary artery disease. Graded exercise testing, stress echocardiography, and stress nuclear imaging have received attention (55–61) and have been reported to be cost-effective and safe (9,13,60,62–67). However, large randomized trials have not tested these modalities in a CPC population. Their predictive values are effected by the pretest probability of disease (68), thus false-positive findings may be a problem in the lowest risk subgroup.

TABLE 7-2. *Recommended early and late marker sampling frequency for the detection of acute myocardial infarction in patients with a nondiagnostic electrocardigram*

Cardiac marker	Admission	2–4 Hours	6–9 Hours	12–24 Hours
Early (<6 h)	X	X	X	(x)
Late (>6 h)	X	X	X	(x)

Early, myoglobin or creatine kinase (CK)-MB isoforms; Late, CK-MB, or cardiac troponin T or I; (x), optional testing.

Adapted from National Academy of Clinical Biochemistry Sixth Conference on Standards of Laboratory Practice Series: *The use of cardiac markers in coronary artery diseases.* Chicago, Illinois: 1998.

Alternatives to the traditional CPC evaluation include discharge after negative serial markers and ECGs (40), immediate exercise ECG testing (66), and rest nuclear imaging (69). Although a patient with negative serial markers over 6 to 10 hours is at very low risk of a cardiac event, the decision to discharge that patient for elective stress testing must be based on the physician's risk tolerance. Because the natural history of UA is not well known, ED discharge before provocative testing or imaging has not been widely accepted.

Certain patients at low risk, based on a nonspecific presentation ECG, clinical findings, initial markers (in most cases), and ability to exercise, have been reported to benefit from immediate ED exercise testing. This management strategy has been suggested to be safe and effective for risk stratification (65,66), even for select patients with known coronary artery disease (70).

Rest nuclear imaging [single photon emission computed tomography (SPECT)] is receiving increased attention as a safe and effective risk stratification tool (69,71–78). Nuclear imaging has a high sensitivity for detection of coronary artery disease (72,73), and patients with a normal study are at low risk for subsequent cardiac events (71,72). Sestamibi or tetrofosmin has the additional advantage of not undergoing rest redistribution, so imaging can occur several hours after injection. They are most sensitive when injected during pain (74), although the time course of sensitivity loss is currently unknown (73). Because a component of silent ischemia with UA likely exists, injection without pain may maintain reasonable sensitivity for several hours (73). If acute (or old) infarction is present, it can be detected by nuclear imaging at any time. Potential disadvantages of nuclear imaging include significant institutional requirements for equipment, prompt injection, and off-hours imaging. Despite these concerns, the technology appears cost-effective (78–80).

A sample protocol and CPC physician orders from the University of Cincinnati are illustrated in Figs. 7-2 and 7-3. This protocol was established as standard of care in 1991. It was based on 9 hours of serial monitoring, followed by exercise ECG testing. Echocardiography was performed before exercise in the first 1,100 patients, but was subsequently discontinued. The protocol was shortened to 6 hours and a rest nuclear imaging option was added in 1998. Use of

nuclear studies has allowed expansion of the protocol to patients who could not exercise. Preferably, injection is done during active pain, typically within a few minutes of the patient's arrival in the ED. If injection is performed in the early hours of the morning, imaging is performed at 6:00 a.m.

A cardiologist interprets exercise ECG or rest nuclear imaging. The treating emergency physician makes disposition decisions. Those who fail to complete the exercise ECG have their disposition determined on an individual basis. Generally, a patient with reasonable exercise capacity for age and state of health, no significant arrhythmias, and no worrisome ECG changes is discharged to follow-up. Otherwise, the patient is admitted for further evaluation.

A review and 30-day follow-up of 2,131 consecutive patients at the University of Cincinnati CPC revealed 1,822 (85.5%) were released home and 309 (14.5%) required admission; 23 cases of acute MI and 63 cases of angina or UA were found in 94 (30%) of these admitted patients. At 30-day follow-up of 1,696 (93% follow-up rate) patients discharged from the ED, findings were 9 cardiac events (0.53%, 95% confidence interval 0.24% to 1.01%), 7 percutaneous transluminal coronary angioplasties, 1 coronary artery bypass graph, and 1 death (81).

The Mayo Clinic reported a similar protocol in a prospective, randomized trial of the safety, efficacy, and cost of a CPC compared with hospital admission (Fig. 7-4). The entry criteria here were based on the Agency for Health Care Policy Research (AHCPR) UA guidelines (22) and final testing (exercise ECG, nuclear stress testing, or stress echo) was individualized. No differences were reported in rate of cardiac events for the 212 patients in each group, and there were no primary cardiac events in the 97 patients discharged from the CPC (16).

The CPC population can be subdivided into a low- and moderate-risk group, based on history, cardiac risk factors, and initial ECG. Botsford General Hospital (Farmington Hills, MI) reported a protocol modified in length according to risk subgroup (Fig. 7-5) (82).

The rest nuclear imaging approach was pioneered at the Medical College of Virginia (MCV). Their protocol, which is used in a geographically separate CPC, divides patients with chest pain into levels based on history and clinical variables.

Heart ER

Admit to the RDTC for rule-out acute coronary syndrome
Allergies:
Vital signs q 2 hours x 2 , then q 4hours
Continuous cardiac monitoring with ST-Guard
Bedrest with assist to bathroom
Diet: cardiac
IV heparin lock
Call physician if:
        SBP >180 or <90
        DBP >110 or <50
        Heart rate >120 or <50
        Respiratory rate >25 or <10
        Chest pain
Labs:
        CK-MB, cTnT, and Myoglobin at 0, 3, and 6 hours
        12-lead ECG at 0, 3, and 6 hours
        Other:
Medications
        Oxygen via NC at ____l/min
        Nitroglycerin paste ____inch(es) q 8 hours
        ASA 325mg po
        Other:
Testing:
        ☐ Patient is on call for first available GXT after successful completion of protocol
        ☐ Patient has been injected for rest nuclear imaging
        ☐ Other testing:

FIG. 7-2. Sample admission orders for the "Heart ER," a chest pain center at the University of Cincinnati Center for Emergency Care. Patients are evaluated in the main treatment area of the emergency department before transfer to the Rapid Diagnosis and Treatment Center (RDTC). ST-Guard is a continuous ST-segment monitoring system (Marquette Electronics; Milwaukee, WI). Three serum markers are obtained at 0, 3, and 6 hours, although the type, timing, and number of markers varies greatly between institutions. A chest radiograph is obtained before transfer to the RDTC. Other medications regimens might include a beta-blocker, alternative nitroglycerin routes, and other antiplatelet agents, if used. GXT, graded exercise test.

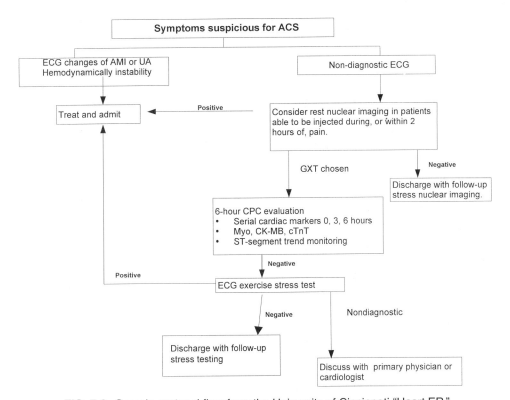

FIG. 7-3. Sample protocol flow from the University of Cincinnati "Heart ER."

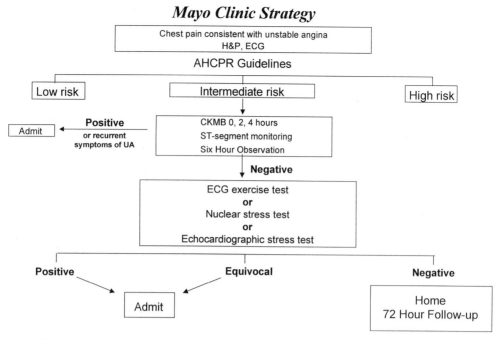

FIG. 7-4. Sample chest pain center (CPC) protocol from the Mayo Clinic. (Adapted from Farkouh ME, Smars PA, Reeder GS. A clinical trial of a chest-pain observation unit for patients with unstable angina. *N Engl J Med* 1999;339:1882–1888.)

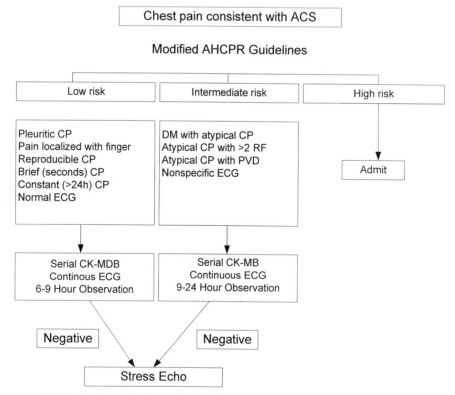

FIG. 7-5. Sample chest pain center (CPC) protocol with modification according to the division of patients into low and intermediate risk. (Adapted from Stomel R, Grant R, Eagle KA. Lessons learned from a community hospital chest pain center. *Am J Cardiol* 1999;83:1033–1037.)

Diagnostic testing is based on the levels. Level 4 patients—the typical CPC population at most centers—receive immediate rest nuclear imaging in the ED. They are typically released for follow-up outpatient stress imaging if this initial test is negative. This strategy was suggested to be an effective and safe method in 1,187 consecutive patients (69).

Education

A patient's presence in a CPC represents an ideal time to provide education regarding cardiac testing procedures and good health habits. Regardless of their final outcome, patients would likely benefit from risk factor modification. At the minimum, an orientation to the CPC should be provided at admission, and instructions on health habits at discharge.

CONCLUSIONS

Chest pain centers, an integral part of many EDs, are likely to play an increasingly unique role in cost containment. They establish the importance and expertise of emergency medicine in ACS management, as well as emphasize the emergency physician's role in managed care. A CPC may also help with the development of ED observation protocols for other conditions.

A protocol-driven approach helps maximize the identification of ACS in a high volume, potentially high risk, and high liability group of patients. Protocols provide emphasis on expedient reperfusion therapy for appropriate patients with MI, while providing a cost-effective way to manage the larger subgroup of patients at risk for ACS.

Important CPC components include a strategy for the diagnosis of myocardial necrosis, rest ischemia, and exercise-induced ischemia. Several approaches are reported to exist for CPC candidate identification, serial ECGs, serial markers, and provocative testing. Attention to local expertise and collaboration between emergency medicine and cardiology will yield the optimal protocol for a specific institution.

REFERENCES

1. Pope JH, Aufderheide TP, Ruthazer R, et al. Missed diagnoses of acute cardiac ischemia in the emergency department. *N Engl J Med* 2000;342:1163–1170.
2. McCarthy BD, Beshansky JR, D'Agostino RB, Selker HP. Missed diagnoses of acute myocardial infarction in the emergency department: results from a multicenter study. *Ann Emerg Med* 1993;22:579–582.
3. Lee TH, Rouan GW, Weisburg MC, et al. Clinical characteristics and natural history of patients with acute myocardial infarction sent home from the emergency room. *Am J Cardiol* 1987;60:219–224.
4. Yeghiazarians Y, Braunstein JB, Askari A, et al. Unstable angina pectoris. *N Engl J Med* 2000;342:101–114.
5. Schroder JS, Lamb IH, Hu M. Do patients in whom myocardial infarction has been ruled out have a better prognosis after hospitalization than those surviving? *N Engl J Med* 1980;303:1–5.
6. Bahr RD. Growth of chest pain emergency departments throughout the United States: a cardiologist's spin on solving the heart attack problem. *Coron Artery Dis* 1995;6:827–838.
7. Graff L, Joseph T, Andelman R, et al. American College of Emergency Physicians information paper: chest pain units in emergency departments—a report from the short-term observation services section. *Am J Cardiol* 1995;76:1036–1039.
8. Zalenski RJ, Rydman RJ, Ting S, et al. A national survey of "chest pain centers" in the United States: structure and characteristics of host emergency departments and hospitals. *Am J Cardiol* 1998;81:1305–1309.
9. Gibler WB, Walsh RA, Levy RC, et al. Rapid diagnostic and treatment center for patients with chest pain in the emergency department. *Ann Emerg Med* 1995;25:1–8.
10. Zalenski RJ, Rydman RJ, McCarren M, et al. Feasibility of a rapid diagnostic protocol for an emergency department chest pain unit. *Ann Emerg Med* 1997;29:99–108.
11. Hoekstra JW, Gibler WB, Levy RC, et al. Emergency-department diagnosis of acute myocardial infarction and ischemia: a cost analysis of two diagnostic protocols. *Acad Emerg Med* 1994;1:103–110.
12. Gomez MA, Anderson JL, Karagounis LA, et al. An emergency department based protocol for rapidly ruling out myocardial ischemia reduces hospital time and expense: results of a randomized study (ROMIO). *J Am Coll Cardiol* 1996;28:25–33.
13. Mikhail MG, Smith FA, Gray M, et al. Cost-effectiveness of mandatory stress testing in chest pain center patients. *Ann Emerg Med* 1997;29:88–98.
14. Roberts RR, Zalenski RJ, Mensah EK, et al. Costs of an emergency department–based accelerated diagnostic protocol vs hospitalization in patients with chest pain: a randomized controlled trial. *JAMA* 1997;278:1670–1676.
15. Gaspoz JM, Lee TH, Weinstein MC, et al. Cost-effectiveness of a new short-stay unit to "rule out" myocardial infarction in low-risk patients. *J Am Coll Cardiol* 1994;24:1249–1259.
16. Farkouh ME, Smars PA, Reeder GS, et al. A clinical trial of a chest pain observation unit for patients with unstable angina. Chest Pain Evaluation in the Emergency Room (CHEER) investigators. *N Engl J Med* 1998;339:1882–1888.
17. Zalenski RJ, Selker HP, Cannon CP, et al. National Heart Attack Alert Program position paper: chest pain centers and programs for the evaluation of acute cardiac ischemia. *Ann Emerg Med* 2000;35:462–471.
18. Zalenski RJ. Risk stratification of patients for chest pain centers. The Third National Congress of Chest Pain Centers [Syllabus]. Detroit, MI: Wayne State University 1998;I:95–98.
19. Storrow AB, Gibler WB. Chest pain centers: diagnosis of acute coronary syndromes. *Ann Emerg Med* 2000;35:449–461.
20. Goldman L, Cook EF, Brand DA, et al. A computer protocol to predict myocardial infarction in emergency department patients with chest pain. *N Engl J Med* 1988;318:797–803.
21. Pozen MW, Agostino RB, Selker HP, et al. A predictive instrument to improve coronary-care-unit admission practices in acute ischemic heart disease: a prospective multicenter clinical trial. *N Engl J Med* 1984;310:1273–1278.
22. Agency for Health Care Policy Research. Unstable angina: diagnosis and management. *Clinical practice guideline #10*; 1998.
23. Kushman SO, Storrow AB, Liu T, Gibler WB. Cocaine-associated chest pain in a chest pain center. *Am J Cardiol* 2000;85:394–396.
24. Gibler WB, Lewis LM, Erb RE, et al. Early detection of acute myocardial infarction in patients presenting with chest pain and nondiagnostic electrocardiograms: serial CK-MB sampling in the emergency department. *Ann Emerg Med* 1990;19:1359–1366.
25. Lee TH, Rouan GW, Weisberg MC, et al. Sensitivity of routine clinical criteria for diagnosing myocardial infarction within 24 hours of hospitalization. *Ann Intern Med* 1987;106:181–186.
26. Fisch C. The clinical electrocardiogram: sensitivity and specificity. In: Fisch C, ed. *American College of Cardiology current journal review*. New York: Elsevier Science, 1997:71–75.
27. Fesmire FM, Percy RF, Bardoner JB, et al. Usefulness of automated serial 12-lead ECG monitoring during the initial emergency department evaluation of patients with chest pain. *Ann Emerg Med* 1998;31:3–11.
28. Wilcox I, Freedman BS, Li J, et al. Comparison of exercise stress testing with ambulatory electrocardiographic monitoring in the detection of myocardial ischemia after unstable angina pectoris. *Am J Cardiol* 1991;67:89–91.
29. Stern S, Tzvoni D. Early detection of silent ischemic heart disease by 24-hour electrocardiographic monitoring of active subjects. *Br Heart J* 1974;36:481–486.

30. Krucoff MW, Green CE, Satler LF, et al. Noninvasive detection of coronary artery patency using continuous ST segment monitoring. *Am J Cardiol* 1986;57:916–922.

31. Gibler WB, Sayre MR, Levy RC, et al. Serial 12-lead electrocardiographic monitoring in patients presenting to the emergency department with chest pain. *J Electrocardiol* 1993;26:238–243.

32. Rude RE, Poole WK, Muller JE, et al. Electrocardiographic and clinical criteria for recognition of acute myocardial infarction based on an analysis of 3,697 patients. *Am J Cardiol* 1983;52:936–942.

33. Hichol G, Walls R, Goldman L, et al. A critical pathway for management of patients with acute chest pain who are at low risk for myocardial ischemia: recommendations and potential impact. *Ann Intern Med* 1997;127:996–1005.

34. Vaidya HC. Myoglobin. *Laboratory Medicine* 1992;23:306–310.

35. Gibler WB, Gibler CD, Weinshenker E, et al. Myoglobin as an early indicator of acute myocardial infarction. *Ann Emerg Med* 1987;16(8):851–856.

36. Brogan GX, Friedman S, McCuskey C, et al. Evaluation of a new rapid quantitative immunoassay for serum myoglobin versus CK-MB for ruling out myocardial infarction in the emergency department. *Ann Emerg Med* 1994;24:665–671.

37. Tucker JF, Collins RA, Anderson AJ, et al. Value of serial myoglobin levels in the early diagnosis of patients admitted for acute myocardial infarction. *Ann Emerg Med* 1994;24:704–708.

38. Hoekstra JW, Hedges JR, Gibler WB, et al. Emergency department CK-MB: a predictor of ischemic complications. *Acad Emerg Med* 1994;1:17–28.

39. Hamm CW, Ravkilde J, Gerhardt W, et al. The prognostic value of serum troponin T in unstable angina. *N Engl J Med* 1992;327:146–150.

40. Hamm CW, Goldmann BU, Heeshcen C, et al. Emergency room triage of patients with acute chest pain by means of rapid testing for cardiac troponin T or troponin I. *N Engl J Med* 1997;337:1648–1653.

41. Adams JE, Bodor GS, Davila-Roman VG, et al. Cardiac troponin I. A marker with high specificity for cardiac injury. *Circulation* 1993;88:101–106.

42. Newby LK, Christenson RH, Ohman EM, et al. Value of serial troponin T measures for early and late risk stratification in patients with acute coronary syndromes. *Circulation* 1998;98:1853–1859.

43. Lindahl B, Venge P, Wallentin L. Relation between troponin T and the risk of subsequent cardiac events in unstable coronary artery disease. *Circulation* 1996;93:1651–1657.

44. Ravkilde J, Nissen H, Horder M, et al. Independent prognostic value of serum creatine kinase isoenzyme MB mass, cardiac troponin T and myosin light chain levels in suspected acute myocardial infarction: analysis of 28 months of follow-up in 196 patients. *J Am Coll Cardiol* 1995;25:574–581.

45. Ohman EM, Armstrong PW, Christenson RH, et al. Cardiac troponin T levels for risk stratification in acute myocardial ischemia. *N Engl J Med* 1996;335:1333–1341.

46. Antman EM, Tanasijevic MJ, Thompson B, et al. Cardiac-specific troponin I levels to predict the risk of mortality in patients with acute coronary syndromes. *N Engl J Med* 1996;335:1342–1349.

47. Polanczyk CA, Lee TH, Cook EFD, et al. Cardiac troponin I as a predictor of major cardiac events in emergency department patients with acute chest pain. *J Am Coll Cardiol* 1998;32:8–14.

48. Antman EM, Sacks DB, Rifai N, et al. Time to positivity of a rapid bedside assay for cardiac-specific troponin T predicts prognosis in acute coronary syndromes: a thrombolysis in myocardial infarction (TIMI) 11A Substudy. *J Am Coll Cardiol* 1998;31:326–330.

49. Wu AHB, Apple FS, Gibler WB, et al. National Academy of Clinical Biochemistry Standards of Laboratory Practice: recommendations for the use of cardiac markers in coronary artery diseases. *Clin Chem* 1999;45:1104–1121.

50. Stryer DB. Cardiac troponins in patients with chest pain [Letter]. *N Engl J Med* 1998;338:1314.

51. Brogan GX, Bock JL, McCuskey CF, et al. Evaluation of cardiac status CK-MB/myoglobin device for rapidly ruling out acute myocardial infarction. *Clin Lab Med* 1997;17:655–668.

52. Baxter MS, Brogan GX, Harchelroad FP, et al. Evaluation of a bedside whole-blood rapid troponin T assay in the emergency department: rapid evaluation by assay of cardiac troponin T (REACTT) Investigators study group. *Acad Emerg Med* 1997;4(11):1018–1024.

53. Baxter MS, Brogan GX, Garvey JL, et al. The impact of bedside whole blood assay of cardiac troponin T testing on clinical decision making. *Acad Emerg Med* 1997;4:398(abst).

54. Panteghini M, Cuccia C, Pagani F, et al. Comparison of the diagnostic performance of two rapid bedside biochemical assays in the early detection of acute myocardial infarction. *Clin Cardiol* 1998;21:394–398.

55. Nagueh SF, Zoghbi WA. Stress echocardiography for the assessment of myocardial ischemia and viability. *Curr Probl Cardiol* 1996;21:445–520.

56. Krivokapich J, Child JS, Gerber R, et al. Prognostic usefulness of positive or negative exercise stress echocardiography for predicting coronary events in ensuing twelve months. *Am J Cardiol* 1993;71:646–651.

57. Marwick TH, Mehta R, Arheart K, et al. Use of exercise echocardiography for prognostic evaluation of patients with known or suspected coronary artery disease. *Am J Cardiol* 1997;30:83–90.

58. Olmos LI, Dakik H, Gordon R, et al. Long term prognostic value of exercise echocardiography compared with exercise ^{201}Tl, ECG, and clinical variables in patients evaluated for coronary artery disease. *Circulation* 1998;98:2679–2686.

59. Boyne TS, Koplan BA, Parsons WJ, et al. Predicting adverse outcome with exercise SPECT technetium-99m sestamibi imaging in patients with suspected or known coronary artery disease. *Am J Cardiol* 1997;79:270–274.

60. Fleishmann KE, Hunink MGM, Kuntz KM, et al. Exercise echocardiography or exercise SPECT imaging? Meta-analysis of diagnostic test performance. *JAMA* 1998;280:913–920.

61. Bilodeau L, Theroux P, Gregorie J, et al. Technetium-99m sestamibi tomography in patients with spontaneous chest pain: correlations with clinical, electrocardiographic and angiographic findings. *Am J Cardiol* 1991;18:1684–1691.

62. Zalenski RJ, McCarren M, Roberts R, et al. An evaluation of a chest pain diagnostic protocol to exclude acute cardiac ischemia in the emergency department. *Arch Intern Med* 1997;157:1085–1091.

63. Malani SK, Roy CP, Nath CS, et al. Complications in 1000 consecutive treadmill tests. *J Assoc Physicians India* 1993;41:516–517.

64. Kerns JR, Shaub TF, Fontanarosa PB. Emergency cardiac stress testing in the evaluation of emergency department patients with atypical chest pain. *Ann Emerg Med* 1993;22:794–798.

65. Kirk JD, Turnipseed S, Lewis WR, et al. Evaluation of chest pain in low risk patients presenting to the emergency department: the role of immediate exercise testing. *Ann Emerg Med* 1998;32:1–7.

66. Lewis WR, Amsterdam EA. Utility and safety of immediate exercise testing of low risk patients admitted to the hospital for suspected acute myocardial infarction. *Am J Cardiol* 1994;74:987–990.

67. Stuart RJ, Ellestad MH. National survey of exercise stress testing facilities. *Chest* 1980;77:94–97.

68. Patterson RE, Horwitz SF. Importance of epidemiology and biostatistics in deciding clinical strategies for using diagnostic tests: a simplified approach using examples of coronary artery disease. *J Am Coll Cardiol* 1989;13:1653–1665.

69. Tatum JL, Jesse RL, Kontos MC, et al. Comprehensive strategy for the evaluation and triage of the chest pain patient. *Ann Emerg Med* 1997;29:116–125.

70. Lewis WR, Amsterdam EA, Turnipseed S, et al. Immediate exercise testing of low risk patients with known coronary artery disease presenting to the emergency department with chest pain. *J Am Coll Cardiol* 1999;33:1843–1847.

71. Varetto T, Cantalupi B, Altieri A, et al. Emergency room technetium-99m sestamibi imaging to rule out acute myocardial ischemic events in patients with nondiagnostic electrocardiograms. *Am J Cardiol* 1993;22:1804–1808.

72. Hilton TC, Thompson RC, Williams HJ, et al. Technetium-99m sestamibi myocardial perfusion imaging in the emergency room evaluation of chest pain. *Am J Cardiol* 1994;23:1016–1022.

73. Gregorie J, Theroux P. Detection and assessment of unstable angina using myocardial perfusion imaging: comparison between technetium-99m sestamibi SPECT and twelve-lead electrocardiogram. *Am J Cardiol* 1990;66:42E–46E.

74. Beller GA. Acute radionuclide perfusion imaging for evaluation of chest pain in the emergency department: need for a large clinical trial [Editorial]. *J Nucl Cardiol* 1996;3:546–549.

75. Heller GV, Stowers SA, Hendel RC, et al. Clinical value of acute rest technetium-99m tetrofosmin tomographic myocardial perfusion

imaging in patients with acute chest pain and nondiagnostic electro-cardiograms. *Am J Cardiol* 1998;31:1011–1017.

76. Hilton TC, Fulmer H, Abuan T, et al. Ninety day follow up of patients in the emergency department with chest pain who undergo initial single photon emission computed tomographic perfusion scintigraphy with technetium-99m labeled sestamibi. *J Nucl Cardiol* 1996;3:308–311.

77. Kontos MC, Jesse RL, Schmidt KL, et al. Value of acute rest sestamibi perfusion imaging for evaluation of patients admitted to the emergency department with chest pain. *Am J Cardiol* 1997;30:976–982.

78. Stowers SA. Myocardial perfusion scintigraphy for assessment of acute ischemic syndromes: can we seize the moment? *J Nucl Cardiol* 1995;3:274–277.

79. Weissman I, Dickinson CZ, Dworkin HJ, et al. Cost effectiveness of myocardial perfusion imaging with SPECT in the emergency department evaluation of patients with unexplained chest pain. *Radiology* 1996;199:353–357.

80. Radenasky PW, Hilton TC, Fulmer H, et al. Potential cost effectiveness of initial myocardial perfusion imaging for assessment of emergency department patients with chest pain. *Am J Cardiol* 1997;79:595–599.

81. Storrow AB, Gibler WB, Walsh RA, et al. An emergency department chest pain rapid diagnosis and treatment unit: results from a six year experience. *Circulation* 1998;98:I-425(abst).

82. Stomel R, Grant R, Eagle KA. Lessons learned from a community hospital chest pain center. *Am J Cardiol* 1999;83:1033–1037.

PART III

Critical Pathways in the Hospital

CHAPTER 8

Thrombolysis Critical Pathway

Christopher P. Cannon

Fibrinolytic therapy for acute ST-segment elevation myocardial infarction (MI) has dramatically reduced the mortality rate. In the prethrombolytic era, the mortality rate was approximately 13% at 1 month (1,2); in the current era of enhanced reperfusion, it has fallen to approximately 6% for trial participants following the use of second or third generation fibrinolytic agents (3–5).

Several factors have emerged in the field of fibrinolytic therapy that are needed to optimize treatment. All of these factors listed below can be incorporated into critical pathways as a means of practicing "evidence-based" medicine in a cost-effective manner.

1. Rapid time to treatment is critical—both overall time to treatment as well as the door-to-drug time.
2. Accurate dosing (i.e., avoiding medication errors) is a recently identified means of ensuring optimal reperfusion and clinical outcomes.
3. Adjunctive therapy with aspirin and heparin (and potentially soon low molecular weight heparin or direct thrombin inhibitors); also the dosing of heparin is critical to minimize bleeding complications.
4. In the treatment of patients with acute MI, other therapies are also important, including beta-blockers and angiotensin converting enzyme (ACE) inhibitors.
5. The use of cardiac procedures is a major determinant of cost in patients with acute MI, and their use should be targeted to those who will derive the most benefit.
6. Length of hospital stay is an area where costs savings can likely be achieved without compromising patient safety.

EVIDENCE-BASED APPROACH TO DEVELOPING THE THROMBOLYSIS CRITICAL PATHWAY

Door-to-Drug Time

In the development of our critical pathway for thrombolysis, we sought to improve all the above-mentioned factors, but first set out to improve the door-to-drug time.

First, time to reperfusion is the critical factor in rescuing jeopardized myocardium and reducing mortality with thrombolysis (or primary angioplasty) (6,7). Accordingly, in 1994 the National Heart, Lung, and Blood Institute initiated the National Heart Attack Alert Program (NHAAP) with a goal of improving morbidity and mortality in acute MI through reductions in time to treatment (8). The first goal was to reduce "door-to-drug time"—the time elapsed from presentation in the emergency department (ED) to initiation of fibrinolysis—through creation of a critical pathway to expedite evaluation and management in the ED (8).

Beginning in November 1993, a pathway designed to reduce our door-to-drug time was developed and implemented (6). An overview of the key steps to starting thrombolytic therapy is shown in Fig. 8-1 (6). Patients with chest pain forego the standard ED registration process and immediately have a 12-lead electrocardiogram (ECG) performed. They undergo a focused history and physical examination to evaluate any contraindication to fibrinolytic therapy (e.g., active bleeding, prior or recent stroke, or confirmed uncontrolled hypertension). Patients with cardiogenic shock or any contraindication to fibrinolysis are triaged for primary angioplasty (as is currently the case for most patients).

A dramatic reduction was observed in door-to-drug time, from an average of 76 minutes before the pathway was implemented to an average of 30 to 35 minutes after the pathway had been started (9) (Fig. 8-2). Of note, as had been observed in the National Registry of Myocardial Infarction (NRMI) (10), women have longer door-to-drug times, which did improve to an even greater extent after implementation of the pathway (Fig. 8-3) (9). Similarly, others have reported improvements in door-to-drug times with other types of critical pathways or "fast-track" algorithms for acute MI (Fig. 8-4) (11–13). Of note, evidence has recently been reported showing a direct relationship between longer door-to-drug times and increased mortality (Fig. 8-5), thereby reinforcing the importance of using critical pathways to

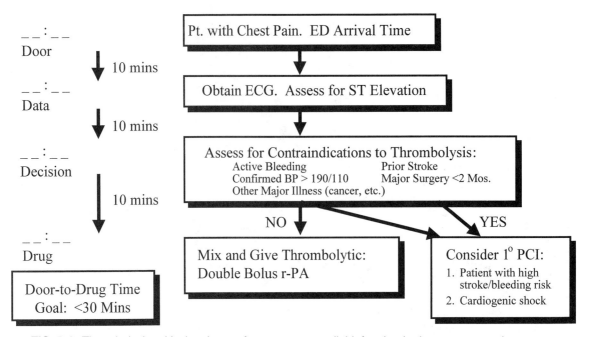

FIG. 8-1. Thrombolysis critical pathways for acute myocardial infarction in the emergency department at Brigham and Women's Hospital. (Adapted from Cannon CP, Antman EM, Walls R, et al. Time as an adjunctive agent to thrombolytic therapy. *J Thromb Thrombolysis* 1994;1:27–34; with permission.)

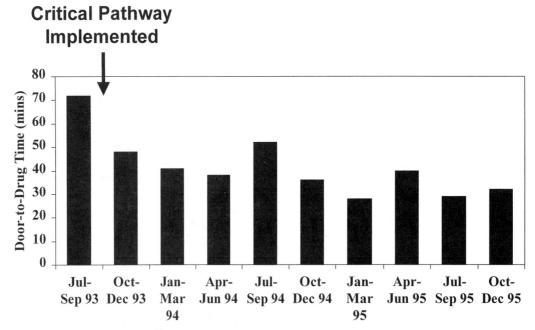

FIG. 8-2. Reduction in door-to-drug time before and after implementation of our thrombolysis critical pathway. (From Cannon CP, Johnson EB, Cermignani M, et al. Emergency department thrombolysis critical pathway reduces door-to-drug times in acute myocardial infarction. *Clin Cardiol* 1999;22:17–22; Sagarin MJ, Cannon CP, Cermignani MS, et al. Delay in thrombolysis administration: causes of extended door-to-drug times and the asymptote effect. *J Emerg Med* 1998;16:557–565; with permission.)

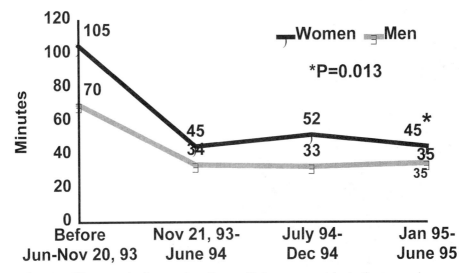

FIG. 8-3. Gender differences in door-to-drug time, with improvement for both men and women. (From Cannon CP, Johnson EB, Cermignani M, et al. Emergency department thrombolysis critical pathway reduces door-to-drug times in acute myocardial infarction. *Clin Cardiol* 1999;22:17–22; with permission.)

ensure that all patients have a door-to-drug time that meets the NHAAP guideline of 30 minutes or less (14).

Choice of Thrombolytic Agent

Initially, our pathway allowed for the use of either tissue plasminogen activator (tPA) or streptokinase, with use being 97% tPA (9). The use of tPA is based on its superiority in achieving early reperfusion and in reducing mortality compared with streptokinase (3,15,16). More recently, however,

bolus fibrinolytic agents have been developed, notably reteplase (4) and tenecteplase (TNK-tPA), which offer two important benefits (16,17). First, administration is greatly facilitated by use of a bolus agent (5,17). The reduction in the time required for preparation and administration of a fibrinolytic agent is a major advantage of bolus fibrinolytic agents. One study documented a 19-minute time savings in door-to-drug time using reteplase as compared with alteplase (18).

Second, simpler dosing can yield one very straightforward clinical benefit—a lower rate of medication errors and

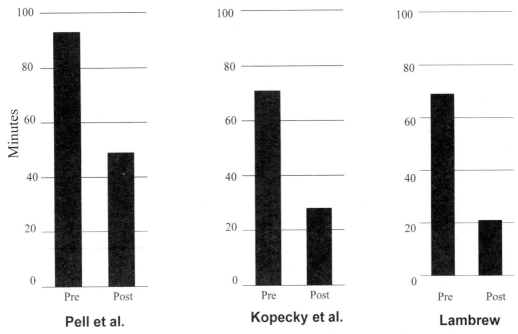

FIG. 8-4. Reduction in door-to-drug time with implementation of thrombolysis critical pathways and protocols (6,11–13,78).

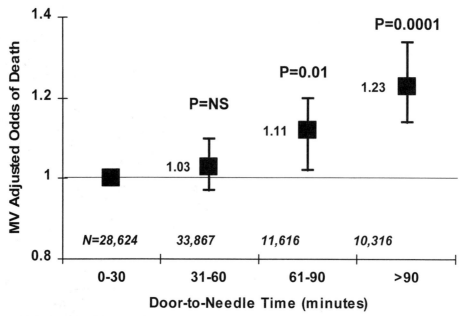

FIG. 8-5. Relationship of door-to-drug time on multivariate adjusted mortality. (Reproduced from Cannon CP, Gibson CM, Lambrew CT, et al. Longer thrombolysis door-to-needle times are associated with increased mortality in acute myocardial infarction: an analysis of 85,589 patients in the National Registry of Myocardial Infarction 2 + 3. *J Am Coll Cardiol* 2000;35[Suppl A]:376A; with permission.)

their potential negative impact on clinical outcome. In one analysis from the Global Use of Streptokinase and tPA for Occluded Coronary Arteries (GUSTO)-I trial, approximately 12% of patients had alteplase or streptokinase administered incorrectly, including the incorrect dose or length of infusion. The 30-day mortality rate for these patients was significantly higher when compared with patients who received the correct dose. The mortality rate for patients

treated with tPA was 5.5% for those correctly dosed versus 7.7% for those who had a medication error ($p < 0.001$) (Fig. 8-6) (19). Similar increased mortality rate and intracranial hemorrhage (ICH) was observed in the Intravenous nPA for Treatment of Infarction Myocardium Early (InTIME) II trial among patients who had medication errors with tPA (10.1% vs. 5.2%) when a correct dose of tPA was administered ($p < 0.0001$) (20,21).

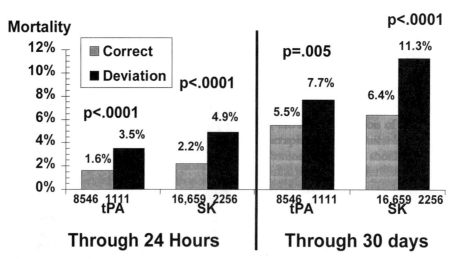

FIG. 8-6. Association of thrombolysis medication errors with increased mortality in the Global Utilization of Streptokinase and tPA for Occluded Coronary Arteries (GUSTO)-I trial. (Data from Vorchheimer DA, Baruch L, Thompson TD, et al. North American vs. non–North American streptokinase use in GUSTO-I: impact of protocol deviation on mortality benefit of tPA. *Circulation* 1997;96[Suppl I]:I-535; reproduced from Cannon CP. Thrombolysis medication errors: benefits of bolus thrombolytic agents. *Am J Cardiol* 2000;85:17C–22C; with permission.)

In the InTIME-II trial, the bolus agent lanoteplase had a modest, but significantly lower rate of dosing errors (5.7% vs. 7.3%) for patients receiving tPA ($p < 0.001$). However, among patients ≤67 kg, when tPA should be weight adjusted, 20% had medication errors with tPA (20). Similarly, another study found significantly fewer patients given reteplase had incomplete doses (1%) compared with those receiving tPA (4%; $p = 0.03$) (18). Thus, emerging, albeit preliminary, evidence from several trials indicates that (a) medication errors with infusion-based thrombolytic agents are relatively common; (b) they appear to be associated with an increased mortality rate; and (c) bolus fibrinolytic agents markedly reduce the incidence of errors, which would improve the safety of fibrinolysis. For these reasons, at Brigham and Women's Hospital we have switched to using bolus fibrinolysis, currently reteplase, but soon TNK.

Reperfusion Therapy

Data from several registries suggest that certain patients appear to be candidates for thrombolysis (or primary angioplasty) who do not receive reperfusion therapy (22–25). In the *TIMI-9 Registry* of ST elevation MI, 69% either received thrombolysis (60%) or underwent primary angioplasty (9%) (24). Of those who presented to the hospital within 12 hours of the onset of pain, 75% received acute reperfusion therapy. Of the 31% of the total group who did not receive reperfusion therapy, one third were from delay in presentation, another third had contraindications to thrombolysis, and the final third had no clearly identifiable reason why thrombolysis was not administered. Similar findings were reported in the much larger NRMI study, where 24% of apparently eligible patients did not receive thrombolysis or primary angioplasty (25). Thus, opportunities for improvement exist, with the ultimate goal of extending the benefits of reperfusion therapy to all patients with ST-segment elevation MI.

Our pathway design focused on ensuring that the attending physician was the person to interpret the ECG. In addition, we have recently added the Acute Cardiac Ischemia—Time Insensitive Predictive Instrument (ACI-TIPI), to assist further in ECG interpretation (26). These two measures are designed to reduce the possibility that diagnostic ST-segment elevation would be missed.

UTILIZATION OF EVIDENCE-BASED, GUIDELINE-RECOMMENDED MEDICATIONS

A major problem in the management of acute MI is that a large proportion of patients do not receive recommended medical therapies. Aspirin has been the first (and perhaps most important) example, with a clear mortality benefit seen in the Second International Study of Infarct Survival (ISIS-2) trial (2). However, in the first NRMI, involving 240,989 patients, only 87% of thrombolytic-treated patients received aspirin (23). Similarly, in the Cooperative Cardiovascular Project,

among patients fully eligible to receive aspirin (i.e., no contraindications such as bleeding ulcer), only 80% received it (27). Indeed, the American Heart Association published a "scientific statement" strongly urging physicians to increase the use of aspirin in appropriate patients (28).

Similarly, beta-blockers are beneficial in patients with acute MI (29,30). ACE inhibitors have been shown to be beneficial after MI in patients with either documented left ventricular (LV) dysfunction or congestive heart failure (CHF), and those with acute MI, especially anterior ST-segment elevation MI (33–35).

Unfortunately, as with aspirin, beta-blockers were given to only 61% in the TIMI-9 Registry (24). In patients who developed CHF or had documented LV dysfunction after MI, only 39% were treated with ACE inhibitors at hospital discharge (24). Although these number are better than these observed in the NRMI, opportunity remains for improvement (23).

HEPARIN

Heparin is an important adjunctive agent following tPA and tPA-derived agents (TNK-tPA and rPA) to maintain infarct-related artery patency (36–38). An important lesson learned in the TIMI-10B and Assessment of the Safety of a New Thrombolytic (ASSENT) I trials, which was also observed in TIMI-9 and GUSTO-II, is that reduced doses of heparin with thrombolysis are associated with reduced rates of ICH and major hemorrhage (39–43). A recent overview of all major thrombolytic trials, and of detailed information from the TIMI trials and the InTIME-II trial confirmed that lower doses of heparin with thrombolysis are associated with reduced ICH (44). Based on the emerging data, the 1999 update to the American College of Cardiology/American Heart Association Guidelines for the Management of Acute MI will recommend a new, lower, weight-based dose of heparin: Bolus of 60 U/kg (maximum 4,000 U), and an initial infusion of 12 U/kg/h (maximum 1,000 U/h) (45).

We list all these evidence-based medications in our pathway to remind the physician to consider them for the patient. As shown in Fig. 8-7, the format is that of a checklist. This design simplifies the procedure so that the busy clinician can quickly be reminded of these key medications and prescribe them. Because the dose for heparin is important for the safety, we have also specified it on the page. Most recently, we have made this pathway into standard order templates in the hospital computer system (see also Chapter 3). All medications and other orders have to be entered electronically; thus, the computerized order template associated with the critical pathway ensures that the physician sees the checklist of orders. The physician simply chooses a pathway based on the clinical diagnosis and clicks on the medications to be ordered. (Note, verbal orders still can be taken, as in the case for administering fibrinolytic therapy, to speed delivery of the drug.) It is hoped that this new system will further increase the use of evidence-based medications.

	Day 0 Emerg. Dept.	Day 0 CCU	Day 1 Stepdown Unit / CCU	Day 2 Stepdown Unit / CCU	Day 3 Stepdown Unit	Day 4 Stepdown Unit	Day 5 Stepdown Unit	Post-Disch.
Goals	○ Door-to-needle<30' Actual __ __ mins ○ LCU Fellow to ED in < 5 mins ○ Consider TIMI 10	○ Admit CCU	○ *Low Risk (Age <70, Small Inferior MI, No prev.MI, Killip I) Transfer to Stepdown* ○ Get ETT/cath slots	○ *Low Risk: Ambulate* ○ **Not LR:** In absence of ischemia/CHF/VT: Transfer to Stepdown	○ *Low risk: am ETT* ○ *If Neg: D/C home If Pos: Cath* ○ Consider TIMI 12	○ ETT ○ *Consider D/C Home* ○ Consider TIMI 12	○ D/C Home in am	
Assessment	○ Vitals ○ Hx:Contraindication ○ Enroll crit. TIMI 10	○ Vitals q 1-2 h ○ Cont. ECG monitor	○ Vitals q 4h ○ Continuous ECG	○ Vitals q 8h ○ *Low Risk: D/C Cont. ECG monitor*	○ Vitals q 8h ○ Not LR: Cont. ECG	○ Vitals q 8h ○ D/C Cont. ECG		
Tests	○ Admit labs: CBC, Chem 20, CK-MB, Lipid Profile, PT/PTT, Clot ○ ECG	○ CK/CK-MB q 8 x2 ○ PTT 6, 12 h ○ ECG on LCU arrival ○ Follow ST's on monitor	○ ECG in am ○ CBC, Chem 7, Mg, PTT in am, 6 h post change	○ Chem 7, Mg ○ PTT, CBC if on hepn ○ Echo (if Ant. / large MI, CHF, prior MI, Qwaves)	○ Not LR: Chem 7			
Medications	○ Thrombolysis ○ ASA 325 chewed ○ Heparin IV (as nec.) ○ Metoprolol IV ○ SL/IV nitro prn ○ Morphine prn	○ Ensure ASA given ○ IV heparin ○ Metoprolol PO ○ IV nitro - wean ○ ACEI (If SBP >100) ○ Consider Magnesium	○ ASA ○ IV heparin ○ Metoprolol ○ IV nitro - D/C ○ Lipid lowering prn ○ ACE inhibitor	○ ASA ○ IV heparin ○ Metoprolol ○ Lipid lowering prn ○ ACE inhibitor	○ ASA ○ D/C heparin ○ Warfarin prn ○ Beta-blocker ○ Lipid lowering prn ○ ACE inhibitor	○ ASA ○ Beta-blocker ○ Lipid low prn ○ ACE inhibitor	○ ASA ○ Beta-blocker ○ Lipid low prn ○ Cont. ACEI if EF<40, CHF, Ant. or prior MI	
Treatments	○ Cont. ECG monitor ○ 20 gauge IV ○ O2 as needed	○ If ischemia, shock, or failed thrombolysis ->cath ○ O2	○ If ischemia/-> Cath ○ D/C Foley ○ O2	○ If ischemia-> Cath ○ D/C O2	○ If ischemia -> Cath	○ If ischemia-> Cath		
Activity/ Rehab	○ Bedrest	○ Bedrest	○ Bedrest	○ Low Risk: Ambulate Not LR: Bedrest	○ Routine activity	○ Routine activity	○ Routine activity	
Diet	○ NPO	○ Heart Healthy Diet	○ Dietary consult	○ Heart Healthy Diet	○ Heart Healthy Diet	○ Heart Healthy	○ HeartHealthy	
Education/Pt/ Fam	○ Family to 12D ○ Explain Dx:Pt./Fam	○ Explain Diagnosis to Pt./ family	○ Discuss with family readiness for D/C	○ Discuss Meds /Risk factors with Pt./Fam.	○ Discharge instructions	○ Disc. Meds/ Risk factors	○ Discharge instructions	
Discharge Planning	○ Book bed in CCU with charge nurse	○ Notify Primary MD ○ Notify Case Manager	○ Soc. Serv. consult prn	○ Arrange VNA prn ○ Lipid manag.plan/clinic prn ○ Exercise plan/Rehab prn ○ Appt to 1°. MD	○ Low Risk: If ETT -: Discharge in am ○ Call 1° MD ○ D/C letter	○ Recheck D/C arrangements	○ D/C in am ○ Call 1° MD ○ D/C letter	○ F/U call 24-48h
Variances								

Instructions for the ○: If completed, mark ●. If not done, record a number in the circle, ①, and in the Variances box, record 1: one-two word reason" (Example: if severe COPD, in the Medications section, record ① for metoprolol PO, and in the Variances section: Write "1: Severe COPD")

FIG. 8-7. Thrombolysis critical pathway at Brigham and Women's Hospital, Boston, MA.

OVERUTILIZATION OF CARDIAC PROCEDURES

Another area having the potential for cost reduction (but not necessarily improvement in clinical outcome) is in the use of cardiac procedures following admission for acute MI. In acute MI, numerous studies have found wide differences in the use of cardiac procedures but no differences in mortality rate (46–52). Such observations have been made when comparing hospitals with on-site cardiac catheterization facilities with those without, and when comparing patients in Canada with those in the United States; many fewer procedures are performed in Canada, but the overall mortality rates for patients in the United States and Canada is similar (46–52). These data suggest that perhaps unnecessary procedures are being performed in some patients.

In the TIMI-IIB randomized trial, 3,339 patients treated with tPA were randomized to either an invasive strategy consisting of cardiac catheterization 18 to 48 hours later, followed by angioplasty [percutaneous transluminal coronary angioplasty (PTCA)] or bypass surgery if the anatomy was suitable, or to a conservative strategy in which catheterization and PTCA were performed only for recurrent spontaneous ischemia or a positive exercise test (53–55).

The 42-day rates of death or MI were similar (10.9% for invasive vs. 9.7% for conservative, $p = NS$) (53). Similarly, no difference between the two strategies was observed through 1 year or 3 years of follow-up (21% death or MI for the invasive strategy vs. 20% for the conservative strategy, $p = NS$) (54,55). In contrast, the rate of revascularization in the two strategies was vastly different: 72.3% of patients having invasive strategy underwent PTCA or coronary artery bypass graft (CABG) by 1 year, compared with only 35.5% in the conservative strategy.

Approximately 750,000 patients with acute MI are admitted to acute care hospitals in the United States annually; estimating that one half have ST-segment elevation, the potential cost savings of following a conservative strategy are astounding. Using a figure of $2,000 for a diagnostic catheterization and $4,000 for a PTCA procedure, this would translate into an annual savings of $1 billion. If a sensitivity analysis were performed, reducing the cost of the procedures by one half, the savings following a conservative strategy still amounts to $500 million annually in the United States. Thus, because both strategies led to similar long-term outcome, this trial established the "watchful waiting" approach as the most cost-effective strategy.

The findings from TIMI-IIB, with the added support of the findings from the Should We Intervene Following Thrombolysis? (SWIFT) trial, and other studies, lend strong support to the notion that coronary angiography can be reserved for patients who demonstrate recurrent ischemia after thrombolysis for ST-segment elevation MI (46–52,56). In the current era of cost containment, close scrutiny of the indications for cardiac catheterization, with more strict adherence to its need in patients with documented recurrent ischemia after MI, may allow reductions in the use of cardiac procedures (and thus costs), without any loss of clinical benefit. In our pathway, we have left the decision regarding catheterization to the discretion of the treating physician, but we generally follow the TIMI-IIB strategy following thrombolytic therapy.

With regard to acute procedures, rescue angioplasty for failed thrombolysis is performed only if patients have evidence of ongoing pain and persistent ST-segment elevation, or in those with hemodynamic compromise. Research is ongoing to identify other ECG criteria and serum markers to assist in this decision (57–60).

Reducing Other Cardiac Testing

Other potential areas of testing overutilization also exist (e.g., laboratory tests and echocardiography). During some admissions, multiple measurements of lipid profiles or liver function are ordered, which may be unnecessary. Our pathway lists what the recommended blood tests are for the house staff. In this fashion, routine ordering of unnecessary blood work can be reduced.

Echocardiography, which is used widely to assess LV function after MI, is the most powerful determinant of subsequent prognosis (61–63). The American College of Cardiology/American Heart Association Guidelines for the Management of Acute MI recommend that LV function be assessed in all patients (30). However, one study, now validated by three other groups, has shown that several clinical features [nonanterior MI, no prior Q waves, total creatine kinase (CK) <1,000 IU, and no evidence of CHF] can be used to predict normal LV function (ejection fraction >40%) with 97% specificity (64–66). Thus, for patients with small non–Q-wave MI, assessment of LV function via echocardiography or ventriculography may not be necessary, a strategy which could have potential implications for more cost-effective care. In our pathway, echocardiography is recommended for most patients, except those with small inferior MI without complications in whom LV function can be inferred to be normal according to the aforementioned clinical prediction rule (64).

REDUCING HOSPITAL (AND INTENSIVE CARE UNIT) LENGTH OF STAY

Reducing lengthy hospitalizations has been the driving force behind the creation of critical pathways. In acute MI, hospitalization was very long just 5 years ago. In GUSTO-I, the median length of stay was 9 days (67). In a follow-up analysis in which patients were divided into those who had an uncomplicated course (no recurrent ischemia, CHF, or any other complication) and those having any one of these complications, the median length of stay for both groups was 9 days. In the 1995 TIMI-9 Registry, for uncomplicated patients with ST-segment elevation MI, the median length of stay was 8 days (24,68). Thus, it appears that hospitalization historically has been lengthy in patients with acute MI, and opportunities exist to reduce it safely, especially in patients at low risk.

Identifying Patients at Low Risk

With the benefit of aggressive reperfusion therapy in acute MI, it has been possible to identify patients who are at low risk of subsequent mortality or morbidity (69). In the TIMI-II trial, a group of patients were prespecified as "low risk" if they had the following characteristics: age <70 years, no prior MI, inferior or lateral MI, normal sinus rhythm, and Killip class 1 at admission (53). This classification was subsequently validated (70). Similar observations have been made in the Thrombolysis and Angioplasty in Acute Myocardial Infarction (TAMI) trials, in GUSTO-I, and, most recently, in the InTIME-II trial (Fig. 8-8) (67,71,72).

Strategy of Early Discharge following Thrombolysis

Identification of patients at low risk has led to the possibility of early hospital discharge for such patients (67,71). A pilot trial of such a strategy in 80 patients suggested that hospital stay and costs could be significantly reduced without an increase in morbidity and mortality rates (73). However, it should be noted that all patients who received reperfusion therapy also underwent immediate coronary angiography, the information from which was used in the triage of the patients. Such a strategy is not applicable to standard practice (73). Recently, the cost-effectiveness of early discharge has been subjected to decision analysis, and it was observed that for patients with an uncomplicated MI treated with thrombolytic therapy, the incremental cost of keeping the patient in the hospital beyond 3 days, ($624/day for hospital and physicians' services), and extending the hospital stay to 4 days would cost $105,629/year of life saved. These data emphasize the cost benefits of early discharge in acute MI. Thus, the strategy of early hospital discharge looks very promising and feasible, although only limited observational data demonstrate its safety.

It should be noted that data regarding the efficacy and safety of early discharge are available from the Primary Angioplasty in Myocardial Infarction (PAMI)-2 trial, in which 471 patients at low risk were randomized to a strategy of early discharge or to conventional hospital discharge (74). Clinical outcomes at 6 months were similar in both groups.

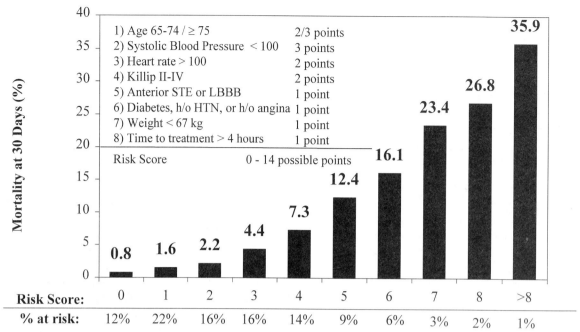

1) Age 65-74 / ≥ 75   2/3 points
2) Systolic Blood Pressure < 100   3 points
3) Heart rate > 100   2 points
4) Killip II-IV   2 points
5) Anterior STE or LBBB   1 point
6) Diabetes, h/o HTN, or h/o angina 1 point
7) Weight < 67 kg   1 point
8) Time to treatment > 4 hours   1 point

Risk Score   0 - 14 possible points

Risk Score:	0	1	2	3	4	5	6	7	8	>8
Mortality	0.8	1.6	2.2	4.4	7.3	12.4	16.1	23.4	26.8	35.9
% at risk:	12%	22%	16%	16%	14%	9%	6%	3%	2%	1%

FIG. 8-8. TIMI risk score for ST-segment elevation myocardial infarction. (Reproduced from Morrow DA, Antman EM, Charlesworth A, et al. The TIMI risk score for ST elevation myocardial infarction: a convenient, bedside, clinical score for risk assessment at presentation. An intravenous nPA for treatment of infarcting myocardium early II trial substudy. *Circulation* 2000;102:2031–2037; with permission.)

The mortality rate was 0.8% versus 0.4% for early discharge versus standard care ($p = 1.0$); unstable angina was 10.1% versus 12.0% ($p = NS$); recurrent MI was 0.8% versus 0.4% ($p = NS$); or the combination of death, unstable angina, MI, CHF, or stroke was 15.2% versus 17.5% $p = 0.49$) (74). On the other hand, for the early discharge critical pathway group, hospitalizations were 3 days shorter (4.2 days vs. 7.1 days, $p = 0.0001$) and hospital costs were lower ($9,658 ± $5,287 vs. $11,604 ± 6,125, $p = 0.002$) (74). Thus, in low-risk primary angioplasty patients, early discharge appears to be safe and result in a substantial reduction in hospital length of stay and cost savings.

Our pathway divides patients by their clinical risk profile (Fig. 8-7), with patients at high risk defined as those with either an anterior MI, a large MI judged by peak CK or echocardiography, those with prior MI, or those presenting in Killip class 1–4 (i.e., with evidence of CHF or cardiogenic shock). In contrast, patients at low risk are those with small inferior MI, without prior MI, who present without evidence of CHF (Fig. 8-7). When the pathway is updated, we will switch to using the TIMI ST-segment elevation MI risk score (Fig. 8-8).

All patients with ST-segment elevation MI are treated in the ED and admitted to the coronary care unit (CCU). Patients at low risk are transferred out of the CCU after 24 hours, whereas others are transferred when their condition allows. The target hospital length of stay is similar to that in the PAMI-II—3 days for low risk patients and 5 days for those at higher risk. Recent registry data from our institution (and paralleling data from the NRMI) have shown a steady decline in length of hospitalizations over recent years, with our current average being 4 to 5 days.

Secondary Prevention and Follow-up

Because follow-up is critical in the overall management of all acute coronary syndromes, the primary care physician receives a phone call, a fax summary or the hospital discharge instructions, a letter from the cardiologist, and the hospital discharge summary (the latter three are also sent to other physicians caring for the patient). These methods of follow-up provide further opportunity for the cardiologist to ensure that the patient receives long-term treatment with key medications such as aspirin, beta-blockers, and cholesterol-lowering medications (75,76). Patient involvement is also critical; thus, patient education regarding diagnosis, prognosis, and risk factor modification begins in-hospital on the first day. This teaching continues with the patient's primary nurse, as well as dietary consultation if needed.

CONCLUSIONS

Our thrombolysis pathway is designed to provide evidence-based cardiac care to our patients. It emphasizes rapid time to treatment, use of guideline-recommended medications, risk stratification, secondary prevention, and patient education. We have documented a significant reduction in door-to-drug time with the use of our pathway. We have not evaluated formally the improvements in other aspects of care, but believe that this approach allows us to meet our goal of improving the quality and cost-effectiveness of patient care.

REFERENCES

1. Gruppo Italiano per lo Studio della Streptochinasi nell'Infarto Miocardico (GISSI). Effectiveness of intravenous thrombolytic treatment in acute myocardial infarction. *Lancet* 1986;1:397–402.
2. ISIS-2 (Second International Study of Infarct Survival) Collaborative Group. Randomised trial of intravenous streptokinase, oral aspirin, both, or neither among 17,187 cases of suspected acute myocardial infarction: ISIS-2. *Lancet* 1988;2:349–360.
3. The GUSTO Investigators. An international randomized trial comparing four thrombolytic strategies for acute myocardial infarction. *N Engl J Med* 1993;329:673–682.
4. The Global Use of Strategies to Open Occluded Coronary Arteries (GUSTO III) Investigators. A comparison of reteplase with alteplase for acute myocardial infarction. *N Engl J Med* 1997;337:1118–1123.
5. Assessment of the Safety and Efficacy of a New Thrombolytic Investigators. Single-bolus tenecteplase compared with front-loaded alteplase in acute myocardial infarction: the ASSENT-2 double-blind randomised trial. *Lancet* 1999;354:716–722.
6. Cannon CP, Antman EM, Walls R, et al. Time as an adjunctive agent to thrombolytic therapy. *J Thromb Thrombolysis* 1994;1:27–34.
7. Goldberg RJ, Mooraad M, Gurwitz JH, et al. Impact of time to treatment with tissue plasminogen activator on morbidity and mortality following acute myocardial infarction (the Second National Registry of Myocardial Infarction). *Am J Cardiol* 1998;82:259–264.
8. National Heart Attack Alert Program Coordinating Committee—60 Minutes to Treatment Working Group. Emergency department: rapid identification and treatment of patients with acute myocardial infarction. *Ann Emerg Med* 1994;23:311–329.
9. Cannon CP, Johnson EB, Cermignani M, et al. Emergency department thrombolysis critical pathway reduces door-to-drug times in acute myocardial infarction. *Clin Cardiol* 1999;22:17–22.
10. Lambrew CT, Bowlby LJ, Rogers WJ, et al. Factors influencing the time to thrombolysis in acute myocardial infarction. Time to Thrombolysis Substudy of the National Registry of Myocardial Infarction-1. *Arch Intern Med* 1997;157:2577–2582.
11. Pell ACH, Miller HC, Robertson CE, et al. Effect of "fast track" admission for acute myocardial infarction on delay to thrombolysis. *BMJ* 1992;304:83–87.
12. Kopecky SL, Siska MJ, Jurek JA, et al. Method of reducing emergency room time to treatment of acute myocardial infarction. *J Am Coll Cardiol* 1995;(Special Issue):206.
13. Lambrew CT. Emergency department triage of patients with nontraumatic chest pain. *Am Curr Cardiol Current Journal Review* 1995;4:61–62.
14. Cannon CP, Gibson CM, Lambrew CT, et al. Longer thrombolysis door-to-needle times are associated with increased mortality in acute myocardial infarction: an analysis of 85,589 patients in the National Registry of Myocardial Infarction 2 + 3. *J Am Coll Cardiol* 2000;35[Suppl A]:376A.
15. The GUSTO Angiographic Investigators. The comparative effects of tissue plasminogen activator, streptokinase, or both on coronary artery patency, ventricular function and survival after acute myocardial infarction. *N Engl J Med* 1993;329:1615–1622.
16. Cannon CP, McCabe CH, Diver DJ, et al. Comparison of front-loaded recombinant tissue–type plasminogen activator, anistreplase and combination thrombolytic therapy for acute myocardial infarction: results of the Thrombolysis in Myocardial Infarction (TIMI) 4 trial. *J Am Coll Cardiol* 1994;24:1602–1610.
17. Cannon CP, Gibson CM, McCabe CH, et al. TNK-tissue plasminogen activator compared with front-loaded alteplase in acute myocardial infarction: results of the TIMI 10B trial. *Circulation* 1998;98:2805–2814.
18. Seyedroudbari A, Kessler ER, Mooss AN, et al. Time to treatment and cost of thrombolysis: a multicenter comparison of tPA and rPA. *J Thromb Thrombolysis* 2000;9:303–308.
19. Vorchheimer DA, Baruch L, Thompson TD, et al. North American vs. non–North American streptokinase use in GUSTO-I: impact of protocol deviation on mortality benefit of TPA. *Circulation* 1997;96[Suppl I]:I-535.

20. Coulter SA, McCabe CH, Giugliano RP, et al. Dosing errors and outcomes in patients receiving single bolus compared with bolus + infusion thrombolytic regimens: an InTIME-II study. *Circulation* 1999;100[Suppl I]:I-791.
21. Cannon CP. Thrombolysis medication errors: benefits of bolus thrombolytic agents. *Am J Cardiol* 2000;85:17C–22C.
22. Granger C, Moffie I, for the GUSTO Investigators. Under use of thrombolytic therapy in North America has been exaggerated: results of the GUSTO MI Registry. *Circulation* 1994;90[Suppl I]:I-324.
23. Rogers WJ, Bowlby LJ, Chandra NC, et al. Treatment of myocardial infarction in the United States (1990 to 1993). Observations from the National Registry of Myocardial Infarction. *Circulation* 1994;90:2103–2114.
24. Cannon CP, Henry TD, Schweiger MJ, et al. Current management of ST elevation myocardial infarction and outcome of thrombolytic ineligible patients: results of the multicenter TIMI 9 registry. *J Am Coll Cardiol* 1995;(Special Issue):231A–232A.
25. Barron HV, Bowlby LJ, Breen T, et al. Use of reperfusion therapy for acute myocardial infarction in the United States: data from the National Registry of Myocardial Infarction 2. *Circulation* 1998;97:1150–1156.
26. Selker HP, Beshansky JR, Griffith JL, et al. Use of the acute cardiac ischemia time-insensitive predictive instrument (ACI-TIPI) to assist with triage of patients with chest pain or other symptoms suggestive of acute cardiac ischemia. A multicenter, controlled clinical trial. *Ann Intern Med* 1998;129:845–855.
27. Ellerbeck EF, Jencks SF, Radford MJ, et al. Quality of care for Medicare patients with acute myocardial infarction. A four-state pilot study from the Cooperative Cardiovascular Project. *JAMA* 1995;273:1509–1514.
28. Hennekens CH, Dyken ML, Fuster V. Aspirin as a therapeutic agent in cardiovascular disease. A statement for healthcare professionals from the American Heart Association. *Circulation* 1997;96:2751–2753.
29. Hjalmarson A, Elmfeldt D, Herlitz J, et al. Effect on mortality of metoprolol in acute myocardial infarction, a double-blind randomized trial. *Lancet* 1981;2:823–827.
30. Ryan TJ, Anderson JL, Antman EM, et al. ACC/AHA guidelines for the management of patients with acute myocardial infarction: a report of the American College of Cardiology/American Heart Association Task Force on Practice Guidelines (Committee on Management of Acute Myocardial Infarction). *J Am Coll Cardiol* 1996;28:1328–1428.
31. Pfeffer MA, Braunwald E, Moye LA, et al. Effect of captopril on mortality and morbidity in patients with left ventricular dysfunction after myocardial infarction. *N Engl J Med* 1992;327:669–677.
32. The Acute Infarction Ramipril Efficacy (AIRE) Study Investigators. Effect of ramipril on mortality and morbidity of survivors of acute myocardial infarction with clinical evidence of heart failure. *Lancet* 1993;342:821–828.
33. GISSI-3: effects of lisinopril and transdermal glyceryl trinitrate singly and together on 6-week mortality and ventricular function after acute myocardial infarction. Gruppo Italiano per lo Studio della Sopravvivenza nell'Infarto Miocardico. *Lancet* 1994;343:1115–1122.
34. ISIS-4 Collaborative Group. ISIS-4: randomized factorial trial assessing early oral captopril, oral mononitrate, and intravenous magnesium sulphate in 58,050 patients with suspected acute myocardial infarction. *Lancet* 1995;345:669–685.
35. Chinese Cardiac Study Collaborative Group. Oral captopril versus placebo among 13,634 patients with suspected myocardial infarction: interim report from the Chinese Cardiac Study (CCS-1). *Lancet* 1995;345:686–687.
36. Hsia J, Hamilton WP, Kleiman N, et al. A comparison between heparin and low-dose aspirin as adjunctive therapy with tissue plasminogen activator for acute myocardial infarction. *N Engl J Med* 1990;323:1433–1437.
37. Bleich SD, Nichols T, Schumacher RR, et al. Effect of heparin on coronary patency after thrombolysis with tissue plasminogen activator in acute myocardial infarction. *Am J Cardiol* 1990;66:1412–1417.
38. de Bono DP, Simoons MI, Tijssen J, et al. Effect of early intravenous heparin on coronary patency, infarct size, and bleeding complications after alteplase thrombolysis: results of a randomized double blind European cooperative study group trial. *Br Heart J* 1992;67:122–128.
39. Giugliano RP, Cannon CP, McCabe CH, et al. Lower dose heparin with thrombolysis is associated with lower rates of intracranial hemorrhage: results from TIMI 10B and ASSENT I. *Circulation* 1997;96[Suppl I]:I-535.

40. Antman EM, for the TIMI 9A Investigators. Hirudin in acute my-ocardial infarction: safety report from the Thrombolysis and Throm-bin Inhibition in Myocardial Infarction (TIMI) 9A trial. *Circulation* 1994;90:1624–1630.

41. Antman EM, for the TIMI 9B Investigators. Hirudin in acute myocar-dial infarction: Thrombolysis and Thrombin Inhibition in Myocardial Infarction (TIMI) 9B trial. *Circulation* 1996;94:911–921.

42. The Global Use of Strategies to Open Occluded Coronary Arteries (GUSTO) IIa Investigators. A randomized trial of intravenous heparin versus recombinant hirudin for acute coronary syndromes. *Circulation* 1994;90:1631–1637.

43. The Global Use of Strategies to Open Occluded Coronary Arteries (GUSTO) IIb Investigators. A comparison of recombinant hirudin with heparin for the treatment of acute coronary syndromes. *N Engl J Med* 1996;335:775–782.

44. Giugliano RP, Cutler SS, Llevadot J. Risk of intracranial hemor-rhage with accelerated tPA: importance of heparin dose. *Circulation* 1999;100[Suppl I]:I-650.

45. Ryan TJ, Antman EM, Brooks NH, et al. 1999 Update: ACC/AHA guidelines for the management of patients with acute myocardial infarction: executive summary and recommendations. *Circulation* 1999;100:1016–1030.

46. Every NR, Larson EB, Litwin PE, et al. The association between on-site cardiac catheterization facilities and the use of coronary angiography after acute myocardial infarction. *N Engl J Med* 1993;329:546–551.

47. Every NR, Parson LS, Fihn SD, et al. Long-term outcome in acute myocardial infarction patients admitted to hospitals with and without on-site cardiac catheterization facilities. *Circulation* 1997;96:1770–1775.

48. Blustein J. High-technology cardiac procedures. The impact of service availability on service use in New York State. *JAMA* 1993;270:344–349.

49. Rouleau JL, Moye LA, Pfeffer MA, et al. A comparison of management patterns after acute myocardial infarction in Canada and the United States. *N Engl J Med* 1993;328:779–784.

50. Pilote L, Califf RM, Sapp S, et al. Regional variation across the United States in the management of acute myocardial infarction. *N Engl J Med* 1995;333:565–572.

51. Mark DB, Naylor CD, Hlatky MA, et al. Use of medical resources and quality of life after acute myocardial infarction in Canada and the United States. *N Engl J Med* 1994;331:1130–1135.

52. Tu JV, Pashos CL, Naylor D, et al. Use of cardiac procedures and outcomes in elderly patients with myocardial infarction in the United States and Canada. *JAMA* 1997;336:1500–1505.

53. TIMI Study Group. Comparison of invasive and conservative strategies after treatment with intravenous tissue plasminogen activator in acute myocardial infarction. Results of the Thrombolysis in Myocardial In-farction (TIMI) phase II trial. *N Engl J Med* 1989;320:618–627.

54. Williams DO, Braunwald E, Knatterud G, et al. One-year results of the Thrombolysis in Myocardial Infarction Investigation (TIMI) phase II trial. *Circulation* 1992;85:533–542.

55. Terrin ML, Williams DO, Kleiman NS, et al. Two- and three-year results of the Thrombolysis in Myocardial Infarction (TIMI) phase II clinical trial. *J Am Coll Cardiol* 1993;22:1763–1772.

56. SWIFT (Should We Intervene Following Thrombolysis?) Trial Study Group. SWIFT trial of delayed elective intervention v. conservative treatment after thrombolysis with anistreplase in acute myocardial in-farction. *BMJ* 1991;302:555–560.

57. Schroder R, Dissmann R, Bruggemann T, et al. Extent of early ST segment elevation resolution: a simple but strong predictor of out-come in patients with acute myocardial infarction. *J Am Coll Cardiol* 1994;24:384–391.

58. Schroder R, Wegscheider K, Schroder K, et al, for the INJECT Trial Group. Extent of early ST segment elevation resolution: a strong pre-dictor of outcome in patients with acute myocardial infarction and a sensitive measure to compare thrombolytic regimens. A substudy of the International Joint Efficacy Comparison of Thrombolytics (INJECT) trial. *J Am Coll Cardiol* 1995;26:1657–1664.

59. Tanasijevic MJ, Cannon CP, Wybenga DR, et al. Myoglobin, creatine kinase MB and cardiac troponin-I to assess reperfusion after thrombol-ysis for acute myocardial infarction: results from TIMI 10A. *Am Heart J* 1997;134:622–630.

60. Tanasijevic M, Cannon CP, Antman EM, et al. Myoglobin, creatine-kinase-MB and cardiac troponin I 60-minute ratios predict infarct-related artery patency after thrombolysis for acute myocardial infarc-tion. Results from the Thrombolysis in Myocardial Infarction study (TIMI) 10B. *J Am Coll Cardiol* 1999;34:739–747.

61. Multicenter Postinfarction Research Group. Risk stratification and sur-vival after myocardial infarction. *N Engl J Med* 1983;309:331–336.

62. Zaret BL, Wackers FJT, Terrin ML, et al. Value of radionuclide rest and exercise left ventricular ejection fraction in assessing survival of patients after thrombolytic therapy for acute myocardial infarction: results of the Thrombolysis in Myocardial Infarction (TIMI) phase II study. *J Am Coll Cardiol* 1995;26:73–79.

63. Nicod P, Gilpin E, Dittrich H, et al. Influence on prognosis and mor-bidity of left ventricular ejection fraction with and without signs of left ventricular failure after acute myocardial infarction. *Am J Cardiol* 1988;61:1165–1171.

64. Silver MT, Rose GA, Paul SD, et al. A clinical rule to predict preserved left ventricular ejection fraction in patients after myocardial infarction. *Ann Intern Med* 1994;121:750–756.

65. Tobin K, Stomel R, Harber D, et al. Validation of a clinical predic-tion rule for predicting left ventricular function post acute myocar-dial infarction in a community hospital setting. *J Am Coll Cardiol* 1996;27[Suppl A]:318A.

66. Krumholtz HM, Howes CJ, Murillo JE, et al. Validation of a clini-cal prediction rule for left ventricular ejection fraction after myocar-dial infarction in patients >65 years old. *Am J Cardiol* 1997;80:11–15.

67. Newby LK, Califf RM, for the GUSTO Investigators. Redefining un-complicated myocardial infarction in the thrombolytic era. *Circulation* 1994;90[pt. 2]:I-110.

68. Cannon CP, Antman EM, Gibson CM, et al. Critical pathway for acute ST segment elevation myocardial infarction: evaluation of the poten-tial impact in the TIMI 9 registry. *J Am Coll Cardiol* 1998;31[Suppl A]:192A.

69. Hillis LD, Forman S, Braunwald E, and the Thrombolysis in Myocar-dial Infarction (TIMI) Phase II Co-Investigators. Risk stratification be-fore thrombolytic therapy in patients with acute myocardial infarction. *J Am Coll Cardiol* 1990;16:313–315.

70. Mueller HS, Cohen LS, Braunwald E, et al. Predictors of early mor-bidity and mortality after thrombolytic therapy of acute myocardial infarction. Analyses of patient subgroups in the Thrombolysis in My-ocardial Infarction (TIMI) trial, phase II. *Circulation* 1992;85:1254–1264.

71. Mark DB, Sigmon K, Topol EJ, et al. Identification of acute myocardial infarction patients suitable for early hospital discharge after aggressive interventional therapy. Results from the Thrombolysis and Angioplasty in Acute Myocardial Infarction Registry. *Circulation* 1991;83:1186–1193.

72. Morrow DA, Antman EM, Charlesworth A, et al. The TIMI risk score for ST elevation myocardial infarction: a convenient, bedside, clin-ical score for risk assessment at presentation. An intravenous nPA treatment of infarcting myocardium early II trial substudy. *Circula-tion* 2000;102:2031–2037.

73. Topol EJ, Bure K, O'Neill WW, et al. A randomized controlled trial of hospital discharge three days after myocardial infarction in the era of reperfusion. *N Engl J Med* 1988;318:1083–1088.

74. Grines CL, Marsalese DL, Brodie B, et al. Safety and cost-effectiveness of early discharge after primary angioplasty in low risk patients with acute myocardial infarction. *J Am Coll Cardiol* 1998;31:967–972.

75. Scandinavian Simvastatin Survival Study Group. Randomised trial of cholesterol lowering in 4444 patients with coronary heart disease: the Scandinavian Simvastatin Survival Study (4S). *Lancet* 1994;344:1383–1389.

76. Sacks RM, Pfeffer MA, Moye LA, et al. The effect of pravastatin on coronary events after myocardial infarction in patients with average cholesterol levels. *N Engl J Med* 1996;335:1001–1009.

77. Sagarin MJ, Cannon CP, Cermignani MS, et al. Delay in thrombolysis administration: causes of extended door-to-drug times and the asymp-tote effect. *J Emerg Med* 1998;16:557–565.

78. Cannon CP, Sayah AJ, Walls RM. Prehospital thrombolysis: an idea whose time has come. *Clin Cardiol* 1999;22[Suppl IV]:IV-10–IV-19.

CHAPTER 9

Critical Pathways for Primary Angioplasty in Acute Myocardial Infarction at Community Hospitals without Cardiac Surgery

Nancy Sinclair McNamara and Thomas P. Wharton, Jr

RATIONALE FOR PRIMARY ANGIOPLASTY AT HOSPITALS WITHOUT CARDIAC SURGERY

The superiority of primary percutaneous transluminal coronary angioplasty (PTCA) as treatment of choice for patients with acute myocardial infarction (MI) at qualified centers in fibrinolytic-eligible patients is now well established (1,2). Primary PTCA results in lower rates of death, stroke, recurrent ischemia, and reinfarction compared to lytic therapy (Table 9-1) (1). In patients with acute MI at low risk, primary PTCA has a very low mortality rate (0.4%), and decreases hospital costs because of safe early discharge (3–4 days) and avoidance of intensive care and predischarge exercise testing (3,4). More importantly, primary PTCA can be applied to the two thirds of patients with acute MI who are ineligible to receive fibrinolytic therapy (5,6): patients without ST-segment elevation (a group at higher risk), patients who present late, patients with bleeding contraindications, patients with cardiogenic shock, and those with prior bypass surgery (7). Patients more than 75 years of age may do worse with lytic therapy than with conservative therapy (8). This group, which may comprise as many as one third of all patients with acute MI (9), has reduced mortality with primary PTCA compared with lytic therapy (10). These patients are at greater risk of death than those eligible to receive lytic therapy (6,11,12), and they need a therapeutic alternative to "morphine and bed rest."

Patients in whom lytic therapy is inappropriate have a considerably lower mortality rate when treated with primary PTCA rather than with conventional or lytic therapy, as demonstrated in Figs. 9-1 and 9-2 (13–15). Most patients with acute MI present to community hospitals that do not have cardiac surgery programs. At these hospitals, patients at high risk, ineligible for lytic therapy, or in whom lytic therapy fails are often transferred to an interventional center.

However, patients transferred for primary PTCA have significantly higher times-to-reperfusion and mortality rates compared with those having primary PTCA at the presenting hospital (Fig. 9-3) (16). A further problem with this approach is that many tertiary centers do not routinely offer primary PTCA and, thus, may hesitate to accept such patients in emergency transfer.

For these reasons, more and more hospitals in the United States that have cardiac catheterization laboratories but not cardiac surgery are starting to routinely perform primary PTCA on site as the treatment of choice for acute MI. These hospitals should have experienced interventionalists who routinely perform elective PTCA at interventional centers, an experienced staff, a well-equipped laboratory, and established protocols for emergent transfer to surgical centers.

Many investigators have demonstrated that hospitals without cardiac surgery can establish safe and effective primary PTCA programs that are not compromised by the lack of on-site surgery (17–27). Figure 9-4 shows pooled outcomes from six studies of primary PTCA at community hospitals without cardiac surgery (18,20–27). As shown in the figure, these outcomes, including reperfusion times and rates of PTCA success, coronary artery bypass graft (CABG) surgery for procedural complication, reinfarction, stroke, and mortality in patients without shock, compare very favorably with the outcomes of patients without cardiogenic shock in the *Primary Angioplasty Registry* of five high-volume cardiac surgery centers (28). In the combined experience of these six community hospital registries, which include a total of 1,679 primary angioplasty procedures, the overall mortality rate was 6.4%. Data on patients with and without shock are available on 1,209 patients in these series. The mortality rate in 1,102 patients without shock was 3.7%. Only 2 of the 1,209 (0.17%) patients for whom data are available required

TABLE 9-1. *Primary PTCA vs. Lytic therapy for acute myocardial infarction: analysis of pooled data in 2,606 patients from 10 randomized trials*

Outcome	Patients (%)	
	Primary PTCA (n, 1,290)	Lytic therapy (n, 1,316)
Mortality	4.4%	6.5%[a]
Death or reinfarction	7.2%	11.9%[b]
Total stroke	0.7%	2.0%[c]
Hemorrhagic stroke	0.1%	1.1%[d]

Data presented are percent of patients.
PTCA, percutaneous transluminal coronary angioplasty;
[a] p-0.02.
[b] $p < 0.001$.
[c] p-0.007.
[d] $p < 0.001$.
From Weaver WD, Simes J, Betriw A, et al. Comparison of primary coronary angioplasty and intravenous thrombolytic therapy for acute myocardial infarction. *JAMA* 1997;278: 2093–2098; with permission.

emergency bypass surgery because of new myocardial jeopardy caused by the angioplasty procedure.

The excellent results in these six series were achieved primarily before stents and IIb/IIIa platelet inhibitors were in common use. These modalities should further improve the safety of the procedure (29–33). In fact, newer-generation stents and glycoprotein (GP) IIb/IIIa platelet inhibitors have lowered the risk of abrupt vessel (re)closure from 2% to 5% to approximately 0.4% (29,30,34,35).

The inherently lower interventional volumes of smaller hospitals may not detract from outcomes if performed by higher-volume interventionalists (≥75 procedures per year) who regularly perform elective intervention. In fact, recent reports from the United States and Canada document either no difference (36) or minimal differences (37) in outcomes between hospitals performing less than 200 procedures per year and those performing more than 400 procedures per year. The current volume-related mortality rate differences (<0.4%) (37) are far less than the mortality difference between primary PTCA and other therapies including fibrinolytic therapy (1), conservative therapy in lytic-ineligible patients (13,15), and transfer to an interventional center (16). In addition, smaller hospitals may be able to perform primary PTCA faster than larger centers (38). Possible reasons for potentially greater efficiency of smaller hospitals may include more direct communication between the emergency physician and the cardiologist with less bureaucracy, decreased travel times if the catheterization team lives nearby, and greater flexibility in a catheterization laboratory schedule that may not be as congested.

A clear need is seen to increase the availability of primary PTCA. Also a clear potential exists to accomplish this, because more than 800 community hospitals in the United States have cardiac catheterization laboratories without

cardiac surgery or interventional programs (39). In this chapter will be proposed standards, critical pathways, and care maps to enable more of these hospitals to set up safe and effective primary PTCA programs. Many small hospitals have initiated interventional programs using standards and protocols that are similar to the ones proposed here. These hospitals have invariably achieved results that are comparable to, or even better than, those of the six community hospital series illustrated in Fig. 9-4.

BUILDING CRITICAL PATHWAYS FOR A SUCCESSFUL COMMUNITY HOSPITAL PRIMARY PTCA PROGRAM

Launching a successful program for primary PTCA at a community hospital requires the commitment and collaboration of all members of the healthcare team. Before starting a PTCA program, cardiologists, emergency department (ED) staff, cardiac catheterization laboratory (CCL) staff, primary care physicians, cardiac nurses, and hospital administrators need to develop a uniform standard of care for patients with acute MI. This program also requires setting up vigorous and ongoing quality improvement processes to ensure a safe and effective program. The common goal is to extend all essential elements of the treatment of acute MI to patients throughout all areas of the hospital.

The essential elements that must be established and developed include:

- An acute MI protocol team
- A primary PTCA critical pathway
- Operator and institutional criteria for primary PTCA
- Position profiles, defined expectations for CCL staff, and staff training programs
- Clinical and angiographic selection criteria for primary PTCA and for emergency transfer for coronary bypass surgery
- A fine-tuned emergency triage system in the ED
- An emergency transfer protocol and formal agreements that ensure rapid transfer to a cardiac surgery center
- A catheterization laboratory primary PTCA protocol and an acuity-based, procedure-bumping protocol
- In-hospital acute MI management pathways, to include the development of patient care protocols, standing orders, and assessment tools from admission to discharge
- Processes and tracking tools for data gathering and analysis, case review, and quality assurance

Let us examine each element of this process individually. Examples are given of critical pathways and care maps for the primary PTCA program at Exeter Hospital, Exeter, NH, which is a small (<100 bed) hospital 15 minutes from the nearest cardiac surgical facility.

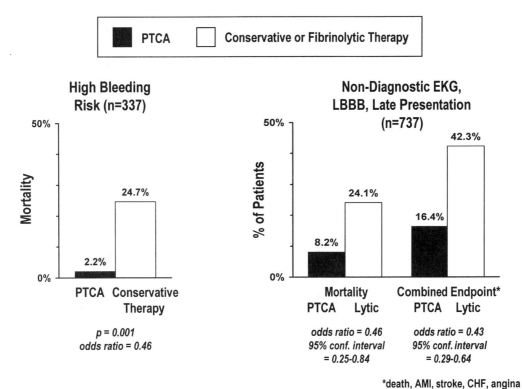

FIG. 9-1. Comparison of the outcomes of primary percutaneous transluminal coronary angioplasty (PTCA) versus other treatments in patients with acute myocardial infarction (AMI) who are inappropriate for fibrinolytic studies in the Maximal Individual Therapy in Acute Myocardial Infarction (MITRA) Study Group Registry from Germany. The graph to the left demonstrates a significant and dramatic reduction in mortality in 337 patients ineligible for fibrinolytics because of bleeding risk who were treated with primary angioplasty versus conservative therapy in the MITRA registry (13). The graph to the right demonstrates a significant reduction in mortality for primary angioplasty compared with fibrinolytics in 737 patients in this registry (14) who are normally excluded from randomized trials: those with nondiagnostic electrocardiogram, left bundle branch block, late presentation >12 hours, or unknown prehospital delay. A significant reduction was also seen in the combined endpoints of death, reinfarction, stroke, advanced CHF, and postinfarction angina for primary angioplasty in this population. *Black bars*: Patients treated with primary PTCA. *White bars*: Patients treated with conservative therapy (left graph) or fibrinolytic therapy (right graph).

Establish an Acute MI Protocol Team

The first step in launching a primary PTCA program is to set up a multidisciplinary acute MI protocol team. The goal of this team is to develop the critical pathways and care plans needed to care for the patient with acute MI from the first prehospital contact all the way through to hospital discharge. These critical pathways and care plans, such as the examples included in this chapter, need to be individualized to fit the circumstances of the hospital, which requires multidisciplinary input. The members of the acute MI protocol team should include physicians, nurses, and technical staff from the cardiology and emergency departments, the emergency medical technicians (EMT), the CCL, the critical care unit (CCU), the telemetry unit, cardiac rehabilitation, the blood laboratory, and case management, along with key members of the hospital administration. The initial commitment of resources to establish an on-call system (if not already in place), to recruit sufficient well-trained CCL personnel, and to fund

the initial stocking of the CCL with interventional equipment requires the full support of an informed hospital administration, who may need to be educated regarding the clinical value of such a program.

Develop a Critical Pathway

The acute MI protocol team should review the current literature and standards on the care of the patient with acute MI and adapt these latest research results to their development of the central critical pathway for primary PTCA. The team should incorporate newer modalities, techniques, and adjunctive medical therapies into this pathway as current standard of care evolves. In addition, the team should review the latest outcomes of the institution in any available databases, such as the National Registry of Myocardial Infarction (NRMI), the Health Care Financing Administration (HCFA) quality indicators, and the results from patient

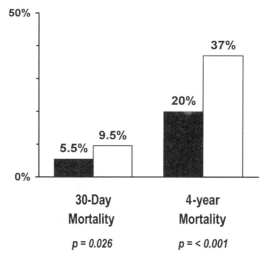

FIG. 9-2. Comparison of the outcomes of patients with non–ST-elevation acute myocardial infarction treated at hospitals that favored an early invasive treatment strategy versus a conservative treatment strategy in the Myocardial Infarction Intervention and Triage (MITI) Registry (15). Significant reductions were seen in both 30-day and 4-year mortality rates for hospitals favoring an early invasive treatment strategy. *Black bars*: Patients with non–ST-elevation acute MI treated at hospitals that favored an early invasive treatment strategy (n = 308). *White bars*: Patients with non–ST-elevation acute MI treated at hospitals that favored a conservative treatment strategy (n = 1,327).

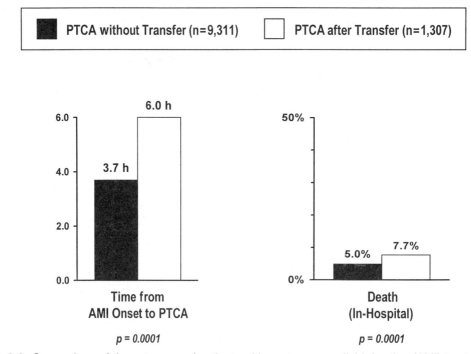

FIG. 9-3. Comparison of the outcomes of patients with acute myocardial infarction (AMI) treated with primary percutaneous transluminal coronary angioplasty (PTCA) at the point of first presentation versus those having primary PTCA after transfer in the Second National Registry of Myocardial Infarction (NRMI-2) (16). Patients transferred for PTCA who underwent the procedure significantly later than patients receiving PTCA at the point of first presentation had a significantly higher mortality rate. *Black bars*: Patients treated with primary PTCA without transfer (n = 9,311). *White bars*: Patients treated with primary PTCA after transfer (n = 1,307).

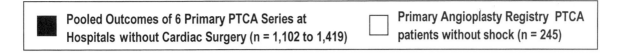

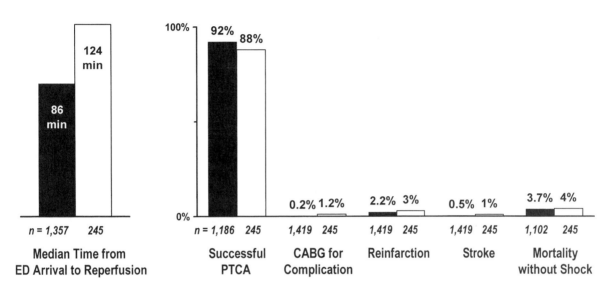

FIG. 9-4. Comparison of the pooled outcomes of patients reported in six studies of primary percutaneous transluminal coronary angioplasty (PTCA) at community hospitals without cardiac surgery (18,21–27) versus 245 patients in the Primary Angioplasty Registry (PAR) of five high-volume cardiac surgery centers (28). The reperfusion times and the rates of PTCA success, coronary artery bypass graft (CABG) surgery for procedural complication, reinfarction, stroke, and mortality were very similar in the nonsurgical community hospitals and the tertiary centers. The number of patients in the community hospital outcomes groups varied from 1,102 to 1,419 because not all studies reported all outcomes. Mortality is shown for patients without cardiogenic shock to allow comparison to the PAR, which excluded patients in shock. (See text for further elaboration.) *Black bars*: Patients treated with primary PTCA in the six studies at community hospitals without cardiac surgery (n = 1,102 to 1,419). *White bars*: Patients without cardiogenic shock treated with primary PTCA in the PAR registry (n = 245).

satisfaction surveys, with a focus on improving the hospital's acute MI care and initiating quality improvement processes. Place special emphasis on examining and improving the hospital's compliance with currently established standards of care, including the percentage of patients (a) offered reperfusion therapy, (b) given medications (e.g., aspirin, beta-blockers, ACE inhibitors, lipid-lowering agents), and (c) offered antismoking advice, cardiac teaching, and rehabilitation. Revise nursing and educational care plans to mirror these objectives. Provide educational sessions for hospital staff to review the pathways and understand the new expectations, procedures, and equipment involved in the development of the PTCA program.

Exeter Hospital's critical pathway for primary PTCA is shown in Fig. 9-5. Key features of Exeter's pathways and care maps include protocols for the emergency medical services (EMS) paramedics in the field and the ED physicians to follow that will optimize treatment and reduce time-to-reperfusion.

The ED physician is empowered to call the interventional cardiologist and CCL team, even before the patient arrives, if the electrocardiogram (ECG) shows diagnostic ST-segment elevation. In the (hopefully infrequent) event that the CCL or interventionalist is not available, the ED will be notified proactively. The ED physician will then be able to administer fibrinolytics promptly to eligible patients, and discuss transfer to another interventional hospital for patients at high risk or ineligible for lytic therapy. The decision regarding which patients with acute MI should be transferred to an interventional center should be individualized and made in conjunction with the cardiologist. In general, because early reperfusion saves lives and saves myocardium, most lytic-ineligible patients with high-risk features, especially cardiogenic shock, should be quickly transferred if the CCL is not available. In addition, because more than 40% of patients treated with fibrinolytics do not achieve brisk [thrombolysis in myocardial infarction (TIMI) grade 3] flow (40), most patients at high risk and eligible for lytic therapy should be transferred after lytic therapy is started, before waiting to determine whether this therapy is going to be effective. For patients in cardiogenic shock, an intraaortic balloon pump (IABP) should be inserted before transfer.

The cardiac catheterization procedure itself is streamlined to assess the coronary anatomy early while attending to the

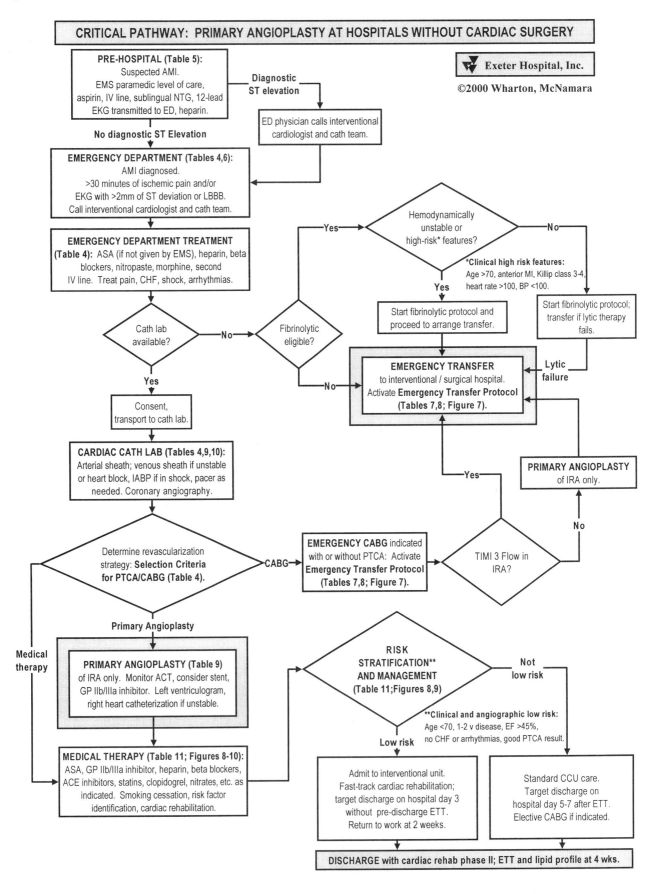

CRITICAL PATHWAY: PRIMARY ANGIOPLASTY AT HOSPITALS WITHOUT CARDIAC SURGERY

PRE-HOSPITAL (Table 5):
Suspected AMI.
EMS paramedic level of care, aspirin, IV line, sublingual NTG, 12-lead EKG transmitted to ED, heparin.

▼ **Exeter Hospital, Inc.**

©2000 Wharton, McNamara

Diagnostic ST elevation

ED physician calls interventional cardiologist and cath team.

No diagnostic ST Elevation

EMERGENCY DEPARTMENT (Tables 4,6):
AMI diagnosed.
>30 minutes of ischemic pain and/or EKG with >2mm of ST deviation or LBBB.
Call interventional cardiologist and cath team.

EMERGENCY DEPARTMENT TREATMENT (Table 4): ASA (if not given by EMS), heparin, beta blockers, nitropaste, morphine, second IV line. Treat pain, CHF, shock, arrhythmias.

Hemodynamically unstable or high-risk* features?

Yes — No

*Clinical high risk features:
Age >70, anterior MI, Killip class 3-4, heart rate >100, BP <100.

Yes

Start fibrinolytic protocol and proceed to arrange transfer.

Start fibrinolytic protocol; transfer if lytic therapy fails.

Cath lab available? — No — Fibrinolytic eligible?

EMERGENCY TRANSFER
to interventional / surgical hospital.
Activate **Emergency Transfer Protocol (Tables 7,8; Figure 7).**

Lytic failure

No

Yes

Consent, transport to cath lab.

CARDIAC CATH LAB (Tables 4,9,10):
Arterial sheath; venous sheath if unstable or heart block, IABP if in shock, pacer as needed. Coronary angiography.

PRIMARY ANGIOPLASTY
of IRA only.

No

Yes

Determine revascularization strategy: **Selection Criteria for PTCA/CABG (Table 4).** — CABG — **EMERGENCY CABG** indicated with or without PTCA: Activate **Emergency Transfer Protocol (Tables 7,8; Figure 7).**

TIMI 3 Flow in IRA?

Primary Angioplasty

Medical therapy

PRIMARY ANGIOPLASTY (Table 9)
of IRA only. Monitor ACT, consider stent, GP IIb/IIIa inhibitor. Left ventriculogram, right heart catheterization if unstable.

RISK STRATIFICATION** AND MANAGEMENT (Table 11; Figures 8,9)

Not low risk

**Clinical and angiographic low risk:
Age <70, 1-2 v disease, EF >45%, no CHF or arrhythmias, good PTCA result.

Low risk

MEDICAL THERAPY (Table 11; Figures 8-10):
ASA, GP IIb/IIIa inhibitor, heparin, beta blockers, ACE inhibitors, statins, clopidogrel, nitrates, etc. as indicated. Smoking cessation, risk factor identification, cardiac rehabilitation.

Admit to interventional unit. Fast-track cardiac rehabilitation; target discharge on hospital day 3 without pre-discharge ETT. Return to work at 2 weeks.

Standard CCU care. Target discharge on hospital day 5-7 after ETT. Elective CABG if indicated.

DISCHARGE with cardiac rehab phase II; ETT and lipid profile at 4 wks.

TABLE 9-2. *Operator, institutional, and angiographic criteria for primary PTCA programs at hospitals without on-site cardiac surgery*

1. The operators must be experienced interventionalists who regularly perform elective intervention.
2. The nursing and technical CCL staff must be experienced in handling acutely ill patients and comfortable with interventional equipment. They must have acquired experience in dedicated interventional laboratories. They participate in a 24-hour, 7-day per week call schedule.
3. The CCL itself must be well equipped, with optimal imaging systems, resuscitative equipment, and IABP support; it must be well stocked with a broad array of interventional equipment.
4. The CCU nurses must be adept in the management of acutely ill cardiac patients, including invasive hemodynamic monitoring and IABP management.
5. The hospital administration must fully support the program and enable the fulfillment of the above institutional requirements.
6. Formalized written protocols must be in place for immediate and efficient transfer of patients to the nearest cardiac surgical facility.
7. Primary PTCA must be performed routinely as the treatment of choice around the clock for a large proportion of patients with AMI, to ensure streamlined care paths and increased case volumes.
8. Clinical and angiographic selection criteria for the performance of primary PTCA and for transfer for emergency CABG must be rigorous (Table 9-4).
9. An ongoing program of outcomes analysis and formalized periodic case review must exist.

AMI, acute myocardial infarction; CABG, coronary artery bypass graft; CCL, cardiac catheterization laboratory; CCU, cardiac care unit; IABP, intraaortic balloon pump; PTCA, percutaneous transluminal coronary angioplasty.
Adapted from Wharton TP Jr, McNamara NS, Fedele FA, et al. Primary angioplasty for the treatment of acute myocardial infarction: experience at two community hospitals without cardiac surgery. *J Am Coll Cardiol* 1999;33:1257–1265; with permission.

medical treatment of the patient. When primary PTCA is chosen as the reperfusion strategy, the goal of intervention is the early establishment of TIMI grade 3 flow.

After the procedure, the patient can be effectively risk-stratified and triaged to appropriate in-hospital management according to clinical and angiographic features as listed in Fig. 9-5 (3). Patients with low-risk clinical and angiographic features can avoid admission to the CCU, avoid predischarge exercise testing, be targeted for discharge on hospital day 3, and return to work within 2 weeks (3).

Develop Operator and Institutional Criteria

The acute MI protocol team should develop operator, institutional, and angiographic criteria such as those listed in Table 9-2 (25). The team should review local state regulations and national and international guidelines for primary PTCA in the treatment of acute MI (41,42). Invasive and noninvasive cardiologists, credentialing staff, and hospital administration should develop credentialing criteria based on national guidelines and regional standards. Fundamental to any interventional program is a state-of-the-art CCL, with

optimal digital imaging systems, equipped with a broad array of interventional and supportive equipment, and staffed by experienced nursing and technical personnel.

A commitment to provide primary PTCA on a 24-hour, 7-day per week basis will avoid inconsistency in following the critical pathway for primary PTCA and prevent a lower standard of care. A single care plan for the treatment of acute MI will minimize "door-to-decision" times, and increased procedural volumes will accelerate the learning curve for ED staff and CCL team members and operators. This will result in decreased times to reperfusion and improvement of procedural outcomes (43). A higher institutional volume of primary PTCA (but not necessarily elective PTCA) (44) correlates with improved mortality rates (43–45), as does a faster door-to-balloon time (43).

Define Position Profiles and Expectations for CCL Staff and Training Programs

Nursing, technical, and paramedic CCL staff must be experienced in handling acutely ill patients and comfortable with interventional equipment. All members of the CCL team will

FIG. 9-5. Critical pathway from prehospital contact through to hospital discharge for the primary angioplasty program at Exeter Hospital, Exeter, NH, which is a small (<100 bed) hospital 15 minutes from the nearest cardiac surgical facility. ACE, angiotensin converting enzyme; ACT, activated clotting time; AMI, acute myocardial infarction; ASA, aspirin; BP, blood pressure; CABG, coronary artery bypass graft; CCU, cardiac care unit; CHF, congestive heart failure; ED, emergency department; EF, ejection fraction; EKG, electrocardiogram; EMS, emergency medical services; ETT, exercise tolerance test; GP, glycoprotein; IABP, intraaortic balloon pump; IRA, infarct-related artery; IV, intravenous; LBBB, left bundle branch block; NTG, nitroglycerin; PTCA, percutaneous transluminal coronary angioplasty; TIMI, thrombolysis in myocardial infarction; v, vessel. (© 2000 Wharton, McNamara. Used with permission.)

TABLE 9-3. *CCL staffing for primary PTCA programs at hospitals without on-site cardiac surgery: personnel requirements for RN, RCIS, radiology technologist, and paramedic*

Requirements

1. Each member will have acquired or will be provided experience in dedicated interventional laboratories.[a]
2. Each member will have ACLS certification and complete i.v. certification, and be competent in cardiac rhythm monitoring and the operation of temporary pacemakers and defibrillators.
3. Each member will be able to monitor the patient's medical condition and administer intravenous medications, including vasoactive drips and conscious sedation, under the direction of the physician.
4. Each member will be able to serve as scrub assistant to the physician, including performing coronary artery injections, panning the table, and handling of interventional equipment.
5. Each member will be competent with the operation of invasive hemodynamic monitoring equipment and the interpretation of data obtained from it.
6. Each member will be competent with the setting up, operation, timing, and troubleshooting of the IABP.
7. Each member will be familiar with the operation of the digital imaging system, including troubleshooting, acquiring and archiving digital images or images on cine film, and preparing angiograms on CD.
8. Each member will be competent with the operation of in-laboratory blood testing equipment including oximeters, ACT measurement devices, and platelet function testing.
9. Each member will reside within 30 minutes of the hospital. Beepers and cell phones will be provided.
10. Each member will participate in a 24-hour, 7-day per week call schedule.
11. Each member will be expected to communicate effectively with families, nursing units, and tertiary referral centers, and to initiate the transfer protocol when needed.
12. Each member will be available to accompany patients requiring transfer to cardiac surgery when the CCTT team is incomplete or unavailable, including serving as the IABP operator.
13. Each member will be expected to continue education to maintain the skills needed in the laboratory. Each member will be given educational opportunities to learn the latest medical and technical modalities for the treatments of the cardiovascular patient.
14. Each member will be familiar with the institution's guidelines and credentialing criteria for invasive and interventional procedures.
15. Each member will participate in reporting of clinical indicators and in quality improvement projects.

ACLS, advanced cardiac life support; ACT, activated clotting time; CCTT, critical care transportation team; CCL, cardiac catheterization laboratory; CD, compact disc; IABP, intraaortic ballon pump; i.v., intravenous; PTCA, percutaneous transluminal coronary angioplasty; RCIS, registered cardiac interventional specialist; RN, registered nurse.

[a]CCL team members not already experienced in interventional procedures should be sent on rotation and by formal arrangement to the referral surgical hospital for observation and "hands-on" experience in a busy interventional laboratory.

Developed by Wharton TP, McNamara NS, Hiett D, CCL staff, and Human Resources Department, Exeter Hospital, Exeter, NH. ©1993 Wharton, McNamara, Exeter Hospital; with permission.

have acquired or will be provided experience in dedicated interventional laboratories. CCL team members not already experienced in interventional procedures should be sent on rotation and by formal arrangement to the referral surgical hospital for observation and "hands-on" experience in a busy interventional laboratory. For maximal flexibility with a small CCL staff, all personnel should be cross trained in all of the CCL skills and responsibilities. Individuals will have their own areas of expertise, and can serve as mentors to others with other skills (Table 9-3).

All members of the team should work toward this goal. Ultimately, every team member should be able to operate diagnostic imaging equipment, hemodynamic monitoring and recording equipment, temporary pacemakers, defibrillators, and the IABP; serve as scrub assistant to the physician performing the procedure; assist in medical monitoring and management of the patient, including administering medications,

providing written documentation of the procedure, and interfacing with families, nursing units, and tertiary referral centers.

Hospital administration, interventional cardiologists, and the CCL staff must invest in and commit fully to providing the resources necessary to launch and maintain effective, state-of-the-art, 24-hour 7-day per week primary PTCA coverage. The delay and staffing limitations for off-hour procedures at community hospitals need not worsen PTCA success rates, complications, or major in-hospital clinical outcomes (46,47).

Intensive Staffing on a Shoestring Budget?

Community hospitals, with only two or three members of a CCL staff of five to six on call, will find it critical to deploy ED and CCU nurses and respiratory therapists to help

TABLE 9-4. *Clinical and angiographic selection criteria for primary PTCA and emergency bypass surgery*

Inclusion criteria
– >30 min of ischemic pain not controlled by conventional medications (ASA, NTG, beta-blockers, and heparin)

and/or
–ECG with ≥2.0 mV of ischemic ST-segment deviation in two or more contiguous leads
–No time limit if patient has ongoing chest pain, ST-segment deviation with preserved R waves in two or more infarct leads, or cardiogenic shock

Clinical exclusion criteria
–Lack of vascular access
–Inability to obtain informed consent
–Dementia or coma (excepting patients with successful cardioversion of out-of-hospital ventricular fibrillation in the field, regardless of acute mental status
–Any serious illness with life expectancy of only a few weeks

Angiographic exclusion criteria (28,48)
–Avoid intervention in hemodynamically stable patients with
  —Significant (≥60%) stenosis of an unprotected LM artery upstream from a culprit lesion in the left coronary system that might be disrupted by the PTCA catheter
  —Extremely long or angulated culprit lesions with TIMI grade 3 flow
  —Culprit lesions with TIMI grade 3 flow in stable patients with three-vessel disease who are suitable candidates for CABG
  —Infarct-related lesions of small or secondary vessels
  —Lesions in areas other than the IRA

Transfer for emergency bypass surgery (Table 9-7)
–Patients with high-grade residual LM or MV CAD and clinical or hemodyamic instability
  —After PTCA of occluded vessels, as appropriate
  —Preferably with intraaortic balloon pump support

ASA, aspirin; CABG, coronary artery bypass graft; CAD, coronary artery disease; ECG, electrocardiogram; IRA, infarct-related artery; LM, left main; MV, multivessel; NTG, nitroglycerin; PTCA, percutaneous transluminal coronary angioplasty; TIMI, thrombolysis in myocardial infarction.
From Wharton TP Jr, McNamara NS, Fedele FA, et al. Primary angioplasty for the treatment of acute myocardial infarction: experience at two community hospitals without cardiac surgery. *J Am Coll Cardiol* 1999;33:1257–1265.
Developed by Wharton TP, Exeter Hospital, Exeter, NH.

at off hours in unstable patients. These highly skilled patient care providers can contribute to the management of medications and drips, assist with documentation during the CCL procedure, assist with airways, and ventilator management and general patient care. Enlisting the participation of these non-CCL personnel improves continuity of care and is cost-effective: these same nurses and therapists would have been involved with the care of these patient whether or not the patient was in the CCL. Hospital staff members interested in helping the CCL team in these off-hours cases should be encouraged to watch patients and given the opportunity for CCL training.

In regions where it is difficult to recruit trained CCL personnel, other interested hospital staff members should be actively recruited and encouraged to join a 6-month CCL training program to ensure viability of the team.

Establish Clinical and Angiographic Selection Criteria for Primary PTCA and Emergency Transfer for CABG

Cardiologists should develop criteria for primary PTCA and emergency bypass surgery such as those listed in Table 9-4;

these criteria should be documented in the patient care standards manual. We recommend immediate coronary angiography in all patients who present with a clinical picture of acute MI, even if ECG changes are not diagnostic, if they have ongoing ischemic pain for more than 30 minutes not controlled by conventional medications. Patients with acute MI without ST-segment elevation on ECG represent a particularly high-risk group and are not appropriate for fibrinolytic therapy (11). These patients have greatly improved outcomes with PTCA compared with conservative therapy (15). Further, because the progression rate of necrosis in acute MI varies considerably with the degree of baseline antegrade flow and collateral flow, and the time of transition between unstable angina and acute MI is sometimes hard to identify, we suggest that there be no time cutoff for reperfusion therapy if symptoms or signs of ongoing myocardial necrosis or cardiogenic shock are present. The clinical and angiographic criteria for PTCA are based on standards in the literature (28,48). The goal of criteria for both angiography and transfer to a surgical institution is to maximize coronary reperfusion opportunities while minimizing the possibility of causing new myocardial jeopardy (a "surgical

TABLE 9-5. *Prehospital protocol for AMI[a]*

---

911 is activated for suspected AMI: *Local response to include activation of **paramedic** level of EMT care[b]*
—Administer O$_2$
—Complete brief history and physical examination, record vital signs
—*Administer four "baby" **ASA** (total 325 mg) chewed*
—Establish i.v.
—**NTG** SL if SBP > 100 mmHg and patient not in shock.
—Report history, physical examination findings, vital signs to ED physician
—*12-lead ECG immediately acquired and transmitted by cell phone to ED physician (49,50)[c]*
—If AMI is confirmed: administer heparin (5,000 U) i.v. bolus
—**ACLS** protocols per routine. No prophylactic lidocaine.
—**Fluids, atropine** for bradycardia with hypotension
—**Morphine** (2–4 mg) i.v. for uncontrolled chest pain
—Avoid intubation by nasal route: this greatly increases the risk of bleeding if GP IIb/IIIa platelet inhibitors or fibrinolytics are used.
—*Document all clinical data including ST-segment elevation, time of pain onset, patient's physical appearance and vital signs on arrival, and interventions in the field.*
—*While patient with ST-segment elevation is en route, paramedic verifies with ED physician that interventionalist and CCL team are available. ED physician calls cardiologist and CCL team and initiates discussion of the use of primary PTCA for AMI on ED arrival.[d]*

ACLS, advanced cardiac life support; AMI, acute myocardial infarction; ASA, aspirin; CCL, cardiac catheterization laboratory; ED, emergency department; ECG, electrocardiogram; EMT, emergency medical technician; GP, glycoprotein; i.v., intravenous; NTG, nitroglycerin; PTCA, percutaneous transluminal coronary angioplasty; SBP, systolic blood pressure; SL, sublingual.

[a]Italics highlight measures that reduce time-to-reperfusion for primary PTCA.

[b]If no paramedic level of care is available in the community, consider establishing a hospital-based paramedic program.

[c]Ambulances should be equipped with ECG system capable of telephonic transmission to ED for all chest pain calls; this can greatly reduce time-to-diagnosis, time-to-reperfusion, and possibly mortality (49, 50). Patient with initial ST-segment elevation may arrive to ED pain free with a normal ECG, because 10% to 15% of AMIs reperfuse with aspirin and other conservative measures. Documenting ST-segment elevation at initial prehospital contact can influence immediate triage.

[d]One of the more correctable causes of delay in "door-to-balloon time" is the time that it takes to call the interventional cardiologist. Do not worry about "false alarms," which are rare.

Developed by Wharton TP, McNamara NS, Mastromarino J, and ED and EMT Committees, Exeter Hospital, Exeter, NH. ©1998 Wharton, McNamara, Exeter Hospital; with permission.

emergency") by procedures performed without on-site cardiac surgery.

Setting Up a Fine-Tuned Emergency Triage System in the Emergency Department

The ED is the command center for the acute MI (Fig. 9-6). Starting with a prehospital protocol for acute MI, such as that shown in Table 9-5, paramedics in the field administer aspirin and heparin, and transmit the ECG to the ED physician by cellular telephone. This prehospital ECG can greatly reduce time-to-diagnosis and, thus, time-to-reperfusion (49,50) effects that may even improve survival (50). Further, because some patients with initial ST-segment elevation arrive to the ED pain free with a normal ECG (10% to 15% of acute MIs reperfuse with aspirin and other conservative measures), documenting ST-segment elevation at initial prehospital contact can influence immediate triage.

The ED is notified of the incoming patient with acute MI and the acute MI critical pathway is initiated (Table 9-6). The ED physician contacts the predesignated interventional cardiologist on call immediately for patients with suspected acute MI and the unit coordinator pages the CCL team. These pages should go out simultaneously, even before the patient arrives, if diagnostic acute ST-segment elevation is present on ECG. One of the more correctable causes of delay in "door-to-balloon time" is the time that it takes to call the interventional cardiologist. The ED physician should call as soon as the clinical diagnosis is suggested, and should not worry about "false alarms," which are rare.

The ED will be notified proactively whenever the interventional cardiologist or CCL will not be available, to enable prompt administration of fibrinolytics and prompt consideration of transfer to an interventional center (see Fig. 9-5 and discussion above under "Develop a Primary PTCA Critical Pathway"). A suggested transfer protocol is shown in Table 9-7.

Treatment protocols for paramedics and ED staff facilitate urgent triage and treatment (Tables 9-5 and 9-6). The use of transdermal rather than intravenous (i.v.) nitroglycerin and the avoidance of a heparin drip after initial bolus are two measures that can simplify nursing care in the

TABLE 9-6. *Emergency department protocol for AMI[a]*

See **prehospital management protocol for AMI** (Table 9-5), which includes
–Paramedic level of care[b]
–Establish i.v., administer O_2
–**NTG** SBP > 100 mmHg and patient not in shock
–**ASA** (325 mg) chewed
–12-lead ECG while en route; transmit to ED[c]
ED physician should page cardiologist and CCL team simultaneously—even before patient arrives—if diagnostic acute ST-segment elevation is present on ECG, even if transmitted from field (49, 50)[d]
In ED
–*Rapid assessment, rapid call to CCL team/cardiologist for all patients with clinical impression of AMI who meet clinical selection criteria (Table 9-4)[d]*
–**ASA** (325 mg) chewed if not given during prehospital management
  Give ASA rectally if intubated
–**NTG** SL/**nitropaste** for ongoing pain or hypertension
  Omit i.v. NTG for simplification; avoid routine multiple doses of NTG.
  (Hypotension is all too common in this scenario.)
–**Heparin** (70–100 U/kg) bolus without continuous infusion. (This much is usually
  required to raise activated clotting time to mid-200s as needed for stenting.)
  Avoid heparin drip for simplification; ACT will be titrated with further heparin in CCL.
–**Clopidogrel** (300 mg) po here or after intervention, at operator discretion
–Establish second i.v.
–**Metoprolol** (5 mg) i.v. q5 min x 3 unless pulse <55, BP <100, or wheezing
–**Morphine** or **fentanyl** p.r.n. pain; may cause nausea (less so for fentanyl)
–**Prochlorperazine** and **atropine** p.r.n.
–**ACLS** protocols per routine. No prophylactic lidocaine.
–**Fluids, atropine** for bradycardia with hypotension; phenylephrine (pure alpha agonist)
  for refractory hypotension
–**GP IIb/IIIa platelet inhibitors** in ED only on advice of cardiologist, and generally only
  if there is a delay in getting to the CCL
–Consider **fibrinolytics** in cases of a delay of over 45 min in transferring the
  patient to the CCL.
–Avoid intubation by nasal route: this greatly increases the risk of bleeding if GP IIb/IIIa
  agents or fibrinolytics are used.
–Document all clinical data and therapy on Emergency Chest Pain Assessment Record
  (Fig. 9-6).

ACLS, advanced cardiac life support; ACT, activated clotting time; AMI, acute myocardial infarction; ASA, aspirin; CCL, cardiac catheterization laboratory; ECG, electrocardiogram; ED, emergency department; GP, glycoprotein; i.v., intravenous; NTG, nitroglycerin; po, by mouth; p.r.n., as needed; PTCA, percutaneous transluminal coronary angioplasty; SBP, systolic blood pressure; SL, sublingual.
[a]Italics highlight measures that reduce time-to-reperfusion for primary PTCA.
[b]If no paramedic level of care is available in the community, consider establishing a hospital-based paramedic program.
[c]Ambulances should be equipped with ECG system capable of telephonic transmission to ED for all chest pain calls; this can greatly reduce time-to-diagnosis, time-to-reperfusion, and possibly mortality (49,50). Patient with initial ST-segment elevation may arrive to ED pain free with a normal ECG, because 10% to 15% of AMIs reperfuse with aspirin and other conservative measures. Documenting ST-segment elevation at initial contact can influence immediate triage.
[d]One of the more correctable causes of delay in "door-to-balloon time" is the time that it takes to call the interventional cardiologist. Do not worry about "false alarms," which are rare.
Developed by Wharton JP, McNamara NS, ED physicians, and EMT and ED Committees, Exeter Hospital, Exeter, NH. ©1996 Wharton, McNamara, Exeter Hospital, with permission.

ED. Creation of an emergency chest pain assessment record (Fig. 9-6) provides an efficient method of documentation for the permanent medical record, avoids duplication of documentation, and decreases questions asked by the CCL staff. This assessment record provides the ED staff and CCL with clinical information, a list of medications given in the ED, and test results, along with documentation of event times. All these data will be useful in outcomes analysis and ongoing cardiology registries and studies.

The ED nursing staff should create a list of all supplies that are likely to be needed in the initial ED treatment of patients with acute MI and organize a portable "AMI box" to contain all of these medications, i.v. equipment and tubing, and other essentials. This should include all documentation

78

Exeter Hospital, Inc.

10 Buzell Avenue
Exeter, NH 03833
603-778-7311

**EMERGENCY CHEST PAIN
ASSESSMENT RECORD**

PAGE 1of 2

RM _____

NAME	D.O.B.

STATUS ☐ I - EMERGENT ☐ II - URGENT

SELF/ EMS TREATMENT ☐ NONE

	ASSESSMENT TIME	ED PHYSICIAN TIME	CARDIOLOGIST TIME

ARRIVED VIA ☐ AMBULANCE ☐ PRIVATE VEHICLE

IMMUNIZATIONS CHILDHOOD ☐ CURRENT ☐ NA
TETANUS ☐ < 5 YR ☐ > 5 YR ☐ _____

HISTORY OF PRESENT ILLNESS/DURATION OF SYMPTOMS

ALLERGIES/REACTIONS
☐ NKA ☐ LATEX ☐ FOODS:
☐ MEDS:

CURRENT MEDICATIONS

DAILY ASA ☐ NO ☐ YES TAKEN TODAY: ☐ NO ☐ YES

MEDICAL HISTORY: ☐ DENIES

☐ RECENT GI BLEED ☐ CAD ☐ CHF ☐ MI ☐ ANGINA ☐ HTN ☐ DM ☐ STROKE

☐ CABG X _____ ☐ OTHER _____

SMOKER ☐ NO ☐ YES _____ YRS _____ PPD

FAMILY HISTORY: ☐ DENIES ☐ CAD ☐ DM
☐ OTHER _____

PAIN HISTORY TIME OF PAIN ONSET: _____

PAIN AT ONSET: 0 1 2 3 4 5 6 7 8 9 10 PAIN ON ARRIVAL: 0 1 2 3 4 5 6 7 8 9 10

DESCRIPTION OF PAIN: _____ ☐ CONSTANT ☐ INTERMITTENT

RADIATION: ☐ NO ☐ YES TO: _____ CHANGES WITH ☐ DEEP BREATH ☐ MOVEMENT ☐ NONE

ASSOCIATED SYMPTOMS: _____ LAST MEAL: _____

TEMP. ☐ T.M. ☐ P.O. ☐ P.R.	PULSE	RESP	BP L R	STATED WEIGHT	O2 SAT _____ % _____ L / MIN

SKIN TEMP ☐ WARM & DRY ☐ _____

COLOR ☐ WNL ☐ _____

MENTAL STATUS
☐ ALERT & ORIENTED ☐ _____

CARDIOVASCULAR
MONITOR RHYTHM _____

PULSES: RADIAL ☐ L ☐ R FEMORAL ☐ L ☐ R

COMMUNICABLE DISEASE ☐ NO KNOWN RISK
☐ AT RISK (reason) _____

Sx: ANOREXIA, FEVER, PERSISTENT COUGH, BLOODY SPUTUM, WEIGHT LOSS, OR NIGHT SWEATS

* ANY ONE RESP. Sx WITH ANY ONE SYSTEMATIC Sx RAISES CONCERN FOR TB. CONSIDER AIRBORNE PRECAUTIONS. NOTIFY MD AND IC.

PSYCHO-SOCIAL/LIVING STATUS: SUPPORT AVAILABLE ☐ YES ☐ NO ☐ N/A
☐ STRESSORS/DOMESTIC ISSUES
☐ SOCIAL SERVICE CONSULT _____

FUNCTIONAL BARRIERS/LEARNING NEEDS
☐ LEARNING NEEDS ASSESSED & ADDRESSED
☐ WNL ☐ SPECIAL NEEDS _____

LUNG ASSESSMENT
☐ CLEAR ☐ _____

ABDOMINAL ASSESSMENT
☐ WNL ☐ _____

PATIENT INVOLVED IN RESEARCH PROTOCOLS ☐ NO ☐ YES
RESEARCH: _____

RN SIGNATURE TIME

FIG. 9-6. Emergency chest pain assessment record developed at Exeter Hospital, Exeter, NH in 1996. A form such as this provides a more efficient method of documentation for the permanent medical record, avoids duplication of documentation, and decreases questions asked by the cardiac catheterization laboratory staff. This assessment record provides the emergency department (ED) staff and catheterization laboratory staff with clinical information, a list of medications given in the ED, and test results, along with documentation of event times. All these data will be useful in outcomes analysis and ongoing cardiology registries and studies. (©1996 Exeter Hospital. Used with permission.)

EMERGENCY CHEST PAIN ASSESSMENT RECORD
PAGE 2 of 2

TIME	IV/PO IN	ABSORB	TIME	OUTPUT	TOTAL
TOTAL INTAKE			TOTAL OUTPUT		

MEDICATION	DOSE	ROUTE	TIME	INTIALS	MEDICATION	DOSE	ROUTE	TIME	INTIALS
ASPIRIN	4 BABY	PO			MORPHINE		IVP		
NITRO	1/	SL			MORPHINE		IVP		
NITRO	1/	SL			MORPHINE		IVP		
NITRO	1/	SL			PLAVIX	300 MG	PO		
NITRO PASTE		DERMAL			IIb IIIa INHIBITOR:				
NITRO DRIP		IVPB					IVPB		
HEP BOLUS	U	IVP			LYTIC BOLUS:				
HEP DRIP	U/HR	IVPB					IVP		
LOPRESSOR		IVP			LYTIC INFUSION:				
LOPRESSOR		IVP					IVPB		
LOPRESSOR		IVP			LOVENOX	1 MG/KG	SC		

ADDITIONAL ORDERS: ☐ PORTABLE CXR ☐ CBC, CP7WB, PT/PTT, CARDED, CARDPT ☐ IF ADMITTED DO LOW DENSITY LIPID PROFILE.

IF PATIENT IS GOING TO THE CATH LAB - PLACE 2 IV"S #1 _____ SITE #2 _____ SITE

SIGNATURE _____ RN SIGNATURE _____ MD TIME _____

CONTINUED NURSING ASSESSMENT
_____
_____
_____
_____
_____
_____
_____
_____
_____
_____
_____
_____
_____
_____

DISCHARGE ☐ PATIENT / GUARDIAN UNDERSTANDS / ACCEPTS PLAN OF CARE
DISPOSITION ☐ HOME ☐ ADMIT TO _____ ☐ EXPIRED ☐ OTHER:_____
CONDITION ☐ STABLE ☐ SERIOUS ☐ _____
VALUABLES ☐ HOME ☐ WITH PATIENT: _____ ☐ VALUABLE RECEIPT# _____

R.N. SIGNATURE _____ TIME _____

FIG. 9-6. Continued.

TABLE 9-7. *Emergency transfer protocol to cardiac surgery center*

CCL circulator initiates rapid transfer protocol on physician decision for immediate transfer, and places the following calls on pages simultaneously:
–Call to cardiac surgeon at receiving cardiac surgery center
–Call to cardiac surgery clinical coordinator at receiving center
–Call ED to activate CCTT[a] and EMS ambulance provider[b]

Cardiologist provides clinical information to cardiac surgeon and obtains agreement to accept patient.
Cardiologist obtains consent from patient or family member for immediate transfer to cardiac surgery center.

In CCL
–Rapid mobilization is initiated (all hands on deck!). Help will be needed from unit coordinator, nursing supervisor, and social worker.
–Sheaths and balloon pumps are sewn in place; i.v.s, pressure lines, and infusion pumps are organized; patient is placed on stretcher.
–Report to CCTT to review patient status. Physician confirms the level of care required for the patient in collaboration with the CCTT: RN and/or paramedic level.
–CCL RN accompanies patient with multiple drips if CCTT RN is unavailable.
–CCL laboratory staff member or unit coordinator assembles necessary transfer information: copy of chart, cine films or CD of angiogram, copy of chest x-ray film, CCL log of procedure, and handwritten catheterization report.
–Nursing report is given to receiving cardiac center, including status of patient, lists of i.v. drips and doses, equipment, and treatments. Admission status is reconfirmed, ETA given, and destination unit in receiving hospital is provided.
–Cardiologists completes Patient Transfer Orders Out of Facility (Fig. 9-8) and Medicare Inter-Facility Patient Transfer form (CC. 204).
–Family is provided with directions to receiving facility and names of contact persons there.
–For medical problems during transfer, the interventionalist or ED physician at the sending institution should be contacted by cell phone from the ambulance unless other formal arrangements are made.
–Five minutes before arrival at cardiac center, CCTT notifies center of ETA and center confirms in-hospital destination: ED, OR, CCU, or CCL.
–Patient is transferred to designated unit.
–Written documentation of all clinical data during transport recorded.

ACLS, advanced cardiac life support; CCL, cardiac catheterization laboratory; CCTT, cardiac care transport team: CCU, cardiac care unit; CD, compact disc; ECG, electrocardiogram; ED, emergency department; EMS, emergency medical services; ETA, estimated time of arrival; IABP, intraaortic balloon pump; i.v., intravenous; OR, operating room; RN, registered nurse.
[a]A hospital-based CCTT, consisting of critical care nurses, paramedics, and CCL personnel, all with IABP expertise, should be established.
[b]EMS ambulance provider must have available and/or be able to accommodate the following: portable cardiac ECG and pressure monitoring, sufficient O_2 supply, suction, multiple drips, ACLS drugs, resuscitation equipment, defibrillator, and IABP.
Developed by Wharton JP, McNamara NS, CCTT, ED, and CCL staff, Exeter Hospital, Exeter, NH. ©1997 Wharton, McNamara, Exeter Hospital; with permission.

tools (Fig. 9-6) to prevent loss or duplication of information and save valuable time. Use of this AMI box will prevent unnecessary distraction in searching for supplies while caring for the acutely ill aute MI patient in the ED.

Conduct Educational Sessions with the EMTs and ED Staff

Explain the acute MI critical pathway, protocols, standing orders, and emergency chest pain assessment record. Reinforce the goal of the critical pathway to improve time to reperfusion to enhance outcomes in patients with acute MI, emphasizing that coronary artery occlusion is causing progressive death of heart muscle: "Time is myocardium."

Schedule periodic ED meetings and CCL conferences to examine current topics in acute MI care and to evaluate cases. Welcome comments, allow time for problem solving and suggestions from ED staff, EMTs, CCL staff, and ED physicians, and involve them in quality improvement processes.

Create an Emergency Transfer Protocol and Establish Formal Agreements

To ensure rapid transfer to a cardiac surgery center, emergency transfer protocols and formal agreements need to be established (Tables 9-7 and 9-8; Fig. 9-7). Approximately 3% to 5% of patients undergoing immediate coronary angiography will need to be transferred for emergency CABG surgery,

TABLE 9-8. *Elements of a cardiac transfer agreement for primary PTCA programs at hospitals without on-site cardiac surgery: a proven plan for rapid access to cardiac surgery*

1. The cardiologist must have developed a good working relationship with the cardiac surgeons at the receiving facility.
2. The cardiac surgeons from the referral cardiac surgery hospital must formally agree to provide cardiac surgery back-up for urgent and emergent cases at all hours.
3. The cardiologist must review with the surgeon the potential needs and risks of the patient being transferred for emergency care.
4. The surgeon will assure that the patient will be accepted for services based on factors such as the patient's medical condition, the capacity of surgeons to provide services at the time of request, and the availability of facility and staff resources.
5. The referring facility must have an established protocol (Table 9-7) for safe and rapid transfer of patients to the receiving cardiac surgery hospital.
6. An EMS ambulance supplier and a CCTT must be formally contracted to be available on site within 20 minutes of a call on a 24-hour, 7-day per week basis.
7. The CCTT should include critical care nurses, paramedics, and CCL personnel, all with IABP expertise.
8. EMS ambulance provider must have available and/or be able to accommodate the following: portable cardiac ECG and pressure monitoring, sufficient O_2 supply, suction, multiple drips, ACLS drugs, resuscitation equipment, defibrillator, and IABP.
9. Transferring physician will obtain consent from patient or representative.
10. Review of transferred patients must be ongoing, and include feedback from referring facility regarding problems in transfer process, teaching opportunities through catheterization conferences, periodic review of the outcomes of the surgical program with special emphasis on the outcomes of transferred patients.
11. Cardiac surgeon credentialed to visit patients and families at referring hospital to review options of intervention if time allows.
12. Hospital administrations from both referring and accepting facilities must endorse the transfer agreement.

ACLS, advanced cardiac life support; CCL, cardiac catheterization laboratory; CCTT, cardiac care transport team; ECG, electrocardiogram; EMS, emergency medical services; IABP, intraaortic balloon pump; PTCA, percutaneous transluminal coronary angioplasty.

Developed by Wharton JP, McNamara NS, Hiett D, and Cresta D, Exeter Hospital, Exeter, NH.
©1993 Exeter Hospital; with permission.

almost always because of critical anatomy discovered by the angiogram rather than because of procedural mishap (18, 21–26). Formal transfer agreements and protocols must be in place for the expeditious transfer of these patients (Tables 9-7 and 9-8; Fig. 9-7), or for the patient at high-risk or ineligible for lytic therapy when the CCL is not available, or for the rare event of a CCL complication (e.g., abrupt vessel closure or coronary perforation). The goal of these emergency transfer protocols is to ensure the fastest possible response once the decision is made to transfer the patient, whether from the ED or the CCL.

The institution should establish a hospital-based critical care transport team (CCTT), consisting of critical care nurses, paramedics, and CCL personnel, all with IABP expertise. The EMS ambulance provider must have available or be able to accommodate the following: portable cardiac ECG and pressure monitoring, sufficient O_2 supply, suction, multiple drips, advanced cardiac life support (ACLS) drugs, resuscitation equipment, defibrillator, and IABP.

Cardiologists and the hospital administration must work with referral hospitals, especially their cardiac surgeons, to develop an atmosphere of collaboration and trust to ensure a seamless transition of care from the community hospital to the surgical center. The cardiac surgeon should be invited to attend cardiac catheterization conferences at the community hospital and it is hoped that surgeon will be credentialed there. This will enable the surgeon to consult on less emergent inpatients and review treatment options with patients and families to help them make decisions on therapy before transfer. An important element of this relationship includes feedback from the surgical center to the community hospital physicians on surgical outcomes and clinical follow-up.

Develop a Catheterization Laboratory Primary PTCA Protocol and an Acuity-Based Procedure-Bumping Protocol

The protocol in the CCL, such as that suggested in Table 9-9, should be directed toward rapid assessment of the coronary anatomy and rapid triage to the most appropriate therapy: primary PTCA, medical therapy, or transfer for CABG surgery (Table 9-4). Simultaneous to this must be intensive attention to the medical treatment of the patient. When primary PTCA is chosen as the reperfusion strategy, the goal of intervention is the early establishment of TIMI grade 3 flow while reducing to an absolute minimum the chance that new myocardial jeopardy could be created by the procedure itself.

Community hospitals with only one CCL are often busy with elective interventions scheduled throughout the day.

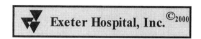

PHYSICIAN ORDERS
Patient Transfer Orders Out of Facility

Allergies (Allergen and Reaction)	Weight

Date/Time	PATIENT TRANSFER ORDERS OUT OF FACILITY
	1. Transfer to: Receiving unit: Receiving physician:
	2. Staff required: ☐ EMT-I (IV Only) ☐ Paramedic or Nurse ☐ Paramedic and Nurse ☐ IABP Team
	3. Cardiac monitor.
	4. ACLS protocols.
	5. Pulse oximetry prn. Titrate O_2 to keep saturation $\geq$ 92%.
	6. Vital signs q 15 minutes.
	7. Maintain current drips, fluids, O_2, ventilator settings.
	8. Medications: NTG 1/150 gr sl q 5 min x3 prn chest pain Prochlorperazine _____ mg IV q _____ prn nausea, vomiting Morphine _____ mg IV q _____ prn pain, anxiety
	9. Other:

Physician Signature   Date   Time

FIG. 9-7. Standing orders for patient transfer out of Exeter Hospital, Exeter, NH. (© 2000 Exeter Hospital. Used with permission.)

TABLE 9-9. *Catheterization laboratory protocol for primary PTCA*

1. Abbreviated history and physical examination in ED. Complete chest pain assessment sheet to send to CCL with patient.
2. Cardiologist to obtain informed consent in the ED from patient or family.
3. CCL team to alert ED as soon as they arrive; plan for patient transfer to CCL within 5 minutes of arrival. (CCL is always left in a state of readiness.)
4. Enforce acuity-based bumping protocol when an elective procedure is in progress in the CCL.
5. Rapid transfer to CCL after informed consent.
6. For off-hours cases with only two CCL team members on call, a CCU or ED nurse or paramedic is predesignated to be available to assist in managing medications, drips, and acute nursing care problems.
7. If patient is intubated or in danger of respiratory compromise, respiratory therapist must stay with patient during procedure.
8. ED nurse, nursing supervisor, or social worker to counsel family during procedure.
9. Uninterrupted ECG monitoring during changeover from portable transport monitor to CCL system.
10. Assure patient has been pretreated with heparin, ASA, and clopidogrel (unless operator prefers deferring clopidogrel until after intervention).
11. Rapid preparation of both groins for bilateral access if IABP is necessary.
12. Administer additional narcotics and sedation if required.
13. Administer i.v. beta-blockers if not given in ED and no contraindications.
14. Continue vigorous medical management, monitoring of oxygen saturation, blood pressure support with fluids and pressors, treatment of congestive heart failure, and so on, as indicated.
15. Place arterial sheath.
16. IABP placement if in shock with introduction of second arterial sheath via opposite groin.
17. Femoral venous sheath placement if hemodynamically unstable or pacemaker likely to be needed.
18. ACT and baseline assessment of platelet function (if aggregometer available). If respiratory or acid-base status is unstable, send arterial blood gasses.
19. Give heparin boluses to assure ACT of 200–300 seconds if stenting or use of GP IIb/IIIa platelet inhibitors is planned. If GP IIb/IIIa platelet inhibitors are not used, aim for ACT of 350–400 seconds.
20. Immediate angiography of both coronary arteries with low-osmolar ionic contrast; limit injections to the minimal number required to define anatomy.
21. Rapid identification and assessment of the IRA.
22. Immediate decision on therapeutic action: PTCA, emergent transfer for surgery (with or without antecedent PTCA as indicated), or initial medical therapy.
23. Open the IRA before LV gram (If IRA has initial TIMI grade 3 flow or the culprit lesion is unclear, performing LV gram before intervention can influence interventional strategy.)
24. Use soft-tipped guidewires and avoid oversized balloons to minimize the chance of coronary artery rupture.
25. Establish coronary flow with guidewire or low-pressure/undersized balloon inflations to define distal anatomy before final selection of balloon or stent stenting.
26. Goal of intervention is early establishment of TIMI grade 3 flow.
27. Flow-limiting lesions in tandem with the culprit lesion in the same arterial segment should also be addressed.
28. Use of stents at discretion of operator. Use of GP IIb/IIIa agents is strongly encouraged in absence of major bleeding contraindications unless immediate transfer for CABG is planned. Consider using platelet aggregometer to titrate level of platelet inhibition to 95% with subsequent partial boluses of GP IIb/IIIa agents as needed (52).
29. If angiographic indications for emergent bypass surgery as present, activate emergency transfer protocol (Table 9-7) while performing any necessary intervention.
30. Avoid intervention in arteries other than the IRA unless lesions appear to be flow-limiting or patient has ongoing ischemia or hemodynamic instability.
31. Right ventricle catheterization with balloon-tipped catheter left indwelling if hemodynamically unstable.
32. LV gram in all cases except severe hemodynamic instability or severe renal insufficiency.

We avoid starting GP IIb/IIIa platelet inhibitors in the ED in patients undergoing immediate coronary angiography, because approximately 5% of these will be found to have coronary lesions that require transfer for emergency CABG.

ACT, activated clotting time; ASA, aspirin; CABG, coronary artery bypass graft; CCL, cardiac catheterization laboratory; CCU, cardiac care unit; ECG; electrocardiogram; ED, emergency department; GP, glycoprotein; IABP, intraaortic balloon pump; IRA, infarct-related artery; i.v., intravenous; LV gram, left ventriculogram; PTCA, percutaneous transluminal coronary angioplasty; TIMI, thrombolysis in myocardial infarction.

Developed by Wharton TP, McNamara NS, and the CCL staff, Exeter Hospital, Exeter, NH. © 1993 Wharton, McNamara; with permission.

TABLE 9-10. *Catheterization laboratory acuity-based procedure bumping protocol*

Purpose: To permit rapid interventional treatment of the most critically ill patients while providing appropriately timed care to less acute patients.

Policy: All physicians, CCL staff, and administration shall agree in advance to adhere to this acuity-based bumping protocol. This may mean the postponement of elective procedures or the interruption of elective procedures already in progress.

Classification of priority: Patients are classified as follows

Class A: Immediate priority
1. Acute high-risk AMI
   a. Hemodynamically compromised (shock or preshock, pulmonary edema)
   b. Heart block
   c. Anterior AMI
   d. Fibrinolytic ineligible
2. Suspected pulmonary embolus with hemodynamic instability
3. Cardiac tamponade
4. Acute aortic dissection requiring angiography

Class B: Emergent priority
1. Hemodynamically stable AMI other than anterior
2. Acute limb ischemia
3. Crescendo TIAs or stroke with abnormal carotid ultrasound

Class C: Urgent priority
1. Unstable angina within 24 hours
2. Inferior vena cava filters or venography for deep venous thrombosis

Procedure

Class A: Immediate transfer to CCL with interruption of elective procedures in progress on stable patients. Interrupted patients with indwelling sheaths will be held in CCU and returned to the CCL after completion of the emergency procedure. Scheduled elective procedures not yet started will be postponed or rescheduled.

Class B: Transfer to CCL within a 30-min window. Procedures in progress will be finished expeditiously.

Class C: Transfer to CCL on completion of the case in progress.

Transfers from other hospitals

Patients being transferred in will be triaged according to the above classification system. Class A patients expected with an estimated time of arrival within 40 min will have the CCL room vacated and held open for direct admission. All others will be evaluated in the ED for transfer to the CCL according to the above system.

AMI, acute myocardial infarction; CCL, cardiac catheterization laboratory; CCU, cardiac care unit; ED, emergency department, TIA, transient ischemic attack.

Developed by Wharton TP, Thomas T (director, cardiovascular specialties), and Sullivan N (vascular surgeon), Exeter Hospital, Exeter, NH. ©1998 Exeter Hospital; with permission.

When initiating a primary PTCA program, all physicians performing procedures in the CCL should mutually develop and agree to follow an acuity-based procedure bumping protocol such as the one we propose in Table 9-10. Having these agreements avoids delays in the immediate treatment of priority patients while lessening dissatisfaction caused by scheduling conflicts.

Create In-Hospital Management Pathways

Risk stratification and management protocols for the patient with acute MI after intervention (Fig. 9-5; Table 9-11) should be developed to provide the team with a clear clinical pathway for each patient.

Interventionalists should institute standing orders that address the care to be provided after primary PTCA (Fig. 9-8). The potential for groin bleeding requires the development of sheath protocols and standing orders (Fig. 9-9) for quick detection and control. Accompany this with education programs in the use of femoral compression devices, hemodynamic monitoring, medication in-services, and IABP modules and training.

Patients at high risk with acute MI admitted to the CCU require intensive care and monitoring. Critical care nurses must learn new skills, because patients often come to the CCU with devices such as femoral sheaths, pulmonary lines, temporary pacemakers, or IABP in place. Cardiac shock patients who might have died without primary PTCA may remain on multiple drips and support technology for several days. Nurses will be continually challenged to maintain their skills at the highest level.

Patients with acute MI at low risk (those <70 years of age with one- or two-vessel coronary artery disease (CAD), ejection fraction (EF) >45%, no congestive heart failure (CHF) or arrhythmias, a good PTCA result, TIMI grade 3 flow, and no major dissection or residual thrombus) can be admitted to an interventional unit, then to telemetry. This group, perhaps one half of all patients with acute MI treated with primary PTCA, has low mortality rate of only 0.3% (3). These patients at low-risk can safely avoid CCU care and predischarge exercise testing, and be discharged on hospital day 3 with return to work in 2 weeks. These measures will save an average of $2,000 per patient in total hospital costs, while decreasing the loss of wages and disability payments.

TABLE 9-11. *In-hospital management and risk stratification protocol after primary PTCA*

1. Communicate with family, primary physician, and ED staff immediately after procedure. Providing photographs of IRA before and after intervention is especially helpful.
2. Stratify patients into **low risk** (those with age <70 yr, 1–2 vessel CAD, EF >45%, no CHF or arrhythmias, good PTCA result with <30% residual stenosis, TIMI grade 3 flow, and no major dissection or residual thrombus) and **high risk** (all others).
3. Patients at low-risk can be transferred to step-down or interventional unit if nurses are able to care for sheaths. Patients at high-risk to CCU.
4. Early sheath removal in 3 h or when ACT is <180 sec.
5. No heparin infusion immediately after procedure if sheaths are to be removed early or if GP IIb/IIIa platelet inhibitors are used. Low-dose weight-adjusted heparin protocol may be started 3 h after sheath removal, at operator discretion.
6. Start maintenance aspirin, clopidogrel, beta-blockers, ACE inhibitors, and statins if no contraindications. Initial dose of clopidogrel should be 300 mg if loading dose has not yet been given.
7. Consider weight-adjusted heparin or enoxaparin after completion of GP IIb/IIIa infusion for patients who have suboptimal interventional result, residual intracoronary thrombus burden, apical left ventricular dyskinesis, CHF, and bedridden status.
8. Follow platelet counts beginning 4–6 h after procedure to assure thrombocytopenia has not been induced by heparin or GP IIb/IIIa platelet inhibitors.
9. Cardiac rehabilitation consultation for all patients.
10. A "fast-track" cardiac rehabilitation program should be established to meet the special needs of patients with low-risk AMI, who are often discharged on day 3 post AMI.
11. Target patients at low-risk for discharge on hospital day 3.
12. Predischarge exercise testing only for high-risk patients.

Positive reinforcement for ED physicians and nurses is particularly important (e.g., providing photographs, report of "door-to-balloon" time, praise of rapid and efficient care, if warranted; constructive troubleshooting if problems occurred).

ACE, angiotensin-converting enzyme; ACT, activated clotting time; AMI, acute myocardial infarction; CAD, coronary artery disease; CCU, coronary care unit; CHF, congestive heart failure; ED, emergency department; EF, ejection fraction; GP, glycoprotein; IRA, infarct-related artery; i.v., intravenous PTCA, percutaneous transluminal coronary angioplasty; TIMI, thrombolysis in myocardial infarction.

Developed by Wharton TP and McNamara NS, Exeter Hospital, Exeter, NH. ©1996 Wharton, McNamara; with permission.

Telemetry and cardiac rehabilitation staff must originate fast-track educational programs for patients at low risk, who are often discharged after only 2 or 3 days in the hospital, and thus may tend to minimize the importance of their MI. Provide a standing order for cardiac rehabilitation phases I and II on the post-MI/post-intervention order sheet (Fig. 9-8). Encourage all patients on discharge to enroll in the phase II cardiac rehabilitation program for risk factor modification and supervised exercise.

Create discharge teaching tools to emphasize established standards of care for patients with acute MI. An example is a risk assessment tool to prompt patients, caregivers, and physicians to recognize risk factors and measures to modify them (Fig. 9-10).

Initiate Processes and Tracking Tools for Data Gathering and Analysis, Case Review, and Quality Assurance

The institution should enroll in a data registry program such as the *American College of Cardiology National Cardiovascular Data Registry* (NCDR), Summit Medical Systems, Inc., or The Northern New England Cardiovascular Disease Study Group. An alternative is to develop a computerized outcomes database, using a case report form such as is shown in Fig. 9-11. Maintaining ongoing data collection and outcomes analysis is particularly important for institutions that are performing unconventional or controversial procedures (e.g., primary PTCA without on-site cardiac surgery). An appropriate data collection tool should include the following information on each patient: demographic information, clinical presentation, initial treatment, times to ED arrival, angiography, reperfusion, coronary anatomy, therapy chosen and reasons, results of PTCA, CCL complications, in-hospital complications, in-hospital mortality, and further procedures or cardiac surgery.

Use of this tracking tool allows identification of areas for improvement, such as suboptimal times to reperfusion and groin bleeding complications. When identified, constructive steps can be taken. For example, at Exeter Hospital we decreased bleeding complications more than fourfold with the initiation of weight-based heparin protocols, postprocedural standing orders (Figs. 9-8 and 9-9), femoral compression devices, and early sheath removal, despite considerably increased use of IIb/IIIa platelet inhibitors. We also discovered that our times-to-reperfusion were suboptimal. This stimulated more streamlined prehospital and ED protocols (Tables 9-5 and 9-6), which resulted in a 17%

(*text continues on page 93*)

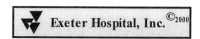

PHYSICIAN ORDERS

Post Myocardial Infarction/Post Intervention

Allergies (Allergen and Reaction)	Weight

Date/Time	POST MYOCARDIAL INFARCTION / POST INTERVENTION ORDERS
	1. Admit to inpatient unit with telemetry monitoring: ☐ CCU, ☐ Interventional Unit, ☐ Telemetry Unit Diagnosis / procedure: Attending physician:
	2. ACLS protocols.
	3. Chest pain protocol.
	4. O2 @ 2L/min. nasal cannula or non-rebreather mask prn. Titrate to maintain O_2 sat > 93%. Pulse oximetry prn..

	5. If post-cath/PTCA/stent:
	  a. Sheath Protocol, draw all bloods from sheath.
	  b. Balloon compression device for any oozing.
	  c. IV normal saline at 150cc/hr. x 1,000cc's or_____
	  d. Foley catheter prn if patient has not voided by 3 h post cath.

	6. Advance to cardiac diet as tolerated.
	7. I&O. ☐ Monitor hourly.

	8. Testing:
	  a. Urinalysis if not already obtained.
	  b. Guaiac all stools; record result in progress notes.
	  c. EKG upon arrival to unit post procedure and q AM x 2 days.
	  d. CPK-MB in 12 with PTT draws; then q AM x 2 days.
	  e. ☐ Portable chest x-ray in AM.
	  f. Chemistry and lipid profile, serum magnesium on admission bloods or in AM.
	  g. AM labs: CBC with diff, lytes, BUN, Creatinine — coordinate with CK-MB, PTT draws.

	9. Medications: ASA 325 mg. po q AM ☐ Heparin protocol (low-dose protocol if on GP IIb/IIIa platelet inhibitor. ☐ IV NTG: titrate to keep BP _____ β-blocker: _____ Statin: _____ K^+: _____ ☐ Fentanyl 50-100 mcg IV q 1 hr prn pain ☐ Prochlorperazine 5-10 mg IV / po q4hrs prn nausea ☐ Diazepam 5-10 mg IV q 4 hrs prn anxiety ☐ Resume all meds previously ordered ☐ Clopidogrel 75mg po qd ☐ Enoxaparin 1mg/kg sc BID GP IIb/IIIa platelet inhibitor: _____ Ace inhibitor: _____ H_2 Blocker: _____ Mg^{++}: _____ ☐ Morphine 5-10 mg IV q1 hr prn pain ☐ Lorazepam 0.5mg-1mg IV / po q 4hrs prn anxiety Hypnotic:
	10. Consult Cardiac Rehabilitation Services.
	11. Other:

_____   _____   _____
Physician Signature   Date   Time

FIG. 9-8. Standing orders for patients admitted with myocardial infarction or postintervention at Exeter Hospital, Exeter, NH. (© 2000 Exeter Hospital. Used with permission.)

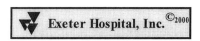

PHYSICIAN ORDERS
Vascular Sheaths / IABP

Allergies (Allergen and Reaction)	Weight

Date/Time	VASCULAR SHEATHS / IABP ORDERS
	(Please refer also to Nursing Care Plan and IABP Policy and Procedure Manual)
	1. VS q 15 min x 4, q 30 min x 2, then q 1 hr.
	2. q 1 hr. Monitoring: VS, Pulse, temp, color mobility of extremity distal to sheath. As applicable: Mean arterial pressure, PA pressure (phasic & mean), PCWedge, CO/CI q shift.

	3. Laboratory testing:
	     a. H & H in 8 hours. (Draw with PTT's whenever possible).
	     b. Complete CBC with platelets QAM.
	     c. U/A QOD.

	4. Heparin Protocol. Low-dose
	5. Change sheath dressing every day. Clean with Betadine and apply dressing.

	6. Bleeding:
	     a. Inspect site q 30 min x 4 hrs, then q 1 hr if no signs of bleeding.
	     b. Watch for concealed trickle of blood down crease in groin. Place 4 x 4 in groin to stanch
	          blood and help quantify oozing. Inspect sheet under patient q 1 hr.
	     c. For oozing: remove dressing; apply Femostop.
	     d. If oozing not controlled in 30 minutes (i.e. rate of one soaked 4 x 4 per hour),
	          call physician to consider Heparin dose, sheath removal, or Femostop.
	     e. Outline hematomas q 2 hrs; call physician if enlarging.

	7. Notify the physician **immediately** for the following:
	     a. Chest pain, flank pain, back pain, or severe pain in or around the puncture site.
	     b. Unstable vital signs
	     a. Bleeding
	     c. Altered color, temperature, sensation or pulses in extremities.
	     d. Urine output < 30 cc / hr or if patient has not voided 3 hours post-cath.
	     b. Hives, dyspnea, itching
	     e. If most recent HCT is above 35 and falls 5 points.
	     f. If most recent HCT is 35 or below and falls 3 points.
	     g. If non-functioning IABP cannot be corrected within 15 minutes.
	     h. Any signs of blood in IABP tubing.

	After sheath removal: 8. Patient to remain in bed for 6 hours. Head of bed may be elevated 30°.
	9. The extremity distal to the puncture site will remain extended straight for 6 hours.
	10. Other:

Physician Signature   Date   Time

FIG. 9-9. Standing orders for patients with vascular sheaths or intraaortic balloon pump (IABP) at Exeter Hospital, Exeter, NH. (© 2000 Exeter Hospital. Used with permission.)

▼ Exeter Hospital, Inc.	Cardiac Risk Assessment Tool With Risk Reduction Recommendations © 1999 McNamara, Exeter Hospital

For diagnosis of: Acute Myocardial Infarction, Stroke, Angina, Bypass Surgery/ Angioplasty/ Stent, Atrial Fibrillation, Congestive Heart Failure [CHF], Coronary Artery Disease [CAD], and CAD Risk Factors

Date: Name: Signature: Risk assessment completed by:	Diagnosis: Procedure: Physician: Cardiologist:

PATIENT SECTION			CARE-GIVER SECTION	
CARDIAC RISK FACTORS:	**ARE YOU AT RISK?** (check all that apply)	**GOAL** (please study/ learn)	**TREATMENT RECOMMENDATIONS**	**PHYSICIAN-PRESCRIBED PLAN**
Smoking	Do you smoke cigarettes, pipes or cigars? Yes☐ No☐	Complete cessation of smoking *QUIT*	☐*Smoking cessation counseling	☐Smoking cessation program Meds:
High Blood Pressure [BP]	Is your BP greater than 140/90? BP_____ Yes☐ No☐	*Lower BP to less than 140/90	☐Diet Teaching ☐Exercise Program ☐*Ace inhibitors ☐Other anti-hypertensive meds	☐Nutrition Consult ☐Low Salt Diet ☐Cardiac Rehab Meds:_____
History of Cardiac or Neurological Disease	Have you had a heart attack, angina, stroke or atrial fibrillation?_____ Yes☐No☐	Aspirin Beta blockers Antiplatelet agent	☐*Aspirin ☐*Beta Blockers ☐*Coumadin ☐Plavix ☐Lovenox	Meds:_____ _____ _____ ☐Cardiac Rehab
Elevated Blood Sugar (Diabetes)	Do you have Diabetes?_____ *Fasting blood glucose_____ ≥ 126 mg/dL HbA1c ≥ 8%_____ Yes☐ No☐	Fasting Blood glucose <110 mg/dL *HbA1c < 7%	☐Diet Education ☐Diabetes Health Reach ☐*Medications to Lower Blood Sugar	☐Nutrition Consult ☐Diet:_____ ☐Diabetes Health Reach Referral Anti diabetic meds: _____
Cardiac dysfunction (CHF)	Do you have a history of CHF or EF<45?_____ Yes☐ No☐	Use of: Ace Inhibitor titrated to therapeutic level Beta Blockers	☐Education: CHF educational booklet ☐Carelink Tele-monitoring referral ☐*ACE Inhibitors ☐*Beta Blockers	Daily wt._____ Meds:_____ _____ _____ _____
High Cholesterol	Do you have high cholesterol?_____ *Fasting Lipid Profile result: Total_____ LDL_____ HDL_____ Triglycerides_____	Total Cholesterol <200 LDL≤ 100 mg/dL HDL≥ 35 mg/dL TG < 200 mg/dL	☐Diet Teaching ☐Exercise Program for weight loss ☐*Cholesterol Lowering Agents	☐Nutritional Consult ☐Cardiac Rehab Meds:_____ _____ _____ _____ _____
Overweight	Are you overweight? (>120% ideal wt)___ Your wt_____	Your ideal body weight_____	☐Weight loss counseling ☐Exercise Program	☐Nutrition consult ☐Cardiac rehab
For more information on your Cardiac Risk Factors, contact: 1-800-xxx-xxxx				

*Indicates treatment standards that are monitored by: Heart Care Partnership, HCFA, HEDAS, NRMI, CCP, NCQA
References and guidelines obtained from: ADA, AHA, ACC, CCP, NCEP, AHCPR
Treatments recommended by The Division of Cardiovascular Specialties at Exeter Hospital 10 Buzell Ave. Exeter, NH. 03833

FIG. 9-10. Cardiac risk assessment tool developed at Exeter Hospital, Exeter, NH as a discharge teaching tool to emphasize established standards of care for patients with acute myocardial infarction. Worksheets such as these prompt patients, caregivers, and physicians to recognize both risk factors and the measures to modify them. (© 1999 McNamara, Exeter Hospital. Used with permission.)

Exeter Hospital, Inc.

CASE REPORT FORM: PRIMARY PTCA

© 1995 McNamara, Wharton

Case No._____

Physician:_____

Patient Name:_____ Research Protocol:_____

Address:_____ Telephone:_____

(street)   (city)   (state)   (zip)

Age:_____   D.O.B.____/____/____   Sex: ☐ Male ☐ Female

Medical Record Number:_____   Social Security Number:_____

Adm. Date:___/___/___   Cath Date:___/___/___   Hospital Billing Number:_____

Date Discharged Home: ___/___/___

Transferred to another hospital: ☐ yes ☐ no   Which One?: _____   Date of transfer:___/___/___

Cardiovascular Risk Factors

YES	NO	UNK		YES	NO	UNK	
☐	☐	☐	Hypertension	☐	☐	☐	Diabetes
☐	☐	☐	Hyperlipidemia (choles. > 240)	☐	☐	☐	If yes, Insulin Dependent?
☐	☐	☐	Peripheral Vasc. Dis., Claudication	☐	☐	☐	Cerebrovascular Disease (stroke, TIA)
☐	☐	☐	Post Menopausal	☐	☐	☐	Current Smoker

Cardiac History Prior to Admission

YES	NO	UNK		YES	NO	UNK	
☐	☐	☐	Prior stable angina (before this illness)	☐	☐	☐	Prior CABG
☐	☐	☐	Prior MI	☐	☐	☐	Prior CHF
☐	☐	☐	Prior PTCA/Stent	☐	☐	☐	HX CAD

Thrombolytic Eligible? ☐ YES ☐ NO ☐ UNK

If No, why not:

YES	NO	UNK		YES	NO	UNK	
☐	☐	☐	Symptom onset unclear	☐	☐	☐	Severe hypertension (>200s or >100 d)
☐	☐	☐	Time> 6 hours	☐	☐	☐	Severe hypotension (≤90 systolic)
☐	☐	☐	Prior or recent TIA/CVA (within 6 mo)	☐	☐	☐	ECG nondiagnostic
☐	☐	☐	Recent GI bleed (within 2 mo)	☐	☐	☐	Pain free
☐	☐	☐	Recent surgery (within 2 mo)	☐	☐	☐	Small infarct
☐	☐	☐	Organ biopsy (within 2 wk)	☐	☐	☐	Other bleeding risk, list
☐	☐	☐	Age (≥ 75 yrs)				(eg. CPR >10m, rib fx, recent cath)

ACUTE PRESENTATION

Date &Time of pain onset: ___/___/___, ___:___   *Note: all times are military

Date &Time of ER arrival: ___/___/___, ___:___   <-------(put N/A if infarct while inpatient)

Cardiologist notified: ___/___/___, ___:___ Cardiologist:_____

Initial Heart Rate:_____   Initial BP:___/___

CHF: Lung rales: ☐ none   ☐ ≤ 1/2 up   ☐ > 1/2 up   Killip Class: _____

YES	NO	UNK		
☐	☐	☐	CHF on Adm. chest X-ray	*1= no rales, no S3 3= rales > 50%, pulm.edema* *2= rales < 50% or S3 4= shock*

EKG: ☐ ☐ ☐ ST elevation >2 mm in >2 contiguous leads ☐ LBBB ☐ Paced Rhythm

Medications Prior to Catheterization

Aspirin Dose:_____mg   Heparin Dose: ___,000 U   Heparin Date, Time: ___/___/___, ___:___   Ticlid/Plavix:_____mg

Pre-Cath Lab Complications (include EMS events)   ☐ If none check here

YES	NO		YES	NO	
☐	☐	Asystole	☐	☐	Sustained hypotension (Req. RX)
☐	☐	Heart block or severe bradycardia requiring pacer or atropine	☐	☐	Respiratory arrest
☐	☐	Sustained VT (>100 / min)	☐	☐	Aspiration
☐	☐	VF	☐	☐	Pulmonary edema / CHF
☐	☐	Transient Hypotension (≤ 90)	☐	☐	Shock
		Other: _____	☐	☐	Death

Out-of-Hospital Procedures   ☐ If none check here

YES	NO		YES	NO	
☐	☐	Temporary pacer	☐	☐	EKG transmission from field
☐	☐	Cardioversion / defibrillation	☐	☐	CPR
☐	☐	Intubation	☐	☐	Other _____

FIG. 9-11. Case report form for primary angioplasty procedures performed at Exeter Hospital, Exeter, NH. (© 1995 McNamara, Wharton. Used with permission.)

Hosptial Procedures Prior to Catheter Insertion ☐ **If none check here**

YES   NO   YES   NO

☐   ☐   Temporary pacer   ☐   ☐   CPR

☐   ☐   Cardioversion / defibrillation   ☐   ☐   Other _____

☐   ☐   Intubation   _____

ACUTE CATHETERIZATION

Acute MI? ☐ yes ☐no   **Acute PTCA?** ☐ **yes** ☐ **no**   Chest Pain on CCL arrival? ☐ yes ☐ no

(I.e., acute occlusion as precipitating event)

Date &Time of arrival in cath lab: ---> ___/___/___, ____:____

Date &Time of first angiogram: ---> ___/___/___, ____:____

Date &Time of 1st ballon inflation: --> ___/___/___, ____:____

Hemodynamics (during LV gram)

HR=_____   Aortic **BP**=____/_____   **LV** End-Diastolic Pressure=_____   **PC W**edge Pressure= _____

                             Mitral Regurgitation Grade _____+   **LV E**jection Fraction= _____%

                                                    (omit EF only if there is no V-Gram)

Contrast Agent: _____   Lytics ≥ 90' _Before_ Cath ☐

Longest ACT in Lab: _____   Lytics in Lab: ☐ I.V. ☐ I.C.

Coronary Anatomy (provide % stenosis _only_ for those vessels with ≥ 50% stenosis - numerical entries only please):

1)_____Left Main   **LCX System**   **RCA System**   **Grafts**

    LAD System   6)_____Prox LCX   11)_____Proximal RCA   17)_____SVG to LAD   30)_____IRA unclear

2)_____Prox. LAD   7)_____Mid LCX   12)_____Mid RCA   18)_____SVG to DIAG   31)_____IRA normal

3)_____Mid LAD   8)_____Distal LCX   13)_____Distal RCA   19)_____SVG to CX/OM

4)_____Distal LAD   9)_____Obtuse marg. 14)_____PDA   20)_____SVG to RCA

5)_____Diagonal   10)____Intermediate 15)_____Posterolateral   21)_____IMA to LAD

                                                      22)_____IMA to DIAG

                                                     23)_____IMA to CX/OM

                                                   24)_____IMA to RCA

Infarct-related artey [IRA] (give _only one number_ from above):_____   (comment if more than one lesion dilated)

(If acute MI and infarct artery unclear or coronaries normal, use #30 or #31)

Stenosis of IRA at 1st angio: _____%   TIMI Flow Grade at first angio: _____   *(eg. 0, 1, 2, 3)*

(If no PTCA, skip to REASONS for no PTCA)

Angioplasty: Success (≤50% stenosis and ≥TIMI 2 flow)?: ☐ yes ☐no IIbIIIa? ☐ yes ☐no

        If NOT SUCCESSFUL, why not?:   Stent? ☐ yes ☐no

          ☐ Unable to pass wire or balloon   _Indication For Stent:_

          ☐ Abrubt closure--dissection   ☐ Planned

          ☐ Abrubt closure-- clot   ☐ PTCA failure (>50% or TIMI 0-1)

          ☐ No reflow   ☐ PTCA suboptimal (30-50% or dissection*)*

          ☐ Stent obstructive or threatening position   _Stent Result:_ ☐ Successful Deployment

          ☐ Other_____   ☐ Not Deployed ☐ Wrong Site

Stenosis post-PTCA:_____%   TIMI Flow Grade post PTCA:_____

Thrombus post-PTCA: ☐yes ☐no   Dissection post PTCA: ☐yes ☐no   TIMI III Flow obtained after I.C.Lytics alone: ☐

Thrombus Size*: _____   Dissection Type*: _____   ***See p.4**

NO PTCA: REASONS (Select the single best reason)   ☐ **N/A**

☐ **Not M.I.** by cath lab diagnosis (i.e., no acute occlusions, with or without CAD)

Acute M.I. with: ☐ Normal coronaries

                 ☐ IRA patent (TIMI III Flow) *note if < 70%:* _____   ☐ IRA unclear   ☐ Small or secondary vessel

                 ☐ Surgical anatomy *(includes Left Main)*, IRA closed   ☐ PTCA not technically feasible, non-surgical

                 ☐ Other (Include diagnosis if not MI:) _____

FIG. 9-11. Continued.

Accessory Cath Lab Procedures   ☐ **If none check here**

YES	NO	
☐	☐	Temp pacemaker
☐	☐	Cardioversion / Defibrillation
☐	☐	Intubation

YES	NO	
☐	☐	CPR
☐	☐	IABP (intra-aortic ballon pump)

Cath Lab Complications   ☐ **If none check here**

YES	NO	
☐	☐	Asystole
☐	☐	Heart block / profound bradycardia (requiring pacer / atropine)
☐	☐	VT (sustained)
☐	☐	VF
☐	☐	Hypotension (req. vasopressors or IABP)
☐	☐	Anaphylaxis
☐	☐	Stroke
☐	☐	TIA

YES	NO	
☐	☐	Aspiration
☐	☐	Respiratory arrest
☐	☐	Pulmonary edema
☐	☐	Coronary perforation
☐	☐	Tamponade
☐	☐	Emergency CABG for failed PTCA
☐	☐	Death
☐	☐	Other_____

POST CATH/PTCA: IN-HOSPITAL CORONARY EVENTS

☐ **If none check here**

Hospital Day (Day 0 = admission)

YES	NO			
☐	☐	Repeat Cath after PTCA *same admission*	Where:_____	_____
☐	☐	*Reinfarction (defined below) "		_____
☐	☐	**Reocculsion (defined below) "		_____
☐	☐	Repeat PTCA/Atherectomy "	Where:_____	_____
☐	☐	Urgent CABG *note on all reg. forms* "	Where:_____Time:_____	_____
☐	☐	Elective CABG *after discharge*	Where:_____	/////////////////////////

* Reinfarction: CPK re-elevation --OR-- chest pain with ST elevation and cath-documented reocclusion . . .
**Reocculsion: >90% restenosis and TIMI 0-1 flow

POST CATH/PTCA NON-HEMORRHAGIC COMPLICATIONS

☐ **If none check here**

Hospital Day (Day 0 = admission)

YES	NO		
Neurologic--->			
☐	☐	Stroke (hemorrhagic)	
☐	☐	Stroke (nonhemorrhagic)	
☐	☐	TIA	
Arrhythmia-->			
☐	☐	Asystole, heart block, or severe bradycardia	
☐	☐	Sustained VT	
☐	☐	VF	
Pump Dysfunction-->			
☐	☐	Pulmonary edema / CHF	
☐	☐	Shock	
Pulmonary			
☐	☐	Respiratory failure (requiring intubation)	
Renal			
	☐	Acute renal failure (requiring dialysis)	
Vascular **(requiring surgery / embolectomy)**			
☐	☐	Loss of pulse	
☐	☐	Pseudo aneurysm or AV fistula	
☐	☐	Perforation	
☐	☐	Other peripheral complications	
Other			
☐	☐	Acute VSD / MR	
☐	☐	Pericarditis	
☐	☐	Deep vein thrombosis	
☐	☐	Sepsis	

☐ *Deficit at discharge, minor*
☐ *Deficit at discharge, disabling*
☐ *Death*

Treatment: ☐ *Pacemaker*
         ☐ *Defibrillation*
         ☐ *CPR*
         ☐ *Intubation*

☐ *Re-cath* ☐ *IABP*
☐ *CPR* ☐ *Intubation*
☐ *Vasopressors* ☐ *Diuretics*

FIG. 9-11. Continued.

POST CATH/PTCA: HEMORRHAGIC COMPLICATIONS

☐ **If none check here**

YES   NO

Bleeding requiring transfusion   Hospital Day (Day 0 = admission)

☐	☐	Groin	_____
☐	☐	Brachial	_____
☐	☐	Retroperitoneal	_____
☐	☐	GU	_____
☐	☐	GI	_____
☐	☐	Unknown	_____
☐	☐	Admission hematocrit of 32 or less	

Total number of units transfused in hospital: _____

IN HOSPITAL DEATH

Did patient die in the hospital: ☐ yes ☐ no

Date &Time: ___/___/___ , _____:_____

Mode of Death:

☐ Reinfarction
☐ Power failure (CHF or shock preceding)
☐ Primary arrhythmia (documented) in absence of power failure
☐ Sudden death (undocumented rhythm)
☐ Stroke, hemorrhagic
☐ Stroke, non hemorrhagic
☐ Other_____

(Make note if death is attributable to Cath/PTCA procedure; see p. 3)

OTHER DATA

YES   NO   UNK

☐	☐	☐	Did patient arrive via ambulance?
☐	☐	☐	Was Cardiac Rehab received?
☐	☐	☐	Was cholesterol lowering agent prescribed?

Total no. days in ICU (being there at midnight counts as one day): _____

Discharge DRG code for primary diagnosis: _____

MI Type ☐ Q-Wave   ☐ Non-Q-Wave

Discharged to: ☐ Home
                ☐ Extended Care Facility
                ☐ Death

THROMBUS SIZE:
Possible: *Haziness only*
Small: *Greatest dimension of the thrombus less than one-half the vessel diameter.*
Moderate: *Greatest linear dimension greater than one-half but less than 2 vessel diameters.*
Large: *Largest dimension greater than 2 vessel diameters.*
Unknown: *Unable to determine due to TIMI 0 flow.*

CORONARY ARTERY DISSECTION / PLAQUE RUPTURE TYPE:
Type 0:   *None*
Type 1:   *Parallel tracts separated by a radiolucent area during contrast injection with minimal or no persistence after dye clearance; does not impinge on lumen.*
Type 2:   *Extraluminal cap with persistence of contrast after dye clearance from the coronary lumen.*
Type 3:   *Spiral luminal filling defects or those impinging on lumen.*

FIG. 9-11. Continued.

improvement in our median "door-to-balloon" time. This process of outcomes analysis can also be used to gauge the effects of new polices and procedures, new equipment and medical therapies, and new educational programs. For example, our rates of reinfarction, reocclusion, and mortality decreased with increased use of stents and GP IIb/IIIa platelet inhibitors (51).

Key members of the acute MI protocol team must take responsibility for spearheading these quality improvement efforts, and for communicating the outcomes of the program to the medical community on an ongoing basis. Continuous quality improvement processes will prevent complacency and continue to stimulate the development of new goals in the care of the patient with acute MI.

CONCLUSIONS

Because of its broader applicability, safety, and efficacy, primary PTCA should be offered as the standard-of-care for patients with acute MI at more well-qualified hospitals that do not have cardiac surgery. Primary PTCA can be provided safely and effectively at such hospitals, with outstanding outcomes that are similar to those reported from high-volume surgical centers.

A uniform commitment to immediate and routine triage of patients with acute MI from the ED to the CCL will improve times-to-reperfusion and increase institutional primary PTCA volumes. These are key factors that positively affect outcomes in patients having primary PTCA (43–45). This approach increases volume, streamlines acute critical care pathways, and ensures optimal emergency management of the patient with acute MI.

Achieving a successful primary PTCA program in a community hospital also requires the intensive collaboration and commitment of all members of the healthcare team. Critical pathways and care plans covering every aspect of management of the acute MI patient—from first contact through discharge—coupled with ongoing assessment of evolving protocols to improve patient care, continuous educational programs, and ongoing data gathering and analysis are required to provide safe and effective interventional treatment of acute MI. These elements are especially imperative for interventional programs at centers without on-site cardiac surgery.

Offering this potentially life-saving therapy to more patients with acute MI in more hospitals throughout the country can provide a substantial healthcare benefit to society.

REFERENCES

1. Weaver WD, Simes J, Betriu A, et al. Comparison of primary coronary angioplasty and intravenous thrombolytic therapy for acute myocardial infarction. *JAMA* 1997;278:2093–2098.
2. Zahn R, Schiele R, Gitt AK, et al. Primary angioplasty is superior to intravenous thrombolysis in all subgroups of patients: results of 9906 patients with acute myocardial infarction. *Circulation* 1999;100:I-359 (abst).
3. Grines CL, Marsalese DL, Brodie B, et al. Safety and cost-effectiveness of early discharge after primary angioplasty in low risk patients with acute myocardial infarction. PAMI-II investigators. Primary angioplasty in myocardial infarction. *J Am Coll Cardiol* 1998;31:967–972.
4. Zijlstra F, Beukema WP, van't Hof AW, et al. Randomized comparison of primary coronary angioplasty with thrombolytic therapy in low risk patients with acute myocardial infarction. *J Am Coll Cardiol* 1997;29:908–912.
5. Rogers WJ. Contemporary management of acute myocardial infarction. *Am J Med* 1995;99:195–206.
6. Rogers WJ, Bowlby LJ, Chandra NC, et al. Treatment of myocardial infarction in the United States (1990 to 1993). Observations from the National Registry of Myocardial Infarction. *Circulation* 1994;90:2103–2114.
7. Grines CL, Booth DC, Nissen SE, et al. Mechanism of acute myocardial infarction in patients with prior coronary artery bypass grafting and therapeutic implications. *Am J Cardiol* 1990;65:1292–1296.
8. Thiemann DR, Coresh J, Schulman SP, et al. Lack of benefit for intravenous thrombolysis in patients with myocardial infarction who are older than 75 years. *Circulation* 2000;101:2239–2246.
9. Ayanian JZ, Braunwald E. Thrombolytic therapy for patients with myocardial infarction who are older than 75 years. *Circulation* 2000;101:2224–2226.
10. Berger AK, Schulman KA, Gersh BJ, et al. Primary coronary angioplasty vs. thrombolysis for the management of acute myocardial infarction in elderly patients. *JAMA* 1999;282:341–348.
11. The TIMI Study Group. Effects of tissue plasminogen activator and a comparison of early invasive and conservative strategies in unstable angina and non–Q-wave myocardial infarction: results of the TIMI IIIB trial. Thrombolysis in myocardial ischemia. *Circulation* 1994;89:1545–1556.
12. Fibrinolytic Therapy Trialists' (FTT) Collaborative Group. Indications for fibrinolytic therapy in suspected acute myocardial infarction: collaborative overview of early mortality and major morbidity results from all randomised trials of more than 1000 patients. *Lancet* 1994;343:311–322.
13. Zahn R, Schuster S, Schielel R, et al. Comparison of primary angioplasty with conservative therapy in patients with acute myocardial infarction and contraindications for thrombolytic therapy. Maximal Individual Therapy in Acute Myocardial Infarction (MITRA) Study Group. *Catheter Cardiovasc Interv* 1999;46:127–133.
14. Zahn R, Schiele R, Schneider S, et al. Primary dilatation versus thrombolysis in patients with acute myocardial infarct, not included in randomized studies. Results of the MITRA study: Maximal Individual Optimized Therapy for Acute Myocardial Infarct. *Z Kardiol* 1999;88:418–425.
15. Scull GS, Martin JS, Weaver WD, et al, for the MITI Investigators. Early angiography versus conservative treatment in patients with non-ST elevation acute myocardial infarction. *J Am Coll Cardiol* 2000;35:895–902.
16. Tiefenbrunn AJ, Chandra NC, Every NR, et al. High mortality in patients with myocardial infarction transferred for primary angioplasty: a report from the National Registry of Myocardial Infarction-2. *Circulation* 1997;96:I-531(abst).
17. Vogel J. Angioplasty in the patient with an evolving myocardial infarction: with and without surgical backup. *Clin Cardiol* 1992;15:880–882.
18. Weaver WD, Litwin PE, Martin JS. Use of direct angioplasty for treatment of patients with acute myocardial infarction in hospitals with and without on-site cardiac surgery. *Circulation* 1993;88:2067–2075.
19. Iannone LA, Anderson SM, Phillips SJ. Coronary angioplasty for acute myocardial infarction in a hospital without cardiac surgery. *Tex Heart Inst J* 1993;20:99–104.
20. Ayres M. Coronary angioplasty for acute myocardial infarction in hospitals without cardiac surgery. *J Invasive Cardiol* 1995;7[Suppl F]:40F–48F.
21. Weaver WD, Parsons L, Every N. Primary coronary angioplasty in hospitals with and without surgery backup. *J Invasive Cardiol* 1995;7[Suppl F]:34F–39F.
22. Brush JE, Thompson S, Ciuffo AA, et al. Retrospective comparison of a strategy of primary coronary angioplasty versus intravenous thrombolytic therapy for acute myocardial infarction in a community hospital without cardiac surgery. *J Invasive Cardiol* 1996;8:91–98.
23. Weaver WD, for the MITI Project Investigators. PTCA in centers without

surgical backup-outcome, logistics, and technical aspects. *J Invasive Cardiol* 1997;9[Suppl B]:20B–23B.

24. Smyth DW, Richards AM, Elliot JM. Direct angioplasty for myocardial infarction: one-year experience in a center with surgical backup 220 miles away. *J Invasive Cardiol* 1997;9:324–332.

25. Wharton TP Jr, McNamara NS, Fedele FA, et al. Primary angioplasty for the treatment of acute myocardial infarction: experience at two community hospitals without cardiac surgery. *J Am Coll Cardiol* 1999;33:1257–1265.

26. Wharton TP Jr, Johnston JD, Turco MA, et al. Primary angioplasty for acute myocardial infarction with no surgery on site: outcomes, core angiographic analysis, and six-month follow-up in the 500-patient prospective PAMI-No SOS. Registry. *J Am Coll Cardiol* 1999;33:352A–353A(abst).

27. Ribichini F, Steffenino G, Dellavalle A, et al. Primary angioplasty without surgical back-up at all. Results of a five years experience in a community hospital in Europe. *J Am Coll Cardiol* 2000;35:364A(abst).

28. O'Neill WW, Brodie BR, Ivanhoe R, et al. Primary coronary angioplasty for acute myocardial infarction (the Primary Angioplasty Registry). *Am J Cardiol* 1994;73:627–634.

29. Stone GW, Brodie BR, Griffin JJ, et al. Prospective, multicenter study of the safety and feasibility of primary stenting in acute myocardial infarction: in-hospital and 30-day results of the PAMI stent pilot trial. Primary Angioplasty in Myocardial Infarction Stent Pilot Trial Investigators. *J Am Coll Cardiol* 1998;31:23–30.

30. Antoniucci D, Santoro GM, Bolognese L, et al. A clinical trial comparing primary stenting of the infarct-related artery with optimal primary angioplasty for acute myocardial infarction. Results of the Florence Randomized Elective Stenting in Acute Coronary Occlusions (FRESCO) trial. *J Am Coll Cardiol* 1998;31:1234–1239.

31. Suryapranata H, van't Hof AW, Hoorntje JCA, et al. Randomized comparison of coronary stenting with balloon angioplasty in selected patients with acute myocardial infarction. *Circulation* 1998;97:2502–2505.

32. The EPISTENT Investigators. Randomised placebo-controlled and balloon-angioplasty-controlled trial to assess safety of coronary stenting with use of platelet glycoprotein-IIb/IIIa blockade. *Lancet* 1998;352:87–92.

33. Brener SJ, Barr LA, Burchenal J, et al. Randomized, placebo-controlled trial of platelet glycoprotein IIb/IIIa blockade with primary angioplasty for acute myocardial infarction. The RAPPORT trial. *Circulation* 1998;98:734–741.

34. Loubeyre C, Morice MC, Berzin B, et al. Emergency coronary artery bypass surgery following coronary angioplasty and stenting: results of a French multicenter registry. *Catheter Cardiovasc Interv* 1999;48:441–448.

35. Stone GW, Brodie B, Griffin J, et al. Role of cardiac surgery in the hospital phase management of patients treated with primary angioplasty for acute myocardial infarction. *Am J Cardiol* 2000;85:1292–1296.

36. Doucet M, Eisenberg MJ, Joseph L, et al. The effect of hospital volume on long-term outcome after percutaneous transluminal coronary angioplasty. *J Am Coll Cardiol* 2000;35:12A(abst).

37. Ho V. Evolution of the volume-outcome relation for hospitals performing coronary angioplasty. *Circulation* 2000;101:1806–1811.

38. Simpson DE, Boura JA, Grines LL, et al. Predictors of delay from ER to cath with primary PTCA for acute MI. *J Am Coll Cardiol* 2000;35:20A(abst).

39. *Directory of cardiac catheterization laboratories in the United States*, 4th ed. Raleigh, NC: The Society for Cardiac Angiography and Interventions, 1997.

40. The TIMI Study Group. The Thrombolysis in Myocardial Infarction (TIMI) trial: phase I findings. *N Engl J Med* 1985;312:932–936.

41. ACC/AHA guidelines for the management of patients with acute myocardial infarction. A report of the American College of Cardiology/American Heart Association Task force on Practice Guidelines (Committee on Management of Acute Myocardial Infarction). *J Am Coll Cardiol* 1996;28:1328–1419.

42. Joint Working Group on Coronary Angioplasty of the British Cardiac Society and British Cardiovascular Intervention Society. Coronary angioplasty: guidelines for good practice and training. *Heart* 2000;83:224–235.

43. Cannon CP, Gibson CM, Lambrew CT, et al. Relationship of symptom-onset-to-balloon time and door-to-balloon time with mortality in patient undergoing angioplasty for acute myocardial infarction. *JAMA* 2000;283:2941–2947.

44. Every NR, Maynard C, Schulman K, et al. The association between institutional primary angioplasty procedure volume and outcome in elderly Americans. *J Invasive Cardiol* 2000;12:303–308.

45. Canto JG, Every NR, Magid DJ, et al. The volume of primary angioplasty procedures and survival after acute myocardial infarction. *N Engl J Med* 2000;342:1573–1580.

46. McNamara NS, Hiett D, Allen B, et al. Can community hospitals provide effective primary PTCA coverage at all hours? *J Am Coll Cardiol* 1997;29:91A(abst).

47. McNamara NS, Wharton TP Jr, Johnston J, et al. Can hospitals with no surgery on site provide effective infarct intervention at all hours? The PAMI-No SOS experience. *Circulation* 1998;98:I-306–I-307(abst).

48. Grines CL, Browne KF, Marco J, et al. A comparison of immediate angioplasty with thrombolytic therapy for acute myocardial infarction: the Primary Angioplasty in Myocardial Infarction Study Group. *N Engl J Med* 1993;328:673–679.

49. Kereiakes DJ, Gibler WB, Martin LH, et al. Relative importance of emergency medical system transport and the prehospital electrocardiogram on reducing hospital time delay to therapy for acute myocardial infarction: a preliminary report from the Cincinnati Heart Project. *Am Heart J* 1992;123:835–840.

50. Canto JG, Rogers WJ, Bowlby LJ, et al. The prehospital electrocardiogram in acute myocardial infarction: is its full potential being realized? *J Am Coll Cardiol* 1997;29:498–505.

51. McNamara NS, Scoggins A, Hiett D, et al. *Improving angioplasty results at hospitals without cardiac surgery using ongoing outcomes monitoring and evaluation*. Transcatheter Cardiovascular Therapeutics Conference, Washington DC, September 23, 1999.

52. Steinhubl S, Talley D, Kereiakes D, et al. A prospective multicenter study to determine the optimal level of platelet inhibition with GPIIb/IIIa inhibitors in patients undergoing coronary intervention—the GOLD study. *J Am Coll Cardiol* 2000;35:44A(abst).

CHAPTER 10

Primary PTCA for Acute MI in the PAMI Trials

Robert Wolyn and Cindy L. Grines

Complete and sustained restoration of coronary flow is the principal mechanism by which reperfusion improves outcomes in patients with acute myocardial infarction (MI). Percutaneous mechanical reperfusion, the preferred method of reperfusion in many centers, has proved to be effective in multiple randomized trials (1). Based on our experience in performing angioplasty as the primary reperfusion strategy and in conducting acute MI trials, we have developed protocols for effective triage, performance, and follow-up care for patients undergoing primary percutaneous transluminal coronary angioplasty (PTCA).

The Primary Angioplasty in Myocardial Infarction (PAMI-1) trial, conducted from 1990 to 1992, compared primary angioplasty with tissue plasminogen activator (tPA) for treatment of acute MI. Angioplasty was superior with regard to in-hospital events. The mortality rate was 2.6% for PTCA- and 6.5% for tPA-treated patients; reinfarction was more than 2.6% for PTCA versus 6.5% for tPA. Intracranial bleeding occurred more frequently in patients who received tPA (2.0% vs. PTCA 0%) (2). This early benefit of primary PTCA was sustained at 2-year follow-up (3).

Primary Angioplasty in Myocardial Infarction-2 (PAMI-2) in which 1,100 patients were enrolled between 1993 and 1995, found that routine use of intraaortic balloon pump (IABP) for 48 hours in patients at high risk did not improve the clinical outcome, reocclusion, or left ventricle (LV) function. However, patients at low risk could be safely triaged to a step-down unit after reperfusion without coronary care unit (CCU) admission. Moreover, these patients could be safely discharged on day 3 without noninvasive testing. Patients at high risk were defined by age >70 years, vein graft culprit occlusion, three-vessel disease, ejection fraction (EF) less than 45%, suboptimal PTCA results, or malignant arrhythmias post PTCA (4,5).

In PAMI-2, we found that residual stenosis more than 30% or dissection was predictive of recurrent ischemia and reocclusion. Coronary stenting could eliminate these problems. Stenting in the setting of thrombus was initially thought to result in high rates of subacute thrombosis. Therefore, the PAMI Stent Pilot study evaluated the feasibility, safety,

and efficacy of primary stenting in acute MI (6,7). For 312 consecutive patients presenting with acute MI and undergoing primary PTCA, stent implantation was feasible in 240 patients (77%) and successful in 98%. The 30-day rates of subacute thrombosis (1.3%), reinfarction (1.7%), and recurrent ischemia (3.8%) were low when compared with historical data from the PAMI trials. The rates of target vessel revascularization (TVR) (12%) and angiographic restenosis at 7.7 months (28%) were also comparatively low. Based on this trial and other encouraging data, a larger, multicenter, randomized trial was initiated.

Stent PAMI (8) randomized 900 patients with acute MI from 1998 to 1999 to routine stent placement or to primary PTCA alone. It showed that stents decrease restenosis and the need for TVR at 1 month and 6 months. No statistical difference was found in the rates of death, stroke, and reinfarction. However, it was disturbing to find the trend for lower rates of thrombolysis in myocardial infarction (TIMI)-3 flow and higher 1-year mortality rate in patients randomized to stenting. Whether this finding could be reproduced in another trial or prevented with glycoprotein (GP) IIb/IIIa blockers is the subject of our recent investigation.

The Controlled Abciximab and Device Investigation to Lower Late Angioplasty Complications (CADILLAC) trial, which enrolled 2,000 patients with acute MI from 1999 to 2000, is now in the follow-up stage. In this trial, patients were randomized in a 2 × 2 factorial design to PTCA versus stent and (open label) abciximab versus placebo. Interim results were presented at the 1999 American Heart Association (AHA) scientific sessions. In-hospital mortality rate was low regardless of the treatment received: PTCA 1.4%, PTCA plus abciximab 1.0%, stent 1.6%, stent plus abciximab 1.6%. Results from the CADILLAC trial will contribute significantly to our fund of knowledge regarding the use of stents and IIb/IIIa inhibitors in the setting of acute MI.

Some registry data have raised doubt that the results from major clinical trials could be replicated in general clinical practice (9). The registry results must be interpreted with caution because data were usually obtained retrospectively and could not account for physician bias to treat sicker patients more aggressively or to determine whether patients were truly thrombolytic eligible. The mortality and cardiac event rates associated with mechanical reperfusion were consistently low in all PAMI trials and lower than in any historical thrombolytic trials. Moreover, we were unable to establish a correlation between hospital or operator volume and patient outcome in the setting of acute MI. If inexperienced operators performed primary PTCA "the PAMI way," good outcomes were achieved.

Lessons learned over the years from PAMI and other trials have been implemented in the routine care of patients presenting with acute MI. The following protocol used in the trials allowed us to achieve excellent results.

TREATMENT OF ACUTE MYOCARDIAL INFARCTION "THE PAMI WAY"

Initial Evaluation

Patients coming to the emergency center (EC) and complaining of chest pain are directed immediately to the Chest Pain Center. Bypassing regular triage, which typically has long waiting lines, allows for rapid evaluation. After a brief history and examination by a nurse, an electrocardiogram (ECG) is performed and presented without delay to an EC physician. If the initial evaluation suggests that the patient is having an acute MI, an interventional cardiologist is contacted (Fig. 10-1).

During business hours, the cardiologist calls the catheterization laboratory (CL) scheduling board which assigns the laboratory and appropriate staffing. If no open CL is available, the elective cases are moved to the holding room (Table 10-1).

During off hours, the EC calls the hospital operator who pages the catheterization team on call. The on-call team designated to cover emergency cases should be composed of a minimum of two people, at least one of whom lives within 20 minutes driving distance of the hospital. All personnel should understand the necessity of rapid response, which offers the patient with an acute MI the best possible outcome. The first team member to arrive at the CL suite should arrange for transportation of the patient from the emergency room (ER) to the CL. Once the second team member has arrived, the attending physician can safely begin the procedure. It must be emphasized to the CL staff that they work quickly. Some hospitals have trays set up in advance. Consideration should be given to have the ER nurse assist in the transfer and preparation of the patient until appropriate CL staff has arrived. An abbreviated history and physical examination should be performed and informed consent obtained. Ancillary medications should be given in the EC or after arrival to CL before the procedure is started (11–21) (Tables 10-2, 10-3).

CATHETERIZATION PROCEDURE

Venous sheaths are placed only if the patient has arrhythmias or hemodynamic problems necessitating temporary pacer or

---

ACUTE MI PATHWAY—The "PAMI Way"

Clinical Indicators
- Chest Pain > 30 minutes, < 24 hours
- ST elevation, new LBBB
- Clinical suspicion of AMI—may need 2 D Echo, Nuclear testing or serology markers
- Cardiogenic shock

EC Interventions
- Standard 12-lead ECG (obtain right-sided with Inferior MI) continuous monitoring: Interventional cardiology consult with notification of cath team lab
- Obtain cardiac panel: CBC, lytes, BUN, glucose, Cr, CK-MB, lipid profile
- EC Medications (preferable order): Aspirin 325 mg Chewed (non-enteric coated); Ticlopidine 500 mg or Clopidogrel 300 mg; Heparin IV bolus 70U/kg (usually 5000U); Beta-blocker IV (Metoprolol 5 mg X 3 every 5 minutes); Nitroglycerin drip (start 33 mcg/min tritate for chest pain); Morphine IV 2-4 mg for persistent chest pain (after obtaining informed consent regarding reperfusion therapy)
- Keep O_2 Sat>95% with O_2 supplement

Catheterization and Intervention
- Arterial access—7 French sheath
- Venous access only for: large proximal RCA occlusions, shock (Swan-Ganz), bradycardia requiring temporary pacemaker
- Check ACT after access achieved
- Ionic, low osmolar contrast (e.g., Hexabrix)
- Visualize non-infarct artery first, use guiding catheter for infarct artery angiograms
- Adjust ACT according to planned strategy
  - Use of GP IIb/IIIa inhibitor—ACT 200-300 sec
  - No GP IIb/IIIa inhibitor—ACT > 350 sec
  - Bail-out GP IIb/IIIa inhibitor—may use Protamine Sulfate to keep ACT 200-300 sec
- "Slow" reperfusion with wire or balloon—wait for arrhythmias
- Upsize balloon (1:1 balloon/artery ratio)
- Treat infarct artery only (in persistent shock, non-infarct artery can be treated)
- Use stents for suboptimal PTCA results
- Consider angiographic and clinical inclusion/exclusion criteria when opting for stent strategy
- Consider GP IIb/IIIa when PTCA only

FIG. 10-1.

Swan-Ganz catheter. After obtaining arterial access, activated clotting time (ACT) should be checked. Selective coronary angiography is performed. In the PAMI studies, ionic contrast was used for all cases. Low osmolar ionic contrast (Hexabrix; Guerbet Laboratories, Cedex, France) was used to reduce the risk of contrast exposure (22–25). The non–infarct-related artery (IRA) should be visualized before PTCA is done to assess collateral flow to the infarct artery. To reduce the time to reperfusion, we use a guiding catheter to visualize the suspected IRA. PTCA is attempted in all patients unless they meet criteria outlined in Table 10-4. We routinely perform PTCA in patients with three-vessel disease, especially if they have an occluded infarct vessel or ongoing pain. We also perform PTCA in most infarct

TABLE 10-1. *Criteria for taking the patient immediately to the catheter laboratory*

Symptoms of AMI <12 h

AMI 12–24 h if continued pain

ECG findings: 1 mm ST-segment elevation in two or more contiguous ECG leads or new LBBB

Nondiagnostic ECG including LBBB, paced rhythm, ST-segment depression, or T-wave inversion when clinical suspicion is high and patient has positive enzyme markers of AMI or additional testing (e.g., 2-D echo) suggests new MI

Cardiogenic shock patients (age <75 yr) within 24 h of shock onset (10)

Lytic failure within 12 h from initial chest pain, especially if anterior MI

Suspected reocclusion after lytic therapy

AMI, acute myocardial infarction; ECG, electrocardiogram; LBBB, left bundle branch block.

vessels with TIMI-3 flow (if thrombolytics have not been given) with excellent angiographic and clinical outcomes (64). This strategy results in 90% of patients with acute MI undergoing primary PTCA, 5% being treated medically and 5% being treated surgically (often 2 or more days after hospital admission). To avoid delays in reperfusion, contrast ventriculography should be performed after the coronary intervention using an angled pigtailed catheter with contrast injections (10–13 ml/sec) for 3 to 4 seconds. We routinely perform left ventriculography because it provides important prognostic information (e.g., EF, regional wall motion, mitral regurgitation, ventricular septal defect), unless the patient has clinical contraindications (e.g., excessive contrast of >250 ml contrast used before left ventriculogram, pulmonary edema, or renal insufficiency).

PTCA PROCEDURE

Ionic Contrast

We use ionic contrast to reduce the risk of abrupt closure and thromboembolic complications. Ionic contrast has been shown to prolong partial thromboplastin and clotting times, inhibit platelet aggregation and degranulation, and shorten the time to thrombolysis. Numerous observational studies, as well as randomized trials, have demonstrated a reduced rate of abrupt closure, and no reflow, recurrent ischemia, or MI with ionic compared with nonionic contrast (22–25). However, recent studies conducted in the setting of stents and IIb/IIIa antagonists suggest that newer nonionic agents can be safely used (26–28).

Heparin

If IIb/IIIa blockers are used, a lower dose of heparin is used (60–70 U/kg; usually already given in EC), and ACT is maintained at 250 seconds.

If IIb/IIIa blockers are not used, additional heparin should be given to achieve an ACT of 350 seconds before intervention. An ACT of 300 seconds does not suppress thrombin activity and results in more platelet aggregation and more abrupt closure compared with higher levels of ACT (29–35). Two studies have suggested that the optimal ACT may be as high as 400 to 500 seconds (34,35). ACT should be monitored every 20 to 30 minutes, with repeat doses of 2,000 to 3,000 U of intravenous (i.v.) heparin administered throughout the procedure to maintain an ACT above 350 seconds.

After reperfusion with the wire, or by passing the balloon, the operator should wait for a few minutes for arrhythmias and hypotension to resolve before inflating the balloon. Balloons

TABLE 10-2. *Medications given in the EC before transfer to catheter laboratory*

Aspirin	Nonenteric coated (325 mg), chewed [enteric-coated aspirin should be avoided, because of delayed absorption and bioavailibility (11,12)]. In patients unable to swallow aspirin, 250 mg can be administered intravenously (available overseas) or rectally.
Ticlopidine	500 mg used in stent PAMI protocols—ticlopidine and aspirin have a synergistic effect on reducing coronary platelet deposition; [ticlopidine 500 mg dose allows earlier anti-platelet effects (13–16)]. More recently, we have been using clopidogrel (300–450 mg) (14).
Heparin	Bolus 70–100 U/kg in EC
i.v. Beta-blockers	Metoprolol (5 mg) i.v. every 5 min for three doses if tolerated and if no contraindications. Additional doses can be given until the heart rate drops to the 60s. *Beta-blockers* are known to decrease arrhythmia in post MI patients (17). In AMI trials prior to thrombolytics, beta-blockers reduced mortality (ISIS-1, MIAMI) (18,19) and when used with thrombolytics (TIMI-2) reduced reinfarction and ischemia when administered on presentation (20,21). Beta-blockers were used in PAMI-2 and showed reduction of ventricular fibrillation (−3.5% vs. 6.7% in PAMI-1).

AMI, acute myocardial infarction; EC, emergency center; ISIS, International Study of Infarct Survival; i.v., intravenous; MIAMI, metoprolol in acute myocardial infarction; PAMI, primary angioplasty in myocardial infarction; TIMI, thrombolysis in myocardial infarction.

TABLE 10-3. *Contraindications to beta-blockers*

Heart rate <60 bpm
Systolic arterial pressure <100 mm Hg
Moderate or severe left ventricular failure
Signs of peripheral hypoperfusion
PR interval >0.24 sec
Second- or third-degree atrioventricular block
Severe chronic obstructive pulmonary disease or history
  of asthma requiring home oxygen or oral steroids

bpm, beats per minute.

should be upsized as necessary as the vessel caliber increases with restoration of flow (a balloon-to-artery ratio of 1:1). Care should be taken not to under dilate the lesion because this predisposes to reocclusion.

PTCA should be performed only in the infarct vessel. Multivessel PTCA should not be attempted. The only possible exception to this rule is cardiogenic shock. If after reperfusion of the infarct artery, the patient is still in shock and the hemodynamic status has not improved, severe stenoses in noninfarct arteries may be attempted in an effort to improve LV function.

Thrombolytics should be avoided because of their procoagulant effect (36–38). Randomized, placebo-controlled trials of thrombolytic drugs used in conjunction with PTCA have demonstrated a significant increase in cardiac events (39–45). However, in the era of newer pharmacotherapies and stents, thrombolytics may be better tolerated (46).

Treatment of no reflow is essential to achieve high rates of TIMI-3 flow. When slow flow occurs in the absence of residual stenosis or dissection, no reflow should be suspected and treated (Table 10-5).

Recurrent thrombosis occasionally happens, particularly in large patulous vessels, such as the right coronary artery (RCA) or a vein graft. Following primary PTCA, the vessel frequently appears hazy. Most of the time, the initiating event is a ruptured plaque; thus, one should not expect the vessel to look normal after primary PTCA. However, when globular filling defects are present, aggressive treatment should be undertaken (Table 10-6) (47–49).

TABLE 10-4. *Angiographic exclusions precluding performance of PTCA*

Unprotected left main coronary stenosis >60%
Infarct vessel with TIMI-3 flow and lesion morphology
  extremely high risk for abrupt closure or no reflow
Multivessel disease in a patient who has TIMI-3 flow, is
  pain-free, and whom the operator believes should
  undergo surgery.
Infarct vessel stenosis <70% with TIMI-3 flow
Infarct vessel with TIMI-3 flow if thrombolytics have been
  given
Infarct vessel supplies a very small amount of myocardium,
  in which the risk of PTCA may outweigh the benefit.
Inability to clearly identify the infarct-related artery.

PTCA, percutaneous transluminal coronary angioplasty;
TIMI, thrombolysis in myocardial infarction.

TABLE 10-5. *Management of no reflow*

May include one or more of the following:
  –Repeated boluses of intracoronary verapamil (100–
    200 μg (watch for bradycardia)
  —Repeated boluses of intracoronary adenosine (50 μg
    boluses until 200–1000 μg have been given). This is the
    favored method of managing no reflow in the patient with
    AMI because it can have the additional benefit of limiting
    infarct size.
  –Intracoronary nitroprusside (50 μg doses up to 200 μg
    total)
  –Abciximab may be potentially useful (47)
  –Placement of intraaortic balloon pump if blood pressure
    is low or multivessel disease is present

AMI, acute myocardial infarction.

Post-PTCA dissection has been found to be predictive of recurrent ischemia and early reocclusion (45). Appropriate management of dissection is essential to reduce these risks (Table 10-7).

STENTS

The indications for coronary stenting in acute MI are still evolving. Previously, an intracoronary thrombus was considered a contraindication to stenting. However, despite concerns about using stents in the setting of thrombus, the initial experience was favorable (6,50–52). These results likely were due to the ability of stents to achieve a large lumen and reduce dissection planes, both of which would reduce shear forces and platelet thrombus deposition. From the PAMI-2 database, we determined that the presence of dissection, or residual stenosis greater than 30% after PTCA was highly predictive of recurrent ischemic events (45,64). Both of these angiographic findings can be eliminated with stenting. Also, routine angiographic follow-up at 6 months has demonstrated reocclusion of an IRA in 10% to 15% and restenosis in 35% to 40% of patients. Given the large lumen achieved after stenting, it is assumed that stenting of patients with acute MI would also reduce these late complications (Table 10-8).

TABLE 10-6. *Management of thrombus*

Recheck activated clotting time to be sure it is >350 sec
  (29–35) or 250 sec if IIb/IIIa agent is used
Avoid nonionic contrast (22–24)
Avoid thrombolytics (39–45)
Perform prolonged, low pressure inflations
  with slightly oversized balloons
Stent if any associated dissection (45), but avoid in
  the setting of heavy thrombus because in myocardial
  infarction flow is generally worse after stenting (8)
Consider transluminal extraction (TEC) atherectomy
  if dissection is absent (48,49)
If dissection is present, consider TEC aspiration without
  cutting (power pack turned off), AngioJet, or aspiration
  with a deeply engaged guiding catheter
Consider bail-out abciximab bolus and infusion (47) or
  intracoronary abciximab

TABLE 10-7. *Management of dissection*

Prolonged, low pressure inflations (up to 15 min) with slightly oversized balloons
Coronary stenting if continued ischemia, slow flow, dissection or if stenosis >30% persists after·prolonged inflations

TABLE 10-9. *Exclusion criteria for stenting in AMI*

Vessel <3.0 mm or >4.5 mm in diameter
If stent would protrude to left main coronary artery
Likely occlusion of large side branch
Lesions longer than 30 mm
No reflow or huge thrombi (globular filling defects with length >2 times coronary diameter)
Vessel tortuosity or heavy calcification that may prohibit tracking or deployment

AMI, acute myocardial infarction.

Stent PAMI was designed to test the hypothesis that routine implantation of a stent versus primary PTCA alone would result in a larger lumen and would be associated with less restenosis and improved clinical outcomes at 6 months (8). The primary endpoint of the study was the composite incidence of death, nonfatal reinfarction, disabling stroke, or ischemia-driven TVR during the 6-month follow-up period. The combined endpoint was lower in the stent group (stent 12.6% vs. PTCA 20.1%, $p < 0.01$) because of the lower rate of revascularization for ischemia (ischemic TVR at 1 month 1.3% stent vs. 3.8% PTCA and at 6 months 7.7% vs. 17%, respectively). No differences were seen in other outcomes. The event rates were low in both groups, again confirming the effectiveness of percutaneous interventions (PCI) to treat acute MI, particularly when bail-out stenting was available in the PTCA arm. An interesting observation was made regarding TIMI flow. After the procedure, TIMI-3 flow was achieved in 89.4% patients in the stent group and 92.7% in PTCA group ($p = 0.1$). Moreover, a trend was seen for a higher mortality rate in the stent arm at 1 year (5.8% vs. 3.1% in the PTCA group; $p = 0.07$) (54). Also in the CADILLAC trial, the only advantage of stenting was reduction in TVR (Table 10-10). Because empiric stenting did not reduce the most important complications of acute MI (mortality, stroke, reinfarction), it would not be unreasonable to withold stent placement after achieving optimal results with PTCA alone (<30% residual stenosis and no dissection) (Table 10-9).

GLYCOPROTEIN IIB/IIIA PLATELET RECEPTOR INHIBITORS

Use of the GP IIb/IIIa antagonist in the setting of acute MI in combination with direct angioplasty was addressed in the ReoPro and Primary PTCA Organization and Randomized Trial (RAPPORT) (53). In this trial, 483 patients with acute MI were randomized to either placebo or abciximab followed by emergency cardiac catheterization with intent to perform direct angioplasty. The combined incidence of death, MI, and ischemia-driven TVR at 30 days was lower in patients treated

TABLE 10-8. *Consider routine stent in patients with high ischemic risk after PTCA for MI*

Residual stenosis $\geq$30%
Dissection refractory to prolonged inflation with slightly oversized balloon
Three-vessel disease

MI, myocardial infarction; PTCA, percutaneous transluminal coronary angioplasty.

with abciximab compared with placebo (5.8% vs. 11.1%; $p = 0.04$). These results were offset by the near doubling of the rate of bleeding. Major bleeding was increased in RAPPORT with abciximab treatment (16.6% in abciximab treated patients vs. 9.5% in controls) and most bleeding occurred at the vascular access site. Rates of transfusion were nearly doubled with abciximab treatment. The higher rate of bleeding relates to the fact that RAPPORT was designed in 1993 before adoption of guidelines for lower dose heparin use and for early vascular sheath removal. However, at 6 months in RAPPORT, the primary endpoint of the study—combined incidence of death, infarction or TVR—was similar in abciximab and placebo groups (28.2% vs. 28.1%; $p = 0.98$).

Adjunctive use of GP IIb/IIIa inhibitors for acute MI with and without routine coronary stent implantation was investigated in the ADMIRAL and CADILLAC trial (55). The CADILLAC study was designed as a 2×2 factorial randomization to abciximab versus placebo and multilink stent versus direct angioplasty alone during acute MI. The primary endpoint of the trial was the 6-month combined incidence of death, infarction, target lesion revascularization, or stroke. The 6 month report from CADILLAC was presented at the 2000 TCT scientific session (Table 10-10). The results demonstrated that abciximab reduced the in-hospital incidence of recurrent ischemia and ischemic TVR after primary PTCA and stenting. In contrast to the stent PAMI trial, stenting in AMI did not result in decreased TIMI-3 flow or survival compared to PTCA. Abciximab use was not associated with major clinical benefit in patients undergoing routine stent implantation. In the primary PTCA group, abciximab enhanced the primary endpoint outcome without reaching statistical significance.

ABCIXIMAB PROTOCOL IN CADILLAC

The abciximab protocol used in CADILLAC is as follows:

- Bolus: 0.25 mg/kg i.v. followed by 0.125 μg/kg/min infusion for 12 hours
- ACT 200–300 seconds in CL
- No postprocedural heparin
- Sheaths removed when ACT <170 seconds

INTRAAORTIC BALLOON PUMP

The multicenter PAMI-2 trial, which involved emergency catheterization and PTCA, stratified patients into high- and

TABLE 10-10. *CADILLAC 6-month events*

Published report	PTCA (%)	PTCA + Abciximab (%)	Stent (%)	Stent + Abciximab (%)
Mortality	4.3	2.3	2.8	3.8
Reinfarction	1.6	2.1	1.2	2.3
Ischemic TVR	14.2	12.1	7.4	5.0
Disabling stroke	0.8	0.8	1.2	1.7
Bleeding (transfusion)	3.1	5.1	3.5	4.5
TIMI-3 flow-final	94.9	96.1	93.8	96.1

CADILLAC, controlled abciximab and device investigation to lower late angioplasty complications; PTCA, percutaneous transluminal coronary angioplasty; TIMI, thrombolysis in myocardial infarction; TVR, target vessel revascularization.

low-risk groups. High-risk required one of the following attributes: Age >70 years, three-vessel disease, EF less than 45%, suboptimal PTCA, vein graft culprit, or persistent serious arrhythmias after angioplasty. Patients at high risk were randomized to receive IABP for 36 to 48 hours (n = 211) versus no IABP (n = 226). Although patients treated with IABP had a reduction in ischemia (11.6% vs. 17.8%; $p = 0.07$) and re-PTCA (8.2% vs. 14.2; $p = 0.05$), no reduction was seen in the predefined endpoints of death, recurrent MI, congestive heart failure (CHF), stroke, or in-hospital reocclusion (6.2% vs. 8%; $p = 0.46$) (4). These differences in recurrent ischemia and re-PTCA are also less important in the era of stenting. Although it has been hypothesized that because IABP placement augments coronary flow and reduces afterload, greater improvement in LV function may be observed. However, LV function at 1 and 6 weeks was similar between the two groups (4). In a post-hoc analysis, we found that if two or more high risk factors were present, IABP reduced the composite endpoint (primarily from a reduction in CHF) (5). Based on these data, we place stents for suboptimal PTCA results (stenosis >30% or dissection) that may predispose patients to recurrent ischemia and reserve IABP placement for other clinical indications (Table 10-11).

REPERFUSION ARRHYTHMIAS

Recanalization of an occluded coronary artery is often associated with cardiac rhythm disturbance. Profound hypotension and bradycardia caused by stimulation of afferent vagal

TABLE 10-11. *Indications for IABP placement*

Continued ischemia after reperfusion
Hypotension or congestive heart failure
Severe left ventricular dysfunction in the presence of
  severe multivessel disease
Mechanical defects—ventricular septal
  defect, severe mitral regurgitation

IABP, intraaortic balloon pump.

fibers (the Bezold-Jarisch reflex) is common during RCA intervention. Sudden ventricular fibrillation is also more frequent with reperfusion of the RCA (56).

In the PAMI-1 trial, ventricular fibrillation occurred in 6.7% of PTCA-treated patients and was more common in patients with inferior versus anterior MI (9.7% vs. 1.4%; $p = 0.03$) (2). Given animal studies showing a higher rate of arrhythmias with rapid versus slow reperfusion, and clinical studies demonstrating the ability of beta-blockers to reduce fatal arrhythmias in postinfarct patients, "slow" reperfusion along with i.v. beta-blockers was adopted in the PAMI-2 study. This resulted in a significant reduction in ventricular fibrillation in PAMI-2 compared with PAMI-1 (3.5% vs. 6.7%; $p = 0.01$). Although data are limited in PTCA reperfusion trials, based on our experience, we recommend the following methods of avoiding and treating reperfusion arrhythmias (Table 10-12):

- Beta-blockade i.v. before PCI
- Low osmolar contrast in patients with arrhythmias or severe LV dysfunction
- Continuous monitoring of O_2 saturation using pulse oximeter
- Adequate hydration before reperfusion of RCA
- Correction of metabolic abnormalities
- "Slow" reperfusion with the wire or dottering with the balloon, allowing reperfusion arrhythmias to resolve before balloon inflation
- 5 F sheath central venous access allowing for rapid temporary pacemaker placement before reperfusion of proximal RCA occlusions if the vessel appears to be large, patulous, or thrombus laden

Data from our studies and others indicate that less than 1% of patients require emergent bypass surgery for failed primary PTCA. Of patients presenting with acute MI, 3% to 5% are referred for surgery for left main or three-vessel coronary disease (58). Because of the low prevalence of emergency surgery when primary PTCA is performed, surgeons are not notified and no formal surgical backup is required. Surgeons are notified only in cases of the above scenario,

TABLE 10-12. *Management of arrhythmias in the catheterization laboratory*

Support head of table if CPR is performed (ineffective CPR can occur due to "diving board effect" of the pedestal table)
Prophylactic lidocaine should not be used[a]
V-fibrillation: Prompt defibrillation and CPR
V-tachycardia: Shock only if associated with hypotension
Bradyarrhythmias: If persistent, use atropine, temporary pacer
Persistent bradycardia and hypotension (Bezold–Jarisch reflex): High-dose atropine (3–5 mg) i.v. push, temporary pacemaker, and metaraminol (Aramine) (0.5–5 mg) i.v. push

Criteria for surgery
　Failed angioplasty with ongoing ischemia
　Severe left main stenosis
　High-risk anatomy not amenable to PTCA

CPR, Cardiopulmonary resuscitation, i.v., intravenous; PTCA, percutaneous transluminal coronary angioplasty.
[a]Metaanalysis of 15 trials evaluating the usefulness of prophylactic lidocaine in 8,745 patients found no benefit. Indeed, mortality was greater in the treated group (57).

and if ischemia cannot be stabilized by other means (i.e., stent, balloon pump, medications). An emerging practice in some community hospitals in the United States is to perform primary PTCA without surgical backup. Reports indicate that the lack of in-house cardiac surgery does not appear to result in worsened outcomes (59–66). The success of these programs depends on having experienced interventionists who routinely perform elective PTCA at tertiary centers, experienced staff, a well-equipped laboratory, and established protocols for transfer to surgical centers.

POSTPROCEDURAL CARE

Admission Route

After coronary intervention patients should be classified into high or low-risk according to PAMI-2 clinical and angiographic criteria (Fig. 10-2). Patients at low risk [age <70 years, EF >45%, <three-vessel CAD, successful intervention, no saphenous vein graft (SVG) occlusion, no persistent ventricular arrhythmias] can be safely transferred to a step-down unit rather than the CCU and discharge targeted to day 3, without predischarge testing. Patients at high risk should be admitted to the CCU, targeting discharge to day 5–7 (Fig. 10-3) (4,5,82).

Vascular Access and Anticoagulation

Vascular sheaths should be removed 4 to 24 hours after the procedure. Early sheath removal is strongly recommended. Approximately four hours before planned removal of vascular sheaths, i.v. heparin should be stopped. An ACT ± 170 seconds or less should be demonstrated just before sheath removal. If the GP IIb/IIIa inhibitors are being used, heparin should not be restarted after the procedure. Anticoagulation can be restarted 1 to 4 hours later at the discretion of the treating physician if the patient has clinical indications for anticoagulation (after larger MI, poor LV function, residual thrombus, prolonged bed rest). Heparin should be discontinued 48 to 72 hours later. Patients who have received heparin for 48 hours are at increased risk of a rebound hypercoaguable state when heparin is discontinued (67–71). We taper to half-dose for 12 hours before discontinuation in hopes of reducing this risk. Alternatively, low molecular weight heparin can be used to avoid the rebound

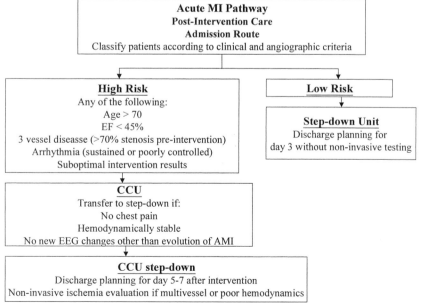

FIG. 10-2.

phenomenon. Longer duration heparin, coumadin, or both are considerations in patients with severe LV dysfunction, mural thrombus, atrial fibrillation, and so on. However, coumadin is not routinely recommended, and given the potential procoagulant effect (72), we are more likely to discharge patients on subcutaneous low molecular weight heparin if post-PTCA anticoagulation is necessary for a short time.

Medications (See Table 10-13)

The benefit of long-term aspirin use in postinfarct patients has been proved in many randomized trials (12).

Platelet ADP inhibitors (ticlopidine and clopidogrel) used with aspirin for 2 to 4 weeks after stent implantation significantly reduce the incidence of stent thrombosis (13,14).

The rationale for the early use of angiotensin converting enzyme (ACE) inhibitors in the course of MI is derived from several large-scale clinical trials. In the ISIS-4 trial, 58,000 patients with suspected acute MI were randomly assigned within the first 24 hours (median 8 hours) to receive either oral captopril or placebo (73). A significant reduction in a 5-week mortality rate was observed among those randomized to captopril. The largest benefit was among those with an anterior infarction. The GISSI-3 trial randomized 19,000 patients with either ST-segment elevation or depression to oral lisinopril or control (74). A significant reduction in 6-week mortality rate was seen, with 60% of the lives saved during the first 5 days of treatment. In the Survival of Myocardial Infarction Long-Term Evaluation (SMILE) study, 1,556

Medical Management Post-Intervention

- Heparin should be stopped post-procedure for sheath removal
- Vascular sheaths should be removed when ACT<170 sec
- Restart Heparin (if indicated) 4 hours after hemostasis achieved for total 48-72 hours (ACT 160-190)
- ½ dose of Heparin drip for 12 hours prior to discontinuation OR low molecular weight Heparin if longer anticoagulation required
- No Heparin post-procedure if GP IIb/IIIa inhibitors given
- Medications for all AMI patients if no contraindications:
  - Aspirin 325 mg po QD
  - Beta-blockers
  - Clopidogrel/Ticlopidine after stent for 4 weeks
  - ACE inhibitor from day one for 6 weeks (then according to EF)
  - HMG-CoA reductase inhibitor for LDL > 100 mg/dl
- 2-D echo if not done in EC
- Teaching/handouts/discharge instructions:
  - MI booklet
  - Activity guidelines
  - Cardiac rehabilitation
  - When to call 911
  - Use of NTG sl
  - Cardiac diet packet
  - Smoking cessation counseling
  - STENT patients: stent booklet

FIG. 10-3.

TABLE 10-13. *Postprocedural care*

Aspirin	325 mg po q.d. should be continued indefinitely (12)
Ticlopidine/clopidogrel	Ticlopidine 250 mg b.i.d. or clopidogrel 75 mg q.d. if stent has been placed or PTCA result is suboptimal for 4 wk (loading dose should be given in EC or CL) (13,14)
Beta-blockers	If no contraindications: —Metoprolol 50 mg po b.i.d. × 2, then 100 mg b.i.d. —Atenolol 100 mg po q.d. —Propranolol 60 mg po t.i.d. —Timolol 20 mg po q.d.
ACE inhibitors	Should be started on day 1 and continued for 6 wk in all AMI patients. At that time, if EF >40% they can be stopped (however in view of HOPE trial results, long-term ramipril 10 mg q.d. should be considered in diabetics or in all patients with CAD) (76). If EF <40%, ACE inhibitors should be continued indefinitely: —Captopril 50 mg po t.i.d. —Lisinopril 10 mg po q.d. —Ramipril 10 mg po q.d.
Calcium blockers and antiarrhythmics	Not routinely recommended
Low molecular weight heparin	If longer anticoagulation is desired Enoxaparin (Lovenox) 1 mg/kg b.i.d. subcutaneously

ACE, angiotension-converting enzyme; AMI, acute myocardial infarction; CAD, coronary artery disease; CL, catheterization laboratory; EC, emergency center; EF, ejection fraction; HOPE, Heart Outcomes Prevention Evaluation; PTCA, percutaneous transluminal coronary angioplasty; b.i.d., twice a day; po, by mouth; q.d., every day; t.i.d., three times a day.

patients with anterior MI who had not received reperfusion therapy were randomly assigned within 24 hours to receive either placebo or zofenopril (75). After 1 year of observation, the mortality rate was still significantly lower in the zofenopril group versus placebo group. All trials in which only oral ACE inhibitors were used demonstrated survival benefit in mortality. Data from these trials indicate that oral ACE inhibitors should generally be started within the first 24 hours, after reperfusion has been completed and blood pressure has stabilized. If tolerated, the ACE inhibitors should be continued for 6 weeks regardless of LV function. ACE inhibitors should not be used if systolic blood pressure is less than 100 mm Hg (unless a high systemic vascular resistance is documented by right ventricle catheterization), if clinically relevant renal failure is present (creatinine >3.0), with a history of bilateral renal arteries stenosis, or a known allergy. ACE inhibitor therapy should start with low-dose oral administration and increase steadily to achieve a full dose within 48 to 72 hours.

Calcium channel blockers have not been shown to reduce mortality after MI. Likewise, nifedipine does not reduce the incidence of reinfarction or mortality when given early (<24 hours) or late after acute MI. Immediate release nifedipine can be hazardous when given to patients with pulmonary congestion (77–81).

INDICATIONS FOR REPEAT CATHETERIZATION

Suspected Reocclusion

Patients with pain relief and resolution of ECG changes who later develop chest pain with reelevation of ST segments should be considered for emergency catheterization.

Recurrent Ischemia

Patients with recurrent ischemia should be considered for emergency catheterization. This is defined as recurrent symptoms lasting more than 20 minutes, despite nitrate therapy and either (a) new ST-segment changes or deep T-wave inversion on a 12-lead ECG; (b) new hypotension, pulmonary edema, or holosystolic murmur; or (c) hemodynamic instability.

REFERENCES

1. Weaver DW, Simes JR, Betriu A, et al. Comparison of primary coronary angioplasty and intravenous thrombolytic therapy for acute myocardial infarction. A quantitative review. *JAMA* 1997;278:2093–2098.
2. Grines CL, Browne KF, Marco J, et al. A comparison of immediate angioplasty with thrombolytic therapy for acute myocardial infarction. *N Engl J Med* 1993;328:673–679.
3. Nunn CM, O'Neill WW, Rothbaum D, et al. Long term outcome after primary angioplasty: report from primary angioplasty in myocardial infarction (PAMI-1) trial. *J Am Coll Cardiol* 1999;33:640–646.
4. Grines CL, Brodie BR, Griffin JJ, et al. Prophylactic intra-aortic balloon pumping for acute myocardial infarction does not improve left ventricular function. *J Am Coll Cardiol* 1996;27:167A.
5. Stone GW, Marsalese D, Brodie BR, et al. The routine use of intra-aortic balloon pumping after primary PTCA improves clinical outcomes in very high-risk patients with acute myocardial infarction—results of the PAMI-2 trial. *Circulation* 1995;92:I-139.
6. Stone GW, Brodie BR, Morice MC, et al. For the PAMI Stent Pilot Trial Investigators. Primary stenting in acute myocardial infarction: design and interim results of the PAMI stent pilot trial. *J Invasive Cardiol* 1997;9[Suppl B]:24B–30B.
7. Stone GW, Brodie BR, Griffin JJ, et al. A prospective, multi-center study of the safety and feasibility of primary stenting in acute myocardial infarction: in hospital and 30 day results of the PAMI stent pilot trial. *J Am Coll Cardiol* 1998;31:23–30.
8. Grines CL, Cox DA, Stone GW, et al. Coronary angioplasty with or without stent implantation for acute myocardial infarction. *N Engl J Med* 1999;341:1949–1956.
9. Every NR, Parsons LS, Hlatky M, et al. A comparison of thrombolytic therapy with primary coronary angioplasty for acute myocardial infarction. Myocardial Infarction Triage and Intervention Investigators. *N Engl J Med* 1996;335:1253–1260.
10. Hochman JS, Sleeper LA, Webb JG, et al., for the SHOCK investigators. Early revascularization in acute myocardial infarction complicated by cardiogenic shock. *N Engl J Med* 1999;341:625–634.
11. Lacoste L, Lam JUT, Letchacovski G. Comparative antithrombotic efficacy of aspirin: 80 mg vs. 325 mg daily. *Circulation* 1994;90:I-552.
12. Becker RC. Antiplatelet therapy in coronary heart disease: emerging strategies for the treatment and prevention of acute myocardial infarction. *Arch Pathol Lab Med* 1993;117:89–96.
13. Leon MB. A clinical trial comparing three antithrombotic drug regimens after coronary artery stenting. STARS investigators. *N Engl J Med* 1998;339:1665–1671.
14. Muller C. A randomized comparison of clopidogrel and aspirin versus ticlopidine and aspirin after the placement of coronary artery stents. *Circulation* 2000;101:590–593.
15. Jeong M, Owen W, Staab M, et al. Does ticlopidine affect platelet deposition and acute stent thrombosis? *Circulation* 1995;92:I-489.
16. Gregorini L, Marco J, Fajadet J, et al. Ticlopidine alternate post-angioplasty thrombin generation. *Circulation* 1995;92:I-608.
17. Deedwania P. *Beta-blockers and cardiac arrhythmia*. New York: Marcel Dekker, 1992.
18. First International Study of Infarct Survival Collaborative Group. Randomized trial of intravenous atenolol among 16,027 cases of suspected acute myocardial infarction: ISIS-1. *Lancet* 1986;2:57–66.
19. The MIAMI Trial Research Group. Metoprolol in acute myocardial infarction: patient population. *Am J Cardiol* 1985;56:1G–57G.
20. The TIMI Study Group. Comparison of invasive and conservative strategies after treatment with intravenous tissue plasminogen activator in acute myocardial infarction: results of the thrombolysis in myocardial infarction (TIMI) phase II trial. *N Engl J Med* 1989;320:618–627.
21. Yusuf S, Peto R, Lewis J, et al. Beta blockade during and after myocardial infarction: an overview of the randomized trials. *Prog Cardiovasc Dis* 1985;27:335–371.
22. Piessens JH, Stammen F, Brolix MC, et al. Effects of an ionic versus a non-ionic low osmolar contrast agent on the thrombotic complications of coronary angioplasty. *Cathet Cardiovasc Diagn* 1993;28:99–105.
23. Aguirre F, Topol EJ, Donohue T. Impact of ionic and non-ionic contrast media on post PTCA ischemic complications: results from the EPIC trial. *J Am Coll Cardiol* 1995;25:8A.
24. Grines CL, Schreiber T, Savas V, et al. A randomized trial of low osmolar ionic versus non-ionic contrast media in patients with acute myocardial infarction or unstable angina undergoing PTCA. *J Am Coll Cardiol* 1996;27:1381–1386.
25. Grines CL. Contrast media: is there a preferable agent for coronary interventions? *J Am Coll Cardiol* 1997;29:1122–1123.
26. Batchelor WB, Granger CB, Kleiman NS. A comparison of ionic versus nonionic contrast medium during primary percutenous transluminal coronary angioplasty for acute myocardial infarction (GUSTO IIb). *Am J Cardiol* 2000;85:692–697.
27. Alexander JH, Kong DF, Cantor WJ. Highlights from the 72nd American Heart Association scientific sessions. Contrast media utilization in high risk PTCA (COURT). *Am Heart J* 1999;137:175–190.
28. Esplugas E, Cequier A, Jara R. Comparison of ionic and nonionic low osmolar contrast media in relation to thrombotic complications of angioplasty in patients with unstable angina. *Am Heart J* 1998;135:1067–1075.
29. Ferguson J, Dougherty K, Gaos C, et al. Relation between procedural activate coagulation time and outcome after percutaneous transluminal coronary angioplasty. *J Am Coll Cardiol* 1994;23:1061–1065.

30. Snitzer R, Hiremath Y, Lee J, et al. Suppression of intracoronary thrombin activity by weight-adjusted administration during coronary interventions. *Circulation* 1995;92:I-609.

31. Winters K, Oltrona L, Hiremath Y, et al. Heparin-resistant thrombin activity is associated with acute ischemic events during high-risk coronary interventions. *Circulation* 1995;92:I-608.

32. Harrington RA, Leimberer JD, Berdan L, et al., for the CAVEAT Investigators. The ACT index: a method for stratifying likelihood of success and risk of acute complications in coronary intervention. *Circulation* 1993;88:I-208.

33. Naqvi T, Ivy P, Linn P, et al. Low dose heparin enhances and high dose heparin suppresses platelet P-selection expression and platelet aggregation. *Circulation* 1995;92:I-693.

34. Ahmed W, Meckel C, Grines CL, et al. Relation between ischemic complications and activated clotting times during coronary angioplasty: different profiles for heparin and hirulog. *Circulation* 1995;92:I-608.

35. Narins CR, Hillegass WG, Nelson CL, et al. Relation between activated clotting time during angioplasty and abrupt closure. *J Am Coll Cardiol* 1994;23:470A.

36. Kerins DM, Roy L, Fitzgerald DJ. Platelet and vascular function during coronary thrombolysis with tissue-type plasminogen activator. *Circulation* 1989;80:1718.

37. Bennet WR, Yawn DH, Miliore PJ, et al. Activation of the complement system by recombinant tissue plasminogen activator. *J Am Coll Cardiol* 1987;10:627.

38. Fitzgerald DJ, Roy L, Wright F, et al. Functional significance of platelet activation following coronary thrombolysis. *Circulation* 1987;76:IV-153.

39. Spielberg C, Schnitzer L, Linderer T, et al. Influence of catheter technology and adjuvant medication on acute complications in percutaneous coronary angioplasty. *Cathet Cardiovasc Diagn* 1990;21:72.

40. Ambrose JA, Torre SR, Sharma SK, et al. Adjuvant urokinase for PTCA in unstable angina: final angiographic results of TAUSA pilot study. *Circulation* 1991;84:II-590.

41. Ambrose JA, Almeida OD, Sharma SK, et al. For the TAUSA Investigators. Adjunctive thrombolytic therapy during angioplasty for ischemic rest angina. Results of the TAUSA trial. *Circulation* 1994;90:69–77.

42. Mehran R, Ambrose JA, Bongu RM, et al. For the TAUSA study group. Angioplasty of complex lesions in ischemic rest angina: results of the thrombolysis and angioplasty in unstable angina (TAUSA) trial. *J Am Coll Cardiol* 1995;26:961–966.

43. Buller CE, Fung AY, Thompson CR, et al. Does pre-treatment with tPA improve safety of coronary angioplasty in acute coronary syndrome? Results from TIMI-IIIB. *Circulation* 1995;90:I-22.

44. O'Neill WW, Weintraub R, Grines CL, et al. A prospective placebo-controlled randomized trial of intravenous streptokinase and angioplasty therapy for acute myocardial infarction. *Circulation* 1992;86:1710–1717.

45. Grines CL, Brodie BR, Griffin J, et al. Which primary PTCA patients may benefit from new technologies? *Circulation* 1995;92:I-146.

46. Ross AM, Coyne KS, Reiner JS, et al. A randomized trial comparing primary angioplasty with a strategy of short-acting thrombolysis and immediate planned rescue angioplasty in acute myocardial infarction: the PACT trial. *J Am Coll Cardiol* 1999;34:1954–1962.

47. Muhlestein JB, Gomez M, Karagounish L, et al. Rescue ReoPro: acute utilization of abciximab for dissolution of coronary thrombus developing as a complication of coronary angioplasty. *Circulation* 1995;92:I-607.

48. Kaplan BM, Safian RD, Grines CL, et al. Usefulness of adjunctive angioplasty and extraction atherectomy before stent implantation in high-risk aortocoronary saphenous vein grafts. *Am J Cardiol* 1995;76:822–824.

49. Kaplan BM, Larkin T, Hoffman M, et al. A prospective clinical trial of extraction atherectomy in high risk acute myocardial infarction patients. *Am J Cardiol* 1996;78:383–388.

50. Levy G, deBoisgelin X, Volpiliere R, et al. Intracoronary stenting in direct infarct angioplasty: is it dangerous? *Circulation* 1995;92:1–139.

51. Neuman F, Walter H, Schmitt C, et al. Coronary stenting as an adjunct to direct balloon angioplasty in acute myocardial infarction. *Circulation* 1992;92:I-609.

52. Monassier JP, Elias J, Meyer P, et al. STENTIMI I: the French Registry of stenting at acute myocardial infarction. *J Am Coll Cardiol* 1996;27:86A.

53. Brener SJ, Barr LA, Burchenal JE, et al. Randomized, placebo-controlled trial of platelet glycoprotein IIb/IIIa blockade with primary angioplasty for acute myocardial infarction: the RAPPORT trial. *Circulation* 1998;98:734–741.

54. Grines CL, Cox DA, Stone GW, et al. Stent PAMI: 12-month results and predictors of mortality. Oral presentation at the ACC 49 Annual Scientific Session, Anaheim, CA. *J Am Coll Cardiol* 2000;35:900–901(abst).

55. Montalscot G, Barragan P, Wittenberg O, et al. Abciximab associated with primary angioplasty and stenting in acute myocardial infarction: the ADMIRAL study, 30-day final results. *Circulation* 1999;100[Suppl I]:I-87a(abst).

56. Kaplan B, Safian RD, Grines CL, et al. Differences in outcome after angioplasty for AMI: the left anterior descending artery vs. the right coronary. *J Am Coll Cardiol* 1996;27:166A.

57. Lau J, Antman EM, Jiminez-Silva J, et al. Cumulative meta-analysis of therapeutic trials for myocardial infarction. *N Engl J Med* 1992;327:248–254.

58. O'Neill WW, Brodie BR, Ivanhoe R, et al. Primary coronary angioplasty for acute myocardial infarction (The Primary Angioplasty Registry). *Am J Cardiol* 1994;73:627–634.

59. Weaver WD, Litwin PE, Martin JS. Use of direct angioplasty for treatment of patients with acute myocardial infarction in hospitals with and without on-site cardiac surgery. *Circulation* 1993:88:2067–2075.

60. Weaver WD, Parsons L, Martin JS, et al. Direct PTCA for treatment of acute myocardial infarction: a community experience in hospitals with and without surgical backup. *Circulation* 1995;92:I-138.

61. Wharton T, McNamara N, Schmitz J, et al. The value of immediate coronary angiography with primary PTCA standby in the triage and treatment of acute myocardial infarction at community hospitals without heart surgery: experience in 305 cases. *J Am Coll Cardiol* 1996;27:250A.

62. Wharton TP, Jhonston JD, Turco MA, et al. Primary angioplasty for acute myocardial infarction at hospitals with no surgery on-site: the prospective multicenter PAMI-No SOS registry. *J Am Coll Cardiol* 1998;31[Suppl A]:210A.

63. Klinke WP, Hui W. Percutaneous transluminal coronary angioplasty without on-site surgical facilities. *Am J Cardiol* 1992;70:1520–1525.

64. Wharton T, Mrasalese D, Brodie B, et al. How often do infarct-related arteries show early perfusion without prior thrombolytic therapy, and should these vessels be dilated acutely? Results from PAMI-2. *Circulation* 1995;92:I-530.

65. Ayres M. Coronary angioplasty for acute myocardial infarction in hospitals without cardiac surgery. *J Invasive Cardiol* 1995;7:40F–46F.

66. Weaver WD, Parsons L, Every N. Primary coronary angioplasty in hospitals with and without surgery backup. *J Invasive Cardiol* 1995;7:34F–39F.

67. Granger C, Armstrong P, for the GUSTO IIa investigators. Reinfarction following discontinuation of intravenous heparin or hirudin for unstable angina and acute myocardial infarction. *Circulation* 1995;92:I-460.

68. Granger C, Miller J, Bovill E, et al. Rebound increase in thrombin generation and activity after cessation of intravenous heparin in patients with acute coronary syndromes. *Circulation* 1995;91:1929–1935.

69. Flather M, Weitz J, Campeau J, et al. Evidence for rebound activation of the coagulation system after cessation of intravenous anticoagulant therapy for acute MI. *Circulation* 1995;92:I485.

70. Stony J, Ahmed W, Meckel C, et al. Clinical evidence for thrombin rebound after stopping heparin but not hirulog. *Circulation* 1995;92:I-609.

71. Khan M, Sepulveda J, Jeroudi M, et al. Rebound increase in thrombin activity with associated decrease in antithrombin III levels after PTCA. *Circulation* 1995;92:I-785.

72. Schomeg A, Neumann FJ, Kastrati A, et al. A randomized comparison of antiplatelet and anticoagulant therapy after the placement of coronary artery stents. *N Engl J Med* 1996;328:1084–1089.

73. ISIS-4: a randomized factorial trial assessing early oral captopril, oral mononitrate, and intravenous magnesium sulphate in 58,050 patients with suspected acute myocardial infarction. ISIS-4 (Fourth International Study of Infarct Survival) Collaborative Group. *Lancet* 1995;345:669–685.

74. GISSI-3: effects of lisinopril and transdermal glyceryl trinitrate singly and together on 6-week mortality and ventricular function after acute myocardial infarction: Gruppo Italiano per lo Studio della Sopravvivenza nelll'infarto Miocardico. *Lancet* 1994;343:1115–1122.

75. Ambrosioni E, Borghi C, Magnani B. The effect of the angiotensin-converting-enzyme inhibitor zofenopril on mortality and morbidity after anterior myocardial infarction: the survival of myocardial infarction: long-term evaluation (SMILE) study investigators. *N Engl J Med* 1995;332:80–85.

76. Yusuf S, Sleight P, Pogue J, et al. Effects of an angiotensin-converting-enzyme inhibitor, ramapril, on cardiovascular events in high-risk patients. The heart outcomes prevention evaluation study investigators. *N Engl J Med* 2000;342:145–153.

77. Furberg CD, Psaty BM, Mayer JV. Nifedipine: dose-related increase in mortality in patients with coronary heart disease. *Circulation* 1995;92:1326–1331.

78. Muller JE, Morrison J, Stone PH, et al. Nifedipine therapy for patients with threatened and acute myocardial infarction: a randomized, double-blind, placebo-controlled comparison. *Circulation* 1984;69:740–747.

79. Sirnes PA, Overskeid K, Pedersen TR, et al. Evolution of infarct size during the early use of nifedipine in patients with acute myocardial infarction: the Norwegian nifedipine multicenter trial. *Circulation* 1984;70:638–644.

80. The Israeli Sprint Study Group. Secondary prevention reinfarction Israeli nifedipine trial (SPRINT): a randomized intervention trial of nifedipine in patients with acute myocardial infarction. *Eur Heart J* 1988;9:354–364.

81. Opie LH, Messerli FH. Nifedipine and mortality: grave defects in the dossier. *Circulation* 1995;92:1068–1073.

82. Brodie BR. Early hospital discharge after acute myocardial infarction. *Journal of Invasive Cardiology* 1995;7[Suppl F]:22F–28F.

CHAPTER 11

Complicated Myocardial Infarction

Richard C. Becker

Acute coronary syndromes (ACS), in general, and acute myocardial infarction (MI), in particular, are best defined as atherothrombotic disorders of the coronary arterial system. Although the underlying pathoanatomic substrate exhibits features of chronicity developing slowly over decades, the defining events of plaque disruption, intraluminal thrombosis, and distal embolization are acute and occur suddenly and often without warning. For this reason, clinicians involved directly in the management of patients with ACS must be well versed in a broad range of diagnostic and treatment strategies to provide rapidly the highest possible level of care and to achieve optimal outcomes.

Acute MI is not infrequently complicated by potentially lethal events that can be categorized as vascular (recurrent coronary thrombosis or mural thromboembolism), myocardial or mechanical (ventricular dilation, aneurysm formation, pump failure, ventricular septal rupture, papillary muscle rupture, free-wall rupture), pericardial (pericarditis), and electrical (heart block, bradyarrhythmias, tachyarrhythmias) (Table 11-1) (Fig. 11-1). Most complications occur within the initial 72 hours of infarction; however, the early risk period extends to include the first 4 to 6 weeks.

Critical pathways, which represent an ideal means to facilitate consistently high levels of care among patients with complicated MI, are highlighted in this chapter.

SETTING THE STAGE FOR COMPLICATIONS

Fundamental Concepts

Acute MI, caused most often by coronary arterial thrombosis that impairs myocardial blood flow and tissue perfusion and less commonly as a result of excessive myocardial oxygen demand, is defined pathologically as an irreversible change or death of an individual cell (myocyte) or, in most cases, group of cells. The necrotic process can be identified approximately 6 hours from the onset of myocardial hypoperfusion and is characterized initially by a heavy infiltration of neutrophils that persists for approximately 48 hours. Within 7 days of infarction, the myocardium thins as necrotic tissue is steadily removed by mononuclear cells and

phagocytes. Granulation tissue infiltrates the involved region 1 week later and, in essence, covers the entire area by 3 to 4 weeks. Over time (typically within 12 to 16 weeks), the zone of infarction contracts to become a thin, white, firm scar (1–4).

Cellular Characteristics of Wound Healing

The infiltration of inflammatory cells, an immediate response to tissue injury in acute MI, includes neutrophils, lymphocytes, macrophages, and fibroblasts. Collagen degradation, also an early response to myocardial necrosis, involves matrix metalloproteases (MMP) that reside within the myocardium in latent forms (5–8). The abrupt release of inflammatory mediators and MMP contribute to coronary arterial thrombosis and plaque instability, respectively, providing, at least in part, one explanation for the heightened propensity for thromboembolic events that persists following the initial event. These same mediators may also play a role in toxic apoptosis (programmed myocyte death). The inflammatory infiltrate coupled with a significant degree of surrounding edema creates a profound effect on electrical conduction and refractory periods. Beyond the "irritability" of necrotic myocardium that can cause automatic ventricular arrhythmias, the differing characteristics of injured and healthy myocardium existing "side-by-side" create "dispersion of refractoriness" and the substrate for reentrant ventricular arrhythmias, including ventricular tachycardia and ventricular fibrillation. Lastly, collagenase activity within the myocardium, although designed to permit "rebuilding" of the damaged area, may initially weaken the infarct zone, increasing the risk of cardiac rupture.

The fibrous stage of wound healing follows the initial inflammatory stage. Increased synthesis of fibrillar type III collagen and, over the subsequent days to weeks, type I collagen, provides an organized scaffold for scar development that follows. It is during this stage that most myocardial remodeling takes place, including expansion of both the infarct- and noninfarct-related zones, leading to aneurysm formation and ventricular dilation.

TABLE 11-1. *Complications of acute myocardial infarction*

Vascular complications
–Recurrent ischemia
–Recurrent infarction

Myocardial complications
–Diastolic dysfunction
–Systolic dysfunction
–Congestive heart failure
–Hypotension/cardiogenic shock
–Right ventricular infarction
–Ventricular cavity dilation
–Aneurysm formation (true, false)

Mechanical complications
–Left ventricular free wall rupture
–Ventricular septal rupture
–Papillary muscle rupture with acute mitral regurgitation

Pericardial complications
–Pericarditis
–Dressler's syndrome
–Pericardial effusion

Thromboembolic complications
–Mural thrombosis
–Systemic thromboembolism
–Deep vein thrombosis
–Pulmonary embolism

Electrical complications
–Ventricular tachycardia
–Ventricular fibrillation
–Supraventricular tachyarrhythmias
–Bradyarrhythmias
–Atrioventricular block (1, 2, or 3 degrees)

In the final stage, fibrillar fibronectin and collagen are deposited and by 4 to 6 weeks most of the necrotic myocardium has been removed and replaced by fibrous scar tissue. As with the initial or inflammatory stage, the late scarring stage is characterized by marked heterogeneity of repolarization and refractory periods, creating a permissive environment for malignant arrhythmias.

EARLY RISK CHARACTERIZATION

A vital component of clinical practice and critical care medicine is an ability to anticipate complications either of the MI itself or of its treatment. The development and utilization of risk assessment scales facilitates a response to potentially life-threatening events and represents the logical "first" step in patient-specific management pathways.

Identification of Patients at High Risk

Early Clinical Phase

Risk stratification schemes for patients with ST-segment elevation MI have been developed by several experienced clinical trial groups, highlighting the importance of patients demographics, medical history, clinical features, and the presenting electrocardiogram (ECG). The Thrombolysis in Myocardial Infarction (TIMI) study investigators (9)

established a risk score that predicted, with considerable accuracy, the occurrence of early morbidity and mortality.

Predictors of early (30-day) mortality were also established by the GUSTO (Global Utilization of Streptokinase and tPA for Occluded Coronary Arteries) investigators (10). In a trial including more than 40,000 patients with acute MI, age was identified as the most significant factor, with death rates of 1.1% in the youngest decile (<45 years) and 20.5% in patients more than 75 years of age. Overall, five characteristics contained 90% of the prognostic information in the baseline clinical data—they included age, lower systolic blood pressure, higher Killip class, elevated heart rate, and anterior site of infarction (Figs. 11-2 and 11-3).

The National Registry of Myocardial Infarction (NRMI) risk assessment assignment was developed as a readily available, bedside clinical "scorecard" for rapid triage and management. Predictors of adverse in-hospital clinical outcomes were identified from more than 100,000 patients with MI (11).

Presenting Surface Electrocardiogram

Clinicians have recognized for some time that the sum of ST-segment "shifts" on the presenting ECG is a reliable marker of infarction size and, as a result, can provide important diagnostic (and prognostic) information. The initial ECG may also contain evidence of a prior MI, identifying patients at increased risk for an early adverse outcome (12) (Fig. 11-4). ST-segment area also provides prognostic information.

Cardiac Enzyme Analysis

Biochemical markers of myocardial necrosis have been used to approximate infarction size and, in general, provide an estimate of outcome. The alteration of pharmacokinetics, particularly for creatine kinase (CK), following coronary reperfusion has complicated the picture somewhat. In essence, when calculated correctly, the "area under the curve" does provide prognostic information, but this measurement requires time (serial CK determinations) and effort.

The prognostic value of cardiac-specific troponin T and I among patients with unstable angina and non–ST-segment elevation MI is recognized; however, data from the Global Use of Strategies To open Occluded Arteries (GUSTO) IIA trial (13) also suggest that an elevated troponin T (>0.1 ng/ml) on hospital presentation correlates strongly and independently with hospital mortality among patients with ST-segment elevation MI.

Inflammatory Markers

The measurement of inflammatory markers represents an important tool that links the triad of atherosclerosis, inflammation, and thrombosis. Recent observations with the acute phase reactant amyloid A protein, in all likelihood will open the door to a vast array of markers that ultimately can be used to determine the "activity" of disease and direct response to treatment (14).

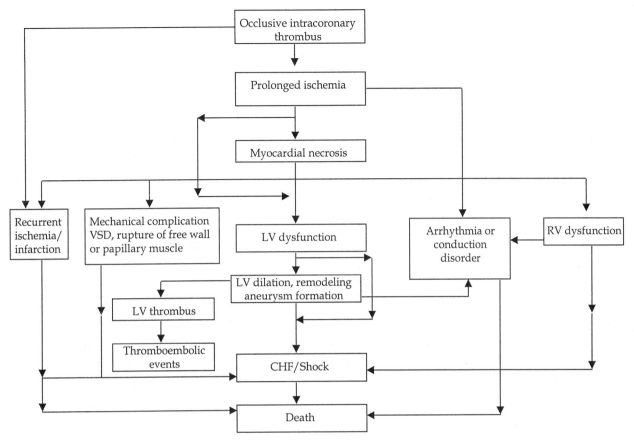

FIG.11-1. Pathobiologic and clinical sequence of events in myocardial infarction.

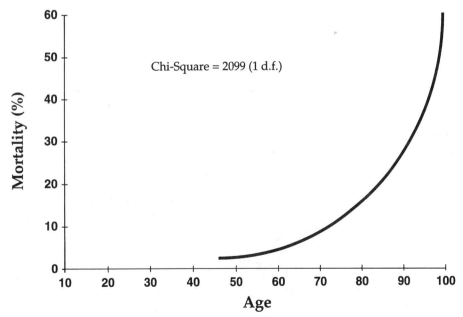

FIG. 11-2. Relationship between age and mortality (30-day) in the Global Utilization of Streptokinase and tPA for Occluded Coronary Arteries (GUSTO)-1 study. (From Anderson RD, Ohman EM. Successful identification and management of high-risk patients with acute myocardial infarction. *J Thromb Thrombolysis* 1996;3:271–278; with permission.)

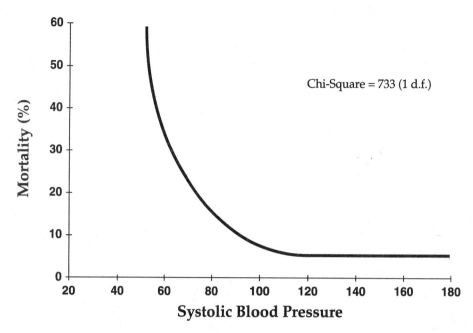

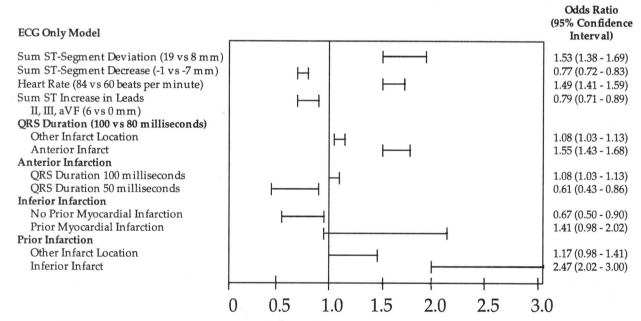

FIG. 11-3. Relationship between presenting systolic blood pressure and mortality (30-day) in the Global Utilization of Streptokinase and tPA for Occluded Coronary Arteries (GUSTO)-1 study. (From Anderson RD, Ohman EM. Successful identification and management of high-risk patients with acute myocardial infarction. *J Thromb Thrombolysis* 1996;3:271–278; with permission.)

FIG. 11-4. Electrocardiographic model to determine risk for 30-day mortality after acute myocardial infarction. The sum of ST-segment deviation was the most predictive. Hathaway WR, Peterson ED, Wagner GS, et al. Prognostic significance of the initial electrocardiogram in patients with acute myocardial infarction. (From GUSTO-I Investigators. Global Utilization of Streptokinase and tPA for Occluded Coronary Arteries. *JAMA* 1998;279:387–391; with permission.)

TABLE 11-2. *Risk factors and predictors of hemorrhagic stroke following thrombolysis: GUSTO-1 trial*

Age
Low body weight
Prior cerebrovascular disease
Diastolic blood pressure
History of hypertension (particularly with increased age)
Combination fibrinolytic therapy
Systolic blood pressure
Tissue plasminogen activator (compared with streptokinase)

GUSTO, Global Utilization of Streptokinase and tPA for Occluded Coronary Arteries: Phase 1 Trial.
From Gore JM, Granger CB, Simoons ML, et al. for the GUSTO-1 Investigators. Stroke after thrombolysis. Mortality and functional outcomes in the GUSTO-1 trial. *Circulation* 1995;92:2811–2818, with permission.

Risk for Stroke

Stroke is the most feared and devastating complication of fibrinolytic therapy (15). Overall, 60% of patients with hemorrhagic stroke die, whereas 25% are left with at least a moderate degree of disability (Table 11-2).

Non–ST-Segment Elevation MI

For nearly two decades, the medical community has placed considerable emphasis on the early management of patients with ST-segment elevation or bundle branch block MI because of the profound impact of early reperfusion on patient outcome. More recently, it has become clear that patients with non–ST-segment elevation MI require careful consideration as well; not solely because of their recognized risk for cardiac events within 6 to 12 months of discharge, but because a sizable number of these patients are at increased risk for in-hospital death.

A total of 183,113 patients with non–ST-segment elevation MI were identified in NRMI-2 (16). Risk factors for in-hospital death included advanced age (odds ratio [OR] 1.51), female sex (OR 1.20), history of diabetes (OR 1.22), prior congestive heart failure (OR 1.30), and Killip class II, III, and IV (OR 1.61, 1.94, and 21.4, respectively) (Table 11-3).

TABLE 11-3. *Predictors of in-hospital death (after 24 h)[a]*

Variable	Odds ratio	95th CI
Aspirin (<24 h)	(0.46)	(0.43–0.48)
Oral beta-blocker (<24 h)	0.59	0.55–0.63
ACE inhibitor (<24 h)	0.66	0.62–0.71
Normal ECG	0.78	0.70–0.85
ST segment depression	1.13	1.06–1.20
Prior stroke	1.39	1.29–1.49
Killip class III or IV	8.72	8.56–8.80

ACE, angiotensin-converting enzyme; CI, confidence interval; ECG, electrocardiogram.
[a]Multivariate logistic regression analysis.

RECURRENT ISCHEMIA AND INFARCTION

Recurrent Ischemia

The two most common cardiac causes of recurrent chest pain among hospitalized patients with acute MI are acute pericarditis and myocardial ischemia; the latter occurs more often and is a marker of poor outcome. Recurrent myocardial ischemia occurs in 15% to 20% of patients and is typically transient (17). It does, however, identify patients with a persistently unstable atherosclerotic plaque as well as those with multivessel coronary artery disease or compromised collateral circulation (18).

Patients with recurrent ischemia can be further stratified according to ECG changes, hemodynamic stability, and overall clinical status. Three distinct categories of patients have been identified as being at increased risk for postinfarction angina and reinfarction: (a) patients with non–ST-segment elevation MI; (b) patients receiving fibrinolytic therapy; and (c) patients with multiple cardiac risk factors (19). The incidence of postinfarction angina is nearly twice as high after non–ST-segment elevation MI (25% to 35%) than after ST-segment elevation or bundle branch block MI (15% to 20%). Patients treated with fibrinolytics have a 20% to 30% incidence of recurrent ischemia and a 4% to 5% incidence of reinfarction even with the concomitant use of aspirin and adjunctive anticoagulant strategies (20).

Management

Recurrent ischemia must be recognized promptly and managed aggressively. Pain relief is best approached in the context of myocardial oxygen supply and demand. Myocardial oxygen demand can be lowered by decreasing heart rate, inotropic state (using intravenous or oral beta-blockers), and by preload (most commonly with nitrate preparations). Morphine sulfate is also useful in early management. A calcium channel blocker can be added, if needed, to control heart rate, prevent episodic coronary vasospasm, or as an alternative to beta-blocker therapy when absolute contraindications exist. Antiplatelet (aspirin ± clopidogrel) therapy should be continued and anticoagulation with intravenous unfractionated heparin or low molecular weight heparin (LMWH) instituted (or continued) for patients with ischemic chest pain at rest. In addition, consideration should be given to the addition of a GP IIb or IIIa antagonist. Anxiolytics such as benzodiazepines can also be used, as needed, to reduce anxiety and provide mild sedation. The goals of therapy are to reduce mean arterial blood pressure and heart rate by approximately 10% to 20%, but not to a level where coronary arterial perfusion pressure is compromised. In clinically unstable patients with evidence of congestive heart failure, volume status must be assessed carefully and treated appropriately.

When aggressive pharmacologic therapy does not alleviate the myocardial ischemia or if concomitant hemodynamic instability exists, early diagnostic coronary angiography is

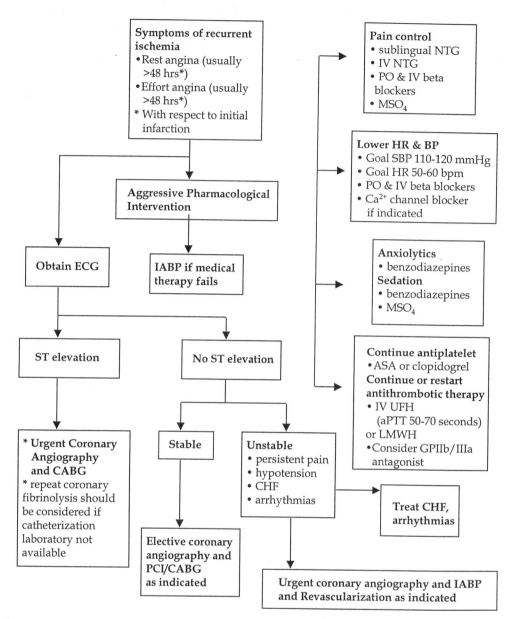

FIG. 11-5. The management of recurrent ischemia is determined by clinical signs and symptoms, electrocardiographic features, hemodynamic status, and angiographic findings. ASA, aspirin; CABG, coronary artery bypass grafting; CHF, congestive heart failure; HR, heart rate; MSO₄, morphine sulfate; NTG, nitroglycerin; PCI, percutaneous coronary intervention; SBP, systolic blood pressure.

recommended. Consideration should also be given to inserting an intraaortic balloon pump to improve myocardial perfusion and serve as a "bridge" to definitive therapy (revascularization, correction of mechanical defects). Serial ECG and clinical assessment are recommended to guide optimal management (Fig. 11-5).

MYOCARDIAL REINFARCTION

Reinfarction represents a recurrent atherothrombotic event with subsequent myocardial necrosis. The diagnosis can be difficult to confirm within the initial 24 hours of the index event because serum cardiac markers have not yet returned

to a normal range. Thus, confirmation must be established in the context of an existing elevation with further (usually twofold) elevation of cardiac enzymes above a prior level (determined within the past 6 hours). Beta-adrenergic blockers have been shown to reduce the risk of reinfarction, whereas fibrinolytic therapy is associated with a slightly increased risk (21,22). Heart rate slowing calcium channel blockers may reduce the rate of reinfarction among patients with preserved left ventricular (LV) function after acute MI, whereas the role of unfractionated heparin is controversial (23). In contrast, the available data strongly support the ability of LMWH and GPIIb/IIIa receptor antagonists to reduce the likelihood of recurrent MI in patients with non–ST-segment elevation MI

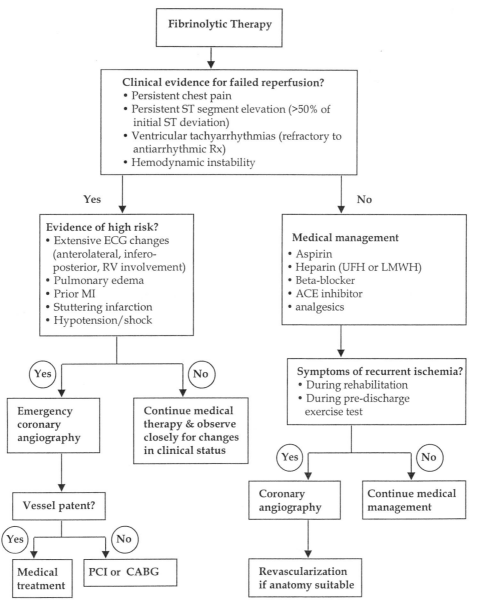

FIG. 11-6. Coronary angiography is recommended for patients with evidence of failed thrombolysis, high risk features, and for those with hemodynamic instability.

and possibly in ST-segment elevation or bundle branch block MI as well (24,25).

Management

The clinical approach to recurrent MI, as with recurrent myocardial ischemia, is determined by the patient's overall clinical status and early indicators of injury (Fig. 11-6).

CORONARY ANGIOGRAPHY AND PERCUTANEOUS CORONARY INTERVENTIONS

Early recurrent myocardial ischemia, persistent ST-segment elevation (>50% of maximal ST-segment deviation), hemodynamic instability, and ventricular tachyarrhythmias

refractory to antiarrhythmic therapy are indications for early coronary angiography (26). The American College of Cardiology/American Heart Association guidelines for coronary angiography and percutaneous coronary intervention are outlined in Table 11-4.

Surgical Revascularization

Although outcomes following emergent surgical revascularization have improved over time as a result of increasing experience, the application of mechanical, hemodynamic or circulatory support measures, and advanced methods of myocardial protection and anesthetic management, the procedure is typically reserved for a carefully selected patient (Table 11-5).

TABLE 11-4. *Early coronary angiography and/or interventional therapy*

Class I
- Patients with persistence of recurrent (stuttering) episodes of symptomatic ischemia, spontaneous or induced, with or without associated ECG changes
- Presence of shock, severe pulmonary congestion, or continuing hypotension

Class IIa
- No recommendation

Class IIb
- No recommendation

Class III
This category applies to patients with AMI who
- Undergo elective angioplasty of a non–infarct-related artery at the time of AMI
- Are beyond 12 h after onset of symptoms and have no evidence of myocardial ischemia
- Have received fibrinolytic therapy and have no symptoms of myocardial ischemia
- Are eligible for thrombolysis and are undergoing primary angioplasty performed by a low-volume operator in a laboratory without surgical capability

AMI, acute myocardial infarction; ECG, electrocardiogram.
From ACC/AHA guidelines for the management of patients with acute myocardial infarction. *J Am Coll Cardiol* 1999; 34:890–911, with permission.

TABLE 11-5. *Emergency or urgent coronary artery bypass graft (CABG) surgery*

Class I
- Failed angioplasty with persistent pain or hemodynamic instability in patients with coronary anatomy suitable for surgery
- AMI with persistent or recurrent ischemia refractory to medical therapy in patients with coronary anatomy suitable for surgery who are not candidates for catheter intervention
- At the time of surgical repair of postinfarction ventricular septal defect (VSD) or mitral valve insufficiency

Class IIa
- Cardiogenic shock with coronary anatomy suitable for surgery

Class IIb
- Failed PCI and small area of myocardium at risk; hemodynamically stable

Class III
- When the expected surgical mortality rate equals or exceeds the mortality rate associated with appropriate medical therapy

AMI, acute myocardial infarction; PCI, percutaneous coronary intervention.
From ACC/AHA guidelines for the management of patients with acute myocardial infarction. *J Am Coll Cardiol* 1996; 28:1328–1428, with permission.

Surgical intervention for mechanical complications of MI and cardiac transplantation will be discussed in a subsequent section.

MYOCARDIAL AND MECHANICAL COMPLICATIONS

Right Ventricular Infarction

Right ventricular (RV) infarction encompasses a complex spectrum of pathologic and clinical presentations, ranging from asymptomatic mild RV dysfunction to overt cardiogenic shock. RV infarction complicates 35% to 50% of inferior MIs which, in turn, make up 40% to 50% of all acute MIs. The diagnosis of RV extension is important because of its association with a higher mortality rate (25% to 30%) (27). Only a small percentage (≈5%) of patients with acute MI present with isolated RV infarction.

The clinical triad of hypotension, clear lung fields, and increased jugular venous pressure in a patient experiencing an inferior MI strongly supports the diagnosis of RV extension. A right-sided S_3 gallop or Kussmaul's sign (distention of the jugular veins during inspiration) may also be present on physical examination. Other potential clinical features of RV infarction include tricuspid regurgitation, sinoatrial (SA) or atrioventricular (AV) nodal conduction disturbances, and AV dissociation. The ECG reveals ST-segment elevation of more than 0.5 mm in V_4R. A Q wave in this lead is considered a nonspecific finding. Other available modalities that can be used to diagnose RV infarction include thallium or sestamibi perfusion imaging, coronary angiography, echocardiography, and hemodynamic measurements with a pulmonary artery catheter.

Complications of acute RV infarction, in most instances, are a manifestation of both LV and RV dysfunction, as well as increased parasympathetic tone (Table 11-6). Overt cardiogenic shock, although occurring rarely, is the most serious complication. High-degree AV block is not uncommon and identifies a patient at particularly high risk. Atrial fibrillation occurs in one third of patients with RV infarction as a result of concomitant right atrial infarction or dilation caused by volume and pressure overload. Other potential complications of RV infarction include ventricular septal rupture (particularly in patients with concomitant transmural posterior septal infarction), RV thrombus formation with subsequent pulmonary embolism, tricuspid regurgitation, and a high incidence of pericarditis, most likely because of the frequent

TABLE 11-6. *Potential complications of right ventricular infarction*

Cardiogenic shock
High degree atrioventricular block
Atrial fibrillation or atrial flutter
Ventricular tachycardia or fibrillation
Ventricular septal rupture
Right ventricular thrombus with or without pulmonary embolism
Tricuspid regurgitation
Pericarditis
Right-to-left shunt via patent foramen ovale

UMMHC	Acute Cardiac Care Interdisciplinary Management Pathway		+ If hemodynamically unstable, refer to Figure 7, 9, and 11 + Refer to Figure 6 ++ Refer to Figure 5 +++ Non-complicated MI			
Diagnosis	**ST Segment Elevation/Bundle Branch Block MI**					

	Day 0 Emergency Department	Day 0 CCU	Day 1 CCU	Day 2+++ Step Down Unit	Day 3+++ Step Down Unit	Pre-Discharge +++
Assessment	• Vitals • Continuous ECG monitoring • Secure venous access	• Vitals q2-4° • Continuous ECG monitoring	• Vitals q4° • Continuous ECG monitoring	• Vitals q8°	• Vitals q8°	• Vitals AM
Benchmark	• Reperfusion Rx* • Salvage myocardium • Treat arrhythmias • Maintain hemodynamic stability	• Pain relief* • Hemodynamically stable • Oxygenating	• Afebrile* • Hemodynamically stable • Oxygenating	• No recurrent chest pain++ • No sign of CHF • No arrhythmias	• Ambulating without difficulty	• Discuss EMS options • Discuss recommendation for seeking medical care
Medication	• ± fibrinolytic + • ß-blocker • Aspirin • Unfractionated Heparin	• Heparin • Aspirin • ß-blocker • ACE-inhibitor • Statin	• Heparin (SC) • Aspirin • ß-blocker • ACE-inhibitor • Statin	• Aspirin • ß-blocker • ACE-inhibitor • Statin	• Aspirin • ß-blocker • ACE-inhibitor • Statin	• Medication education • Prescriptions (including sublingual nitroglycerin)
Laboratory Tests	• CBC • Chem-20 • CK, CK-MB ± Troponin • Lipid profile • INR, aPTT	• CBC • Chem-6 • CK, CK-MB q8° X 3 • APTT	• CBC • Chem-7	• **Chem-7**	• Chem-7	• Fasting lipid profile • CRP 4 weeks post-discharge
Diagnostic/ Interventional Procedures	• 12-lead ECG • ± echocardiogram • ± coronary angiography • ± IABP (for shock)	• 12-lead ECG • ± echocardiogram • ± coronary angiography • ± IABP (for shock)	• 12-lead ECG	• 12-lead ECG	• Modified ETT • ± coronary angiography	• Standard ETT 2 weeks post-discharge • ± echocardiogram
Nutrition	• NPO	• NPO	• AHA Step II	• AHA Step II	• AHA Step II	• AHA Step II
Activity	• Bed rest	• Bed rest	• Bed to chair	• Ambulate.	• Routine activity	• Routine activity
Case Management	• Notify primary care physician • Notify case manager	• Notify social services	• Cardiac rehabilitation consult	• Lipid management • Family education • Smoking cessation	• Nutrition consult	• Discuss medication/ insurance coverage • Notify primary care physician • Schedule return visit

FIG. 11-7. Acute cardiac care-interdisciplinary management pathway.

transmural injury pattern of the thin-walled RV. The development of a right-to-left shunt through a patent foramen ovale is a complication unique to RV infarction and should be suspected when severe hypoxia is not responsive to supplemental oxygen therapy (28).

Management

As with all ST-segment elevation infarctions, the initial approach to patients with RV infarction must address the need for early reperfusion therapy directed at limiting infarct size (Fig. 11-7). Fibrinolytic therapy and primary angioplasty, when successful, improve RV ejection fraction and reduce the incidence of complete heart block. If hemodynamic compromise is present, measures should be implemented to maintain RV preload, reduce RV afterload, and support the dysfunctional RV with pharmacologic inotropic agents. The requirement for volume (preload-dependent state) differentiates the treatment of RV infarction from that of "pure" LV infarction. Volume expansion is the mainstay of therapy, with the goal of maintaining a right atrial or central venous pressure between 12 and 15 mm Hg. Normal saline (250 to 500 ml) given as a bolus should be used acutely, with an appreciation that a large volume of fluid may be required to sufficiently increase RV filling pressure, LV preload, and cardiac output. If volume support does not produce hemodynamic improvement, a pulmonary artery catheter may be required to guide further management.

Patients with persistent hypotension (despite volume resuscitation) may benefit from inotropic support with either dobutamine or dopamine. Because of their potential to reduce preload, vasodilators, including nitroglycerin and morphine sulfate, routinely used in the management of LV infarctions, should be used with great caution in patients with RV infarction. Another crucial factor in sustaining adequate preload is the maintenance of AV synchrony. In patients with high degree AV block, dual chamber pacing may be required, particularly if ventricular pacing does not cause an improvement in the patient's overall clinical status (29). Atrial fibrillation can cause profound hemodynamic deterioration, necessitating prompt cardioversion. In patients with biventricular failure, circulatory support using intraaortic balloon

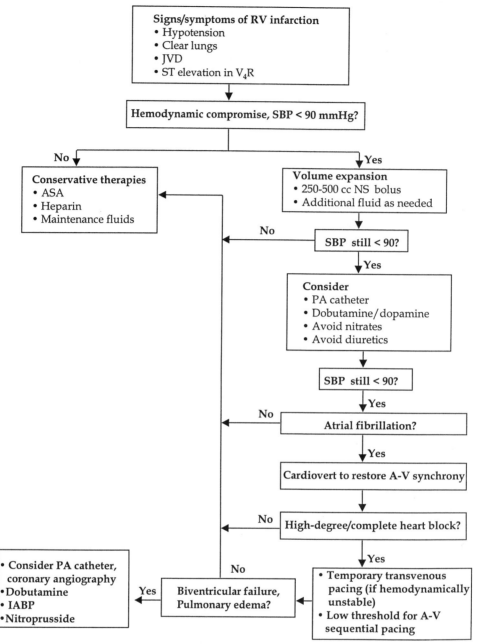

FIG. 11-8. Management algorithm for right ventricular infarction. ASA, aspirin; IABP, intraaortic balloon pump; JVD, jugular venous distention; NS, normal saline; PA, pulmonary artery; SBP, systolic blood pressure.

counterpulsation may be required followed by coronary angiography and either percutaneous or surgical intervention as the findings and clinical status dictate (Fig. 11-8).

Left Ventricular Dysfunction

The extent of LV compromise, which correlates directly with the extent of myocardial damage, is a major determinant of clinical outcome (Fig. 11-9). Anterior site of infarction is commonly associated with extensive LV damage, reduced ventricular performance, and reduced survival. The Killip classification separates patients into four distinct groups based on existing clinical signs and symptoms of LV failure. Increasing Killip class, which represents progressively severe LV compromise, is associated strongly with a poor prognosis (Table 11-7).

The immediate functional consequences of acute myocardial ischemia and infarction include both systolic and diastolic ventricular dysfunction; either can compromise ventricular performance and lead to congestive heart failure.

Relationship Between Left Ventricular Ejection Fraction (EF)
Determined Before Hospital Discharge and 1-Year Mortality

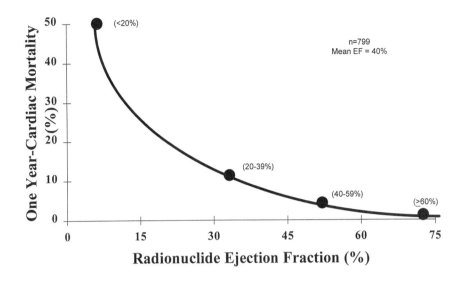

FIG. 11-9. Left ventricular performance is the strongest independent predictor of long-term mortality following acute myocardial infarction. (From Multicenter Postinfarction Research Group. Risk stratification and survival after myocardial infarction. *N Engl J Med* 1983;309:331.)

Diastolic dysfunction (impaired ventricular relaxation) occurs uniformly in patients with acute MI, but is clinically evident in only 20% to 30% of patients. When it does occur, diastolic dysfunction often precedes systolic dysfunction and is the most common early cause of congestive heart failure. Systolic dysfunction, also known as pump failure, is a serious complication of acute MI. The sudden loss of contractile function decreases stroke volume and increases end-systolic volume, end-diastolic volume, and diastolic filling pressure. The clinical manifestations of systolic dysfunction include decreased forward flow (perfusion) and increased backward flow (pulmonary congestion and edema).

The loss of contractile function in the initial minutes to hours of MI is potentially reversible, particularly with successful coronary reperfusion. Myocardial "stunning" as a cause for systolic dysfunction is also a reversible component of myocardial dysfunction (30). Stunned myocardium,

in some instances, responds to pharmacologic inotropic stimulation (31).

Hemodynamic instability associated with LV systolic dysfunction is an indication for placement of a pulmonary artery catheter to determine intracardiac pressures, cardiac output, and systemic vascular resistance, and to guide patient management. A diagnosis of LV failure is supported by increased pulmonary artery (particularly diastolic) and pulmonary capillary wedge pressures (PCWP), decreased cardiac index, and an elevated systemic vascular resistance.

Cardiogenic shock complicates 5% to 15% of all infarctions (32) and typically occurs when myocardial necrosis involves more than 40% of the LV (33). It is the most common cause of in-hospital death among patients with MI, with a mortality rate approaching 80%. Clinically, cardiogenic shock is characterized by hypotension and hypoperfusion of vital organs. Hemodynamic disturbances as measured by a pulmonary artery catheter include elevated PCWP and a markedly reduced cardiac output (Tables 11-8, 11-9). Complications of acute MI other than severe LV dysfunction can also cause cardiogenic shock, including extensive RV infarction, ventricular septal rupture, papillary muscle rupture or ischemic papillary muscle dysfunction with severe mitral regurgitation, and ventricular free-wall rupture with cardiac tamponade.

Diastolic Dysfunction

The comprehensive management of LV diastolic dysfunction must concomitantly address ongoing myocardial ischemia and pulmonary congestion. Intravenous furosemide is considered the diuretic of choice for patients not previously receiving diuretics. Larger doses may be required among patients previously on diuretic therapy and for those with compromised renal function. Excessive diuresis should be

TABLE 11-7. *Killip classification of patients with acute myocardial infarction*

Class	Clinical definition	Patients at hospital admission (%)	Mortality[a] (%)
I	No clinical signs of heart failure	30–40	8
II	Rales over ≤ 50% of lungs, S_3 gallop	30–50	30
III	Rales over ≥ 50% of lungs, pulmonary edema	5–10	44
IV	Cardiogenic shock	10	80–100

[a]Pre-reperfusion or intervention era.
From Killip T, Kimball JT. Treatment of myocardial infarction in a coronary care unit. A two year experience with 250 patients. *Am J Cardiol* 1967;20:457–464.

TABLE 11-8. *Signs, symptoms, and common characteristics of cardiogenic shock*

Clinical
  –Evidence of hypoperfusion
    —Cold, clammy, or mottled skin (livedo reticularus)
    —Impaired mentation (agitation, obtundation, confusion)
    —Oliguria (<30 ml/h)
  –Evidence of primary cardiac abnormality
Hemodynamic
  –Systolic blood pressure <90 mm Hg (mean arterial pressure <70 mm Hg or >20% decrease from baseline)
  –PCWP ≥20 mm Hg
  –CI <2.0 L/min/m^2

CI, cardiac index; PCWP, pulmonary capillary wedge pressure.

TABLE 11-9. *Hemodynamic parameters in commonly encountered clinical situations (idealized)[a]*

CI	SVR	RA	PVR	RV	PA	PAWP	AO
Normal							
≥2.5	1,500	0–6	≤250	25/0–6	25/6–12	6–12	130/80
Hypovolemic shock							
<2.0	>1,500	0–2	≤250	15–20/0–2	15–20/2–6	2–6	≤90/60
Cardiogenic shock							
<2.0	>1,500	8	≤20	50/8	50/35	35	≤90/60
Septic shock							
Early							
≥2.5	<1,500	0–2	<250	20–25/0–2	20–25/0–2	0–6	≤90/60
Late							
<2.0	>1,500	0–4	>250	25/4–10	25/4–10	4–10	≤90/60
Acute massive pulmonary embolism							
<2.0	>1,500	8–12	>450	50/12	50/12–15	≤12	≤90/60
Cardiac tamponade							
<2.0	>1,500	12–18	≤250	25/12–18	25/12–18	12–18	≤90/60
AMI without LVF							
≤2.5	1,500	0–6	≤250	25/0–6	25/12–18	≤18	140/90
AMI with LVF							
>2.0	>1,500	0–6	>250	30–40/0–6	30–40/18–25	>18	140/90
Biventricular failure secondary to LVF							
~2.0	>1,500	>6	>250	50–60/>6	50–60/25	18–25	120/80
RVF secondary to RVI							
<2.0	>1,500	12–20	>250	30/12–20	30/12	<12	≤90/60
Cor pulmonale							
<2.0	>1,500	>6	>500	80/>6	80/35	<12	100/60
Idiopathic pulmonary hypertension							
<2.0	>1,500	0–6	>500	80–100/0–6	80–100/40	<12	100/60
Acute VSR[b]							
<2.0	>1,500	6	>250	60/6-8	60/35	30	≤90/60

AMI, acute myocardial infarction; AO, aortic; CI, cardiac index; LVF, left ventricular failure; PA, pulmonary artery; PAWP, pulmonary artery wedge pressure; PVR, pulmonary vascular resistance; RA, right atrium; RV, right ventricle; RVI, right ventricular infarction; RVF, right ventricular failure; SVR, systemic vascular resistance; VSR, ventricular septal rupture.
[a]Hemodynamic profile seen in approximately one-third of patients in late septic shock.
[b]Confirmed by appropriate RA-PA oxygen saturation step-up.
From Voyce S. *Intensive care medicine.* Philadelphia: Lippincott-Raven Publishers, 1999; with permission.

avoided to prevent a decline in coronary arterial perfusion pressure.

Beta-blockade is an important treatment consideration in patients with isolated ischemic diastolic dysfunction. Beta-blockers not only reduce myocardial oxygen demand, but also improve LV compliance and reduce LV filling pressures, lessening pulmonary congestion. Caution is recommended when systolic and diastolic dysfunction coexist. In this setting, diuresis should be achieved before initiating beta-blocker therapy.

Preload and afterload reducing agents can be used to reduce pulmonary venous pressures. Nitroprusside is both an arteriolar- and venodilator and, as a result, reduces both afterload and preload. This agent is most useful in situations where ischemic diastolic dysfunction complicates existing systolic dysfunction. Nitroglycerin reduces preload and improves both coronary arterial blood flow and myocardial perfusion. For this reason, it is an important therapeutic adjunct in patients with ischemia-mediated congestive heart failure. Because of rapid titratability, intravenous administration is preferred in the coronary care unit setting.

The management of LV systolic dysfunction, when severe, is dictated by specific hemodynamic disturbances as reflected in PCWP, cardiac output (CO), systemic vascular resistance, and systemic blood pressure (BP) (Table 11-10). However, in most patients with uncomplicated MI and mild LV failure, invasive hemodynamic monitoring is not required. Frequent assessment is needed of the patient's cardiopulmonary status, mental status, skin and mucous membranes, cardiac rhythm and heart rate, oxygenation, and urine output. In most patients with systolic dysfunction that is mild in severity, conventional therapy with morphine, nasal oxygen; intravenous, oral, or transdermal nitrates; and gentle diuresis will yield clinical improvement.

The initial management of patients with severe congestive heart failure must include a careful evaluation of oxygenation and acid-base balance; occasionally, endotracheal intubation with ventilatory support is necessary. In the setting of severe LV dysfunction associated with hypotension, intravenous inotropic agents (e.g., dopamine and dobutamine) should be administered. In addition to inotropic support, preload and afterload reduction may be required to augment forward flow and reduce pulmonary congestion. Diuretics and nitrates will diminish pulmonary congestion; however, overall improvement in CO may not occur and, in fact, systemic BP may decrease. Nitroprusside, through a reduction of both preload and afterload, will commonly increase CO, reduce LV end-diastolic pressure, and alleviate pulmonary congestion. In the early hours of acute MI, when ischemia often contributes substantially to LV dysfunction, nitroglycerin is a preferred agent as it causes a greater degree of venodilation than does nitroprusside. The phosphodiesterase inhibitors amrinone and milrinone exhibit inotropic and vasodilating properties and, for this reason, should be considered, particularly in patients with reduced LV systolic function who have been treated previously with beta-blockers. Inotropic and vasodilator therapies must be carefully titrated to maintain a systemic BP of at least 90 mm Hg (mean arterial pressure ≥70 mm Hg). Once BP has remained stable for 60 to 90 minutes, diuresis can be initiated safely.

Patients with severe LV dysfunction, depressed CO, elevated LV diastolic pressure, a mean systemic BP less than 65 mm Hg (or reduced by ≥30% of baseline), and evidence of vital organ hypoperfusion, by definition, have cardiogenic shock. Hypoxemia is common in this setting and should be corrected using supplemental oxygen with a low threshold for endotracheal intubation in the setting of progressive hemodynamic deterioration and severe acidemia. Although intravenous vasopressors including norepinephrine may be required to achieve a mean systemic BP of 70 mm Hg or greater, mechanical circulatory support is a preferred management adjunct in patients with cardiogenic shock and features of active myocardial ischemia. Early angiography followed by revascularization is a particularly attractive management strategy in patients less than 75 years of age (34) (Fig. 11-10).

MECHANICAL COMPLICATIONS

The most commonly encountered mechanical complications of acute MI include ventricular septal rupture (VSR), LV free-wall rupture, mitral regurgitation (MR), and LV aneurysm formation. Papillary muscle and chordal rupture (causing acute MR), VSR, and free-wall rupture, when they occur, commonly do so suddenly within the first week of infarction, whereas aneurysm formation is slow and progressive in nature. In general, patients with acute mechanical complications have smaller infarctions than patients who develop pump failure or malignant ventricular arrhythmias (1). Sudden or rapidly progressive hemodynamic deterioration with systemic hypotension, congestive heart failure, and hypoperfusion should raise suspicion of an acute mechanical

TABLE 11-10. *Indications for hemodynamic monitoring*

Balloon flotation right-heart catheter monitoring

Class I
  −Severe or progressive CHF or pulmonary edema
  −Cardiogenic shock or progressive hypotension
  −Suspected mechanical complications of acute infarction (i.e., VSD, papillary muscle rupture, or pericardial tamponade)

Class IIa
  −Hypotension that does not respond promptly to fluid administration in a patient without pulmonary congestion

Class III
  −Patients with acute infarction without evidence of cardiac or pulmonary complications

CHF, congestive heart failure; VSD, ventricular septal defect.
From ACC/AHA guidelines for the management of patients with acute myocardial infarction. *J Am Coll Cardiol* 1996;28:1328–1428; with permission.

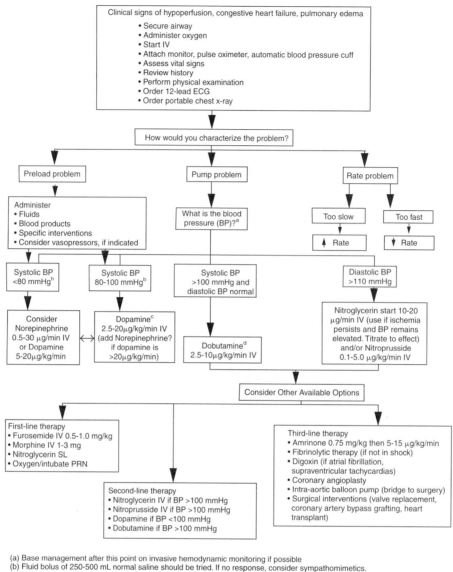

FIG. 11-10. Step-wise approach to cardiogenic shock.

defect. The echocardiogram (transthoracic, transesophageal) is an important diagnostic tool that should be used early in the evaluation of patients suspected of having mechanical defects (Fig. 11-11).

Ventricular Septal Rupture

Rupture of the ventricular septum occurs in 2% to 4% of patients with MI and is responsible for 5% of all in-hospital deaths. Although VSR usually occurs between 3 and 5 days postinfarction, the greatest risk is actually within the first 24 hours. Early occurrence is particularly common among patients who have received fibrinolytic therapy. Risk factors for VSR include first infarction, advanced age, history of hypertension, and female sex. Inferior wall infarction is most often associated with posterior septal rupture, whereas distal septal and apical ruptures are more likely to occur following an anterior site of infarction.

Clinically, acute VSR is characterized by new onset congestive heart failure in the presence of a new, harsh holosystolic murmur; however, patients may exhibit a relatively small degree of pulmonary congestion because of left-to-right shunting. The extent of hemodynamic compromise is determined by the combined defect size and reduced ventricular performance. A diagnosis of VSR can be made using Doppler echocardiography or detection of an oxygen saturation "step-up" between the right atrium and the RV or pulmonary artery during RV catheterization. An oxygen step-up of greater than 10% indicates a significant left-to-right shunt at the ventricular level.

Potential Sites of Cardiac Rupture After Acute Myocardial Infarction

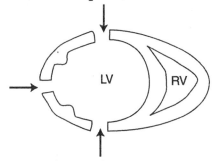

A. Left Ventricular Free Wall Rupture

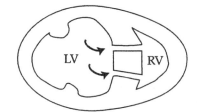

B. Ventricular Septal Rupture

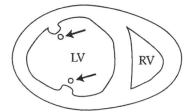

C. Papillary Muscle Rupture

FIG. 11-11. Cardiac rupture, a potentially lethal complication of myocardial infarction, can involve the **(A)** left ventricular free wall, **(B)** ventricular septum, or **(C)** papillary muscle.

Management

The immediate supportive treatment of VSR includes intravenous fluid administration and inotropic therapy (dopamine or dobutamine) in combination with afterload reduction using nitroprusside or, more commonly, intraaortic balloon counterpulsation. Although surgical repair represents the definitive treatment, operative mortality is high, ranging from 20% to 70%. Preoperative shock and inferoposterior infarction, particularly with RV dysfunction, are risk factors for a poor surgical outcome following surgery. Emergency repair should be considered when either pulmonary edema or cardiogenic shock is present, but deferred repair is preferable among hemodynamically stable patients. Although aggressive and early surgery leads to the highest survival rates, many patients have a complicated postoperative course and prolonged hospitalization (34a).

When VSR is suspected, echocardiography with color flow Doppler imaging should be performed as soon as possible to confirm the diagnosis, establish the coexistence of other cardiac abnormalities (mitral regurgitation, pericardial effusion), and provide estimates of both RV and LV systolic function. If a decision is made to proceed with surgical repair, coronary angiography should be performed in anticipation of concomitant revascularization. Left ventriculography may not be necessary if echocardiography provides adequate information on LV performance and the existence of concomitant valvular abnormalities.

Left Ventricular Free-Wall Rupture

Rupture of the LV free wall occurs in 1% to 2% of patients, but is responsible for 10% to 15% of in-hospital deaths. After cardiogenic shock and ventricular arrhythmias, it is the most common cause of death. In addition, rupture of the LV free wall occurs 8 to 10 times more frequently than rupture of either a papillary muscle or the ventricular septum. Autopsy series have shown that the lateral wall is the most common site of rupture. Similar to acute VSR, risk factors for free-wall rupture include age more than 70 years, female sex, hypertension, first MI, and transmural infarction in the absence of collateral vessels (35,36).

The clinical presentation among patients with ventricular free-wall rupture ranges from sudden hypotension with electromechanical dissociation and death from cardiac tamponade to transient chest discomfort and bradyarrhythmias. The patient frequently develops signs of systemic hypoperfusion, jugular venous distention, pulsus paradoxus, and distant heart sounds. Episodes of chest pain with diaphoresis and nausea can herald subacute or impending, free-wall rupture. The diagnosis is most often suggested clinically and confirmed by echocardiography or pericardiocentesis, or at the time of emergent surgery.

Management

Patients suspected of having LV free-wall rupture and systemic hypotension should receive intravenous fluid. A large volume is commonly required to increase ventricular preload and maintain CO. Vasopressor support must follow without delay if the hemodynamic status does not improve. Emergent pericardiocentesis can be a life-saving maneuver in patients with abrupt electromechanical dissociation; however, surgical intervention remains the definitive treatment (37).

Mitral Regurgitation

Acute MR is associated with a poor prognosis (38). With moderate to severe MR, the 1-year survival rate is approximately 50%. Although the diagnosis is typically suggested by the presence of a new holosystolic murmur, up to 50% of the patients with severe MR do not have an audible murmur. Because of the frequency of "silent" MR, the clinician must maintain a high index of suspicion in patients with unexplained hypotension or pulmonary edema.

The papillary muscle is the cardiac structure that ruptures least frequently; however, this event is associated with rapid hemodynamic deterioration because the compromised LV is unable to compensate for the excessive volume load imposed by the incompetent mitral valve. Because the posteromedial papillary muscle receives its blood supply solely from the posterior descending artery (usually as a branch of the right coronary artery), it is susceptible to ischemia, necrosis, and rupture. The anterolateral papillary muscle has a dual blood supply provided by the left anterior descending and left circumflex coronary arteries and, therefore, is less susceptible to ischemic dysfunction and injury.

Management

Patients with acute MR causing congestive heart failure or overt cardiogenic shock require hemodynamic monitoring and pharmacologic inotropic or vasopressor therapy. Intraaortic balloon counterpulsation should be considered for hemodynamic support and to serve as a bridge to coronary angiography and surgical intervention. Serial echocardiography can be used to determine progression and to assess overall LV compensation in relatively stable patients. Moderate to severe MR, particularly when unresponsive to pharmacologic and supportive measures, should be addressed surgically (39);

however, concomitant mitral valve replacement (or repair if feasible) and bypass grafting, even in experienced hands, are associated with a high surgical mortality rate.

The management of patients with mechanical complications of acute MI are summarized in Fig. 11-12.

Left Ventricular Dilation and Aneurysm Formation

Infarct "expansion" occurs acutely (in the first few days following MI) and results in dilation and thinning of the infarcted segment (40). This event must be distinguished from infarct "extension" (or reinfarction). Clinically, these two complications of MI may present similarly (electrocardiographic ST-segment changes and hemodynamic disturbances); however, infarct expansion is not accompanied by reelevation of cardiac enzymes as is the case with infarct extension. Infarct expansion usually occurs in the setting of transmural, anterior infarction; it is proportional to the size of the MI and portends a greater likelihood of death.

LV dilation and remodeling, which occurs more insidiously, is a progressive process that begins shortly after the acute event and continues over the subsequent weeks to months. Following acute injury, the ventricle dilates in an effort to maintain CO. Unfortunately, progressive dilation causes increased wall stress which, in turn, leads to further cavity enlargement, decompensation, and impaired performance.

Management

Efforts to reduce wall stress through reductions in preload and afterload are important. Early treatment with intravenous nitroglycerin and angiotensin converting enzyme (ACE) inhibitors is effective, particularly the latter (41,42), which exerts most of its effects at the tissue level. The potential added benefit of combined ACE inhibition and angiotensin II receptor antagonists is under investigation.

At the extreme end of a spectrum that characterizes LV remodeling is aneurysm formation. The prevalence of LV aneurysms following MI, as estimated from postmortem studies, is between 3% and 15%. The location is typically anterior, anteroapical, or apical. Aneurysms can be asymptomatic or associated with angina pectoris, arrhythmias (including malignant ventricular dysrhythmias), cardioembolism, or congestive heart failure. A diagnosis is most often confirmed by two-dimensional echocardiography or contrast ventriculography.

Patients developing ventricular aneurysms should be treated in a manner similar to others with MI (beta-blocker, ACE inhibitor, aspirin). Pharmacologic therapies should not be based solely on the presence of an aneurysm, but according to the presence of congestive heart failure, mural thrombi, or life-threatening ventricular arrhythmias. Occasionally, surgical resection is indicated to correct refractory heart failure, recurrent life-threatening arrhythmias, and recurrent systemic emboli despite anticoagulant therapy. Aneurysmectomy

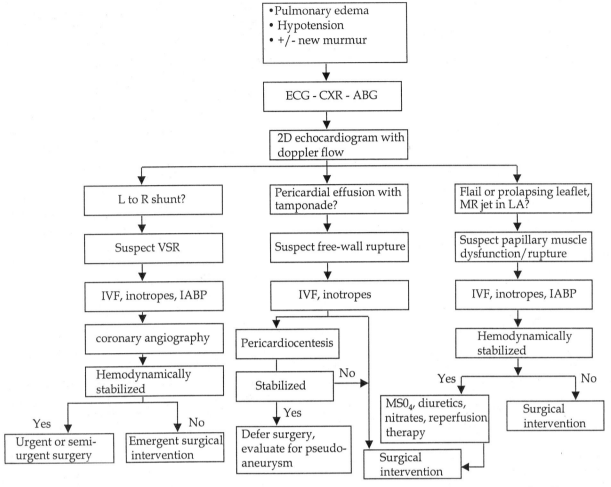

FIG. 11-12. The management of patients with postinfarction mechanical complications is determined by the site of the involvement and the degree of hemodynamic compromise.

is usually combined with coronary bypass grafting and, in patients with concomitant ventricular arrhythmias, the line of resection should be guided by electrophysiologic mapping.

Pseudoaneurysm

Pseudoaneurysms are a rare complication of acute MI and, in essence, represent a "contained rupture" of the ventricular free wall. Clot forms in the pericardial space and an aneurysmal wall consisting of organized thrombus and pericardium prevents hemorrhage within the mediastinum. Unlike a true ventricular aneurysm, a pseudoaneurysm (false aneurysm) has a narrow base (neck) and the risk of rupture (recurrent rupture) is high. The pseudoaneurysm, which has the potential to progressively expand, is clinically silent in most instances, but can cause congestive heart failure, an abnormal bulge on the cardiac silhouette, persistent ST-segment elevation within the region of infarction, or systolic murmurs (43).

The diagnosis of LV pseudoaneurysm can be established by two-dimensional echocardiography, ventriculographic radionuclide studies, magnetic resonance imaging, or contrast left ventriculography.

Management

In addition to the pharmacologic management of congestive heart failure and life-threatening arrhythmias, anticoagulation should be discontinued because of the risk of rupture. Surgical resection with or without bypass grafting is recommended.

PERICARDIAL COMPLICATIONS

Pericarditis

Pericardial inflammation, which is common following acute MI, typically manifests in either an acute or subacute form. Although pericarditis is less common with the advent of reperfusion therapy, it nevertheless must be recognized and diagnosed promptly.

Early Postinfarction Pericarditis

The most common manifestation of pericarditis is chest pain that characteristically is aggravated by inspiration, swallowing, coughing, and lying flat, and lessened when the patient sits up and leans forward. Fever, generally less than 38.6°C, can accompany postinfarction pericarditis and typically lasts for several days (44). A scratchy one, two- or three-component pericardial friction rub is often appreciated along the left sternal border. Concave upward ST-segment elevation in five or more ECG leads supports the diagnosis. Although sinus tachycardia is the most common rhythm abnormality, a wide variety of dysrhythmias, including atrial fibrillation, have been described (45). A pericardial effusion, identified by echocardiography, is not uncommon following MI and its presence or absence neither confirms nor excludes the diagnosis of pericarditis.

Management

The pain of pericarditis usually responds promptly to aspirin or a nonsteroidal antiinflammatory agent, which should be administered for approximately 5 to 7 days. Aspirin represents the treatment of choice and is given at a dose of 650 mg every 4 to 6 hours. Indomethacin also provides effective symptom relief; however, it can cause increased coronary vascular resistance and, in experimental animal models, causes thinning of the infarct. Corticosteroids should be avoided whenever possible because of their association with myocardial rupture and recurrent symptoms after discontinuation. Although anticoagulant therapy is not an absolute contraindication, it must be used cautiously to minimize the risk of hemorrhagic progression (46) (Table 11-11).

Postmyocardial Infarction Syndrome (Dressler's Syndrome)

Dressler's syndrome typically occurs between 2 and 12 weeks after the initial event and may follow either ST-segment elevation or non–ST-segment elevation MI (although it is rare following the latter). The overall frequency of Dressler's syndrome has diminished substantially with the advent of reperfusion therapy.

The clinical features of Dressler's syndrome are fever, pleuritic chest pain, and polyserositis. Pleural and pericardial friction rubs, lasting from several days to weeks, can be appreciated. Pericardial and pleural effusions are present in most patients and, although they are typically small, large hemorrhagic effusions have been described. Dressler's syndrome is an immune-mediated phenomenon.

Management

The pharmacologic approach to Dressler's syndrome is similar to that of early postinfarction pericarditis; however, a course of oral corticosteroid therapy more often is needed for complete symptom relief. Nevertheless, treatment should begin with aspirin or nonsteroidal antiinflammatory agents and, if steroids are used, they should be gradually tapered over 1 to 4 weeks. Unfortunately, recurrences are common, often requiring reinstitution of corticosteroids with a more gradual tapering. Drainage procedures may be necessary for large pleural effusions that compromise overall pulmonary performance.

Thromboembolic Complications

Thromboembolism, a recognized complication of acute MI, occurs in 5% to 10% of patients. Both arterial and venous events can occur, with LV mural thrombi accounting for most systemic emboli, and RV or deep vein thrombi serving as a nidus for pulmonary emboli.

Pulmonary Embolism

The prevalence of deep venous thrombosis (DVT) among patients with acute MI is reported to be between 18% and 38% (47). Risk factors in this setting include large infarctions in any location, anterior infarctions, congestive heart failure, and complicated infarctions—each associated with a systemic inflammatory response, prolonged immobilization, and venous stasis. In addition to traditional risk factors, reduced CO also predisposes to DVT. The diagnosis is particularly challenging in critically ill patients who typically suffer from a variety of active medical problems. Early reports suggested that 10% to 15% of all patients with DVT experienced a pulmonary embolism and 3% to 6% had fatal events. More recent estimates are less impressive but still concerning, with rates of 3% to 5% and 1%, respectively.

Early mobilization, as clinical status permits, and prophylactic anticoagulation are recommended for all patients experiencing acute MI, particularly those with prior events or known thrombophilias. The management of venous thromboembolism is outlined in chapter 19.

Systemic Embolism

The prevalence of systemic embolism in patients with MI is approximately 5% (48). Emboli to the cerebral, renal, mesenteric, iliofemoral, or other arterial beds can occur, typically originating from mural thrombi within the LV (49). Left atrial appendage thrombi are a potential source of emboli in patients with atrial fibrillation. The predilection of the

TABLE 11-11. *Management of early postinfarction pericarditis and Dressler's syndrome*

Distinguish postinfarction pericarditis from recurrent myocardial ischemia or infarction
Aspirin: 160–325 mg daily, as high as 650 mg every 4 to 6 h if required, with decreasing doses as symptoms permit
Indomethacin 25–50 mg three times daily, to be used in severe cases
Morphine sulfate or other oral analgesia for severe pain
Avoid corticosteroids whenever possible

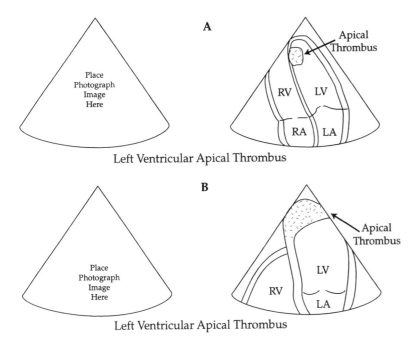

FIG. 11-13. Thrombi developing within the left ventricular apex can be **(A)** well-defined and partially mobile, or **(B)** laminated to the endocardial surface. LA, left atrium; LV, left ventricle; RA, right atrium; RV, right ventricle.

ventricular apex for thrombus development is caused by localized inflammation (from the infarction) and stagnant blood flow. Although depressed LV function and chamber dilation are not absolute prerequisites for thrombus formation, both contribute substantially to the process (50).

Left ventricular thrombi typically develop within the first three postinfarction days, but can form later. Systemic embolization occurs, on average, 14 days after infarction and is relatively rare after 6 weeks in the absence of clinical heart failure and LV chamber dilation. The diagnosis is most often made by two dimensional echocardiography (Fig. 11-13).

Management

Patients with systemic embolism, particularly those with a documented cardiac source or in whom a high index of suspicion for cardioembolism is seen, should be systemically anticoagulated with unfractionated or LMWH heparin, followed by warfarin (target INR 2 to 3) for 6 to 12 months. A longer treatment duration may be indicated for patients with persistently depressed ejection fractions (<30%). Long-term anticoagulation is recommended for patients with chronic atrial fibrillation and those with prior cardioembolism.

ELECTRICAL COMPLICATIONS

Rhythm and Conduction Disturbances

Abnormalities of cardiac rhythm and conduction, which are common following MI, can be life-threatening. Before hospital arrival, ventricular tachycardia and fibrillation account for most sudden cardiac deaths. Both tachyarrhythmias and bradyarrhythmias are encountered in the hospital phase of acute MI and most patients experience one or more conduction abnormalities (25%) or rhythm disturbances (90%) in the first 24 hours. The cause of electrical complications is multifactorial, including myocardial ischemia, necrosis, altered autonomic tone, hypoxia, electrolyte and acid-base disturbances, and adverse drug effects.

Management

The general goal of therapy in the setting of rhythm and conduction disturbances is to return heart rate and AV synchrony to their normal state (Tables 11-12, 11-13, 11-14).

The use of temporary transvenous pacing in the setting of acute MI is determined by the specific bradyarrhythmia or conduction disturbance, the presence of hemodynamic compromise, and the site of infarction. Transcutaneous pacing systems are suitable for stable patients judged to be at low to moderate risk for progressive AV block. Transcutaneous modalities are also attractive among patients who have received fibrinolytic therapy, given their added risk for vascular and hemorrhagic complications. Recommendations for placement of transcutaneous pacing patches and temporary transvenous pacing wires are detailed in Tables 11-15 and 11-16.

Temporary pacing in the early stages of MI does not automatically translate to a requirement for permanent pacemaker placement. Indications for permanent pacing after acute MI are summarized in Table 11-17.

TREATMENT COMPLICATIONS

Hemorrhage

Antithrombotic and fibrinolytic therapy, by design but not by intention, impair both thrombotic potential (a goal of treatment) and hemostatic capacity (an unwanted effect).

TABLE 11-12. *Management of ventricular tachycardia/ventricular fibrillation*

Class I

VF should be treated with an unsynchronized electric shock with an initial energy of 200 J; if unsuccessful, a second shock of 200 to 300 J should be given, and, if necessary, a third shock of 360 J.

Sustained (>30 seconds or causing hemodynamic collapse) polymorphic VT should be treated with an unsynchronized electric shock using an initial energy of 200 J; if unsuccessful, a second shock of 200 to 300 J should be given, and, if necessary, a third shock of 360 J.

Episodes of sustained monomorphic VT associated with angina, pulmonary edema, or hypotension (blood pressure <90 mm Hg) should be treated with a synchronized electric shock of 100 J initial energy. Increasing energies may be used if not initially successful.

Sustained monomorphic VT not associated with angina, pulmonary edema, or hypotension (blood pressure <90 mm Hg) should be treated with one of the following regimens

    Lidocaine: bolus 1.0 to 1.5 mg/kg. Supplemental boluses of 0.5 to 0.75 mg/kg every 5 to 10 min to a maximum of 3 mg/kg total loading dose may be given as needed. Loading is followed by infusion of 2 to 4 mg/min (30 to 50 μg/kg/min).

    Procainamide: 20 to 30 mg/min loading infusion, up to 12 to 17 mg/kg. This may be followed by an infusion of 1 to 4 mg/min.

    Amiodarone: 150 mg infused over 10 min followed by constant infusion of 1.0 mg/min for 6 h and then a maintenance infusion of 0.5 mg/min.

    Synchronized electrical cardioversion starting at 50 J (brief anesthesia is necessary).

Class IIa

Infusions of antiarrhythmic drugs may be used after an episode of VT/VF but should be discontinued after 6 to 24 h and the need for further arrhythmia management assessed.

Electrolyte and acid-based disturbances should be corrected to prevent recurrent episodes of VF when an initial episode of VF has been treated.

Class III

Treatment of isolated ventricular premature beats, couplets, runs of accelerated idioventricular rhythm, and nonsustained VT.

Prophylactic administration of antiarrythmic therapy when using fibrinolytic agents.

VF, ventricular fibrillation; VT, ventricular tachycardia.
From ACC/AHA guidelines for the management of patients with acute myocardial infarction. *J Am Coll Cardiol* 1996;28:1328–1428; with permission.

Antiplatelet Therapy

Bleeding events associated with disorders of primary hemostasis most often involve the skin, joint spaces, and mucous membranes; however, the gastrointestinal and genitourinary tracts and central nervous system are occasionally involved. Bleeding severity is directly related to the degree of platelet dysfunction, integrity of the vasculature, and status of both the

TABLE 11-13. *Management of atrial fibrillation*

Class I

−Electrical cardioversion for patients with severe hemodynamic compromise or intractable ischemia

−Rapid digitalization to slow a rapid ventricular response and improve left ventricular function

−Intravenous beta-adrenoceptor blockers to slow rapid ventricular response in patients without clinical left ventricular dysfunction, bronchospastic disease, or atrioventricular block

−Heparin should be given

Class IIa

−Either diltiazem or verapamil intravenously to slow a rapid ventricular response if beta-adrenoceptor blocking agents are contraindicated or ineffective

From ACC/AHA guidelines for the management of patients with acute myocardial infarction. *J Am Coll Cardiol* 1996;28:1328–1428; with permission.

intrinsic and extrinsic coagulation pathways. In general, an isolated platelet defect is rarely the cause of life-threatening hemorrhage.

The template bleeding time has been employed as a general estimate of platelet function; however, it is nonspecific and vulnerable to technical errors. Laboratory-based platelet aggregation studies can also be performed if time allows. The evolution of bedside assays and point-of-care platelet aggregometers provide a readily available means to diagnose rapidly platelet abnormalities, particularly those related to pharmacologic inhibition.

For the most part, treatment of bleeding is nonspecific. As with any hemorrhage, the source should be identified, the offending agent discontinued (when feasible), and local measures (manual pressure, suturing) explored first. Thereafter, treatment is dictated by the severity of the event. Platelet

TABLE 11-14. *Management of bradyarrhythmias and heart block*

Atropine

Class I

−Symptomatic sinus bradycardia (generally, heart rate <50 bpm associated with hypotension, ischemia, or escape ventricular arrhythmia)

−Ventricular asystole

−Symptomatic AV block occurring at the AV nodal level (second-degree type I or third-degree with a narrow-complex escape rhythm)

Class IIa

−None

Class III

−AV block occurring at an infranodal level (usually associated with anterior myocardial infarction with a wide-complex escape rhythm)

−Asymptomatic sinus bradycardia

AV, atrioventricular; bpm beats per minute.
From ACC/AHA guidelines for the management of patients with acute myocardial infarction. *J Am Coll Cardiol* 1996;28:1328–1428; with permission.

TABLE 11-15. *Indications for temporary pacing: placement of transcutaneous patches—and active (demand) transcutaneous pacing*

Class I
Sinus bradycardia (rate <50 bpm) with symptoms of hypotension (systolic blood pressure <80 mm Hg) unresponsive to drug therapy
Mobitz type II second-degree AV block
Third-degree heart block
Bilateral BBB (alternating BBB, or RBBB and alternating LAFB, LPFB) (irrespective of time onset)
Newly acquired or age indeterminate LBBB, LBBB and LAFB, RBBB, and LPFB
RBBB or LBBB and first-degree AV block

Class IIa
Stable bradycardia (systolic blood pressure >90 mm Hg, no hemodynamic compromise, or compromise responsive to initial drug therapy)

Class IIb
Newly acquired or age-determinate first-degree AV block

Class III
Uncomplicated myocardial infarction without evidence of conduction disease

AV, atrioventricular; BBB, bundle branch block; bpm, beats per minute; LAFB, left anterior fascicular block; LBBB, left bundle branch block; LPFB, left posterior fascicular block; RBBB, right bundle branch block.
From ACC/AHA 1996 guidelines.

TABLE 11-16. *Indications for temporary transvenous pacing*

Class I
Asystole
Symptomatic bradycardia (includes sinus bradycardia with hypotension and type I second-degree AV block with hypotension unresponsive to atropine)
Bilateral BBB (alternating BBB or RBBB) with alternating LAFB/LPFB (any age)
New or indeterminate-age bifascicular block (RBBB with LAFB or LPFB) with first-degree AV block
Mobitz type II second-degree AV block

Class IIa
RBBB and LAFB or LPFB (new or indeterminate)
RBBB with first-degree AV block
LBBB, new or indeterminate
Incessant VT, for atrial or ventricular overdriving pacing
Recurrent sinus pauses (>3 sec) unresponsive to atropine

Class IIb
Bifascicular block of indeterminate age
New or age-indeterminate isolated RBBB

Class III
First-degree heart block
Type I second-degree AV block with normal hemodynamics
Accelerated idioventricular rhythm
BBB or fascicular block known to exist before AMI

AMI, acute myocardial infarction; AV, atrioventricular; BBB, bundle branch block; LAFB, left anterior fascicular block; LBBB, left bundle branch block; LPFB, left posterior fascicular block; RBBB, right bundle branch block; VT, ventricular tachycardia.
From ACC/AHA 1996 guidelines.

TABLE 11-17. *Indications for permanent pacing after myocardial infarction*

Class I
−Persistent second-degree AV block in the His–Purkinje system with bilateral BBB or complete heart block after AMI
−Transient advanced (second- or third-degree) AV block and associated BBB
−Symptomatic AV block at any level

Class IIb
−Persistent advanced (second- or third-degree) block at the AV node level

Class III
−Transient AV conduction disturbances in the absence of intraventricular conduction defects
−Transient AV block
−Acquired LAFB in the absence of AV block
−Persistent first-degree AV block in the presence of BBB that is old or age indeterminate

AMI, acute myocardial infarction; AV, atrioventricular; BBB, bundle branch block; LAFB, left anterior fascicular block.
From ACC/AHA 1996 guidelines.

transfusions, either with or without DDAVP, should be given for serious or life-threatening hemorrhage.

Profound thrombocytopenia (platelet counts <2,000/mm³) has been observed with the GP IIb/IIIa antagonists. The largest experience is with abciximab. Most patients have responded to discontinuation of the medication and platelet transfusions. Intravenous immunoglobulin and corticosteroid therapy have not had an impact on the natural history of the acute disorder; however, delayed thrombocytopenia (>2 weeks after exposure) has been described (after abciximab administration) and may be immune mediated. Accordingly, immunosuppressive therapy and platelet transfusion should be considered. Fibrinogen supplementation with cryoprecipitate or fresh frozen plasma represents an important first-line treatment when major hemorrhage occurs during administration of the small molecule competitive inhibitors, tirofiban and eptifibatide.

Heparin Compounds

Mild to moderate bleeding should initially prompt a reduction in the unfractionated heparin dose (particularly if the activated partial thromboplastin time is excessively prolonged) or an interruption of the infusion for a brief period of time (30–60 minutes). More severe hemorrhage may require complete discontinuation or, with life-threatening hemorrhage, neutralization with protamine sulfate (1 mg/100 U heparin administered in the preceding 4 hours). However, in patients with active coronary heart disease, a careful risk-to-benefit assessment must be undertaken, considering the risks of coronary thrombosis versus those of bleeding. It may be in the patient's best interest to continue systemic anticoagulation, particularly if the bleeding is not serious or life-threatening

TABLE 11-18. *Suggested dose of protamine to neutralize anticoagulant effects of enoxaparin[a]*

	Last dose of enoxaparin (1.0 mg/kg)		
	≤8h	>8 h and ≤12 h	>12 h
Protamine dose[b]	1 mg protamine/1 mg enoxaparin	0.5 mg protamine/1 mg enoxaparin	May not be required

Fresh frozen plasma may be required in patients with life-threatening hemorrhage.
[a]The potential risk of rapid neutralization must be weighed against the perceived benefit.
[b]Protamine neutralizes the anti-IIa effects of enoxaparin (and other low molecular weight heparins).

TABLE 11-19. *Management of prolonged INR associated with warfarin therapy[a]*

INR	<6.0	6.0–10.0	>10.0	>20.0
Clinical profile[a] Recommended approach	No bleeding Omit next 1–2 doses of warfarin	No bleeding Vitamin K 1–2 mg s.c. ↓ Repeat INR in 8 h ↓ Consider additional vitamin K	No bleeding Vitamin K 3–5 mg s.c. ↓ Repeat INR in 6 h ↓ Consider additional vitamin K	No bleeding Vitamin K 5–10 mg s.c. ↓ Repeat INR in 6 h ↓ Consider additional vitamin K

INR, international normalized ratio; i.v., intravenous; s.c., subcutaneous.
[a]For rapid reversal of anticoagulant effect because of life-threatening hemorrhage, fresh frozen plasma or prothrombin concentrates should be administered. Concomitant administration of vitamin K (3–5 mg IV) is also recommended.

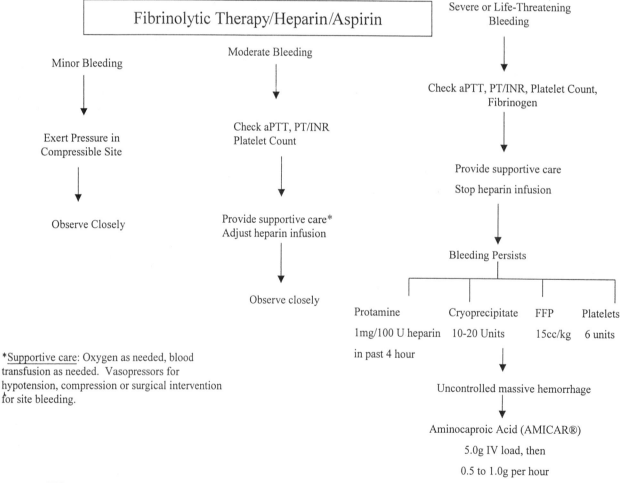

FIG. 11-14. A recommended approach to the management of patients with hemorrhagic complications following fibrinolytic (and adjunctive antithrombotic) therapy.

and can be controlled adequately with local measures (e.g., manual pressure over a site of vascular trauma).

Protamine sulfate (1 mg/100 U anti-Xa) can also be administered to neutralize partially the anticoagulant effects of LMWH. It is important to be aware that the neutralization is incomplete (≈60%). Fresh-frozen plasma should be administered in the setting of life-threatening bleeding to correct any residual hemostatic impairment (Table 11-18).

The neutralization of heparinoids (danaparoid sodium) is even more challenging, given their long circulating half-life and poor response to protamine. As with LMWH preparations, fresh-frozen plasma should be administered for serious or life-threatening bleeding complications. Plasmapheresis has been used successfully to remove the circulating anticoagulant in several patients following bypass surgery complicated by uncontrolled hemorrhage.

Hirudin and Other Direct Thrombin Antagonists

No antidotes are known for hirudin and other direct thrombin antagonists, creating potentially serious challenges when bleeding occurs. Beyond immediate discontinuation of the drug, fresh-frozen plasma should be considered as a source of clotting factors. Plasmapheresis should be considered for life-threatening hemorrhage.

Warfarin

The anticoagulant effect of warfarin can be reduced or entirely reversed by lowering the dose, discontinuing treatment, administering vitamin K, or replacing the defective coagulation factors with fresh-frozen plasma or prothrombin concentrate. The severity of bleeding and inherent risks of reduced anticoagulation should dictate the course of action (Table 11-19).

Fibrinolytic Therapy

Even with careful patient selection and close monitoring, hemorrhagic events do occur. Routine management includes volume and BP support as well as a prompt and thorough search for the site of bleeding. Abdominopelvic or head computed tomography scans may be useful in the diagnosis and management of major hemorrhagic events. Life-threatening hemorrhage warrants prompt intervention. Heparin should be discontinued and neutralized with protamine sulfate. Fresh-frozen plasma is an excellent source of factors V and VIII, α_2-antiplasmin, and plasminogen-activator inhibitor. Cryoprecipitate (8–10 U) is the preferred source of fibrinogen (200–250 mg/10–15 ml) and factor VIII (80 U/10–15 ml). If the platelet count is low (<80,000/mm^3), platelets (6 U random donor) should be given. If indicated, DDAVP (0.3 g/kg i.v. over 20 minutes) can be used to correct qualitative platelet abnormalities. Persistent and potentially life-threatening hemorrhage unresponsive to standard measures (outlined previously) may require antifibrinolytic therapy.

This intervention should be used with caution because serious thrombotic complications can be precipitated. Alpha-aminocaproic acid (Amicar) and tranexamic acid are the most frequently used agents (Fig. 11-14).

REFERENCES

1. Braunwald E. *Heart disease: a textbook of cardiovascular medicine*, Vol. 2. Philadelphia: WB Saunders, 1984:1262–1300.
2. Buja LM, Willerson JT. Clinicopathological correlates of acute ischemic heart disease syndromes. *Am J Cardiol* 1981;47:343–356.
3. Fishbein MC, Maclean D, Maroko PR. The histopathological evolution of myocardial infarction. *Chest* 1978;73:843–849.
4. Henson DE, Najafi H, Callaghan R, et al. Myocardial lesions following open heart surgery. *Arch Pathol* 1969;88:423–430.
5. Tyagi SC, Ratajska A, Weber KT. Myocardial matrix metalloproteinase(s): localization and activation. *Mol Cell Biochem* 1993;126:49–59.
6. Cleutjens JPM, Kandala JC, Guarda E, et al. Regulation of collagen degradation in the rat myocardium after infarction. *J Mol Cell Cardiol* 1995;27:1281–1292.
7. McCormick RJ, Musch TI, Bergman BC, et al. Regional differences in LV collagen accumulation and mature cross-linking after myocardial infarction in rats. *Am J Physiol* 1994;266:H354–H359.
8. Finesmith TH, Broadley KN, Davidson JM. Fibroblasts from wounds of different stages of repair vary in their ability to contract a collagen gel in response to growth factors. *J Cell Physiol* 1990;144:97–107.
9. Mueller HS, Cohen LS, Braunwald E, et al., for the TIMI Investigators. Predictors of early morbidity and mortality after thrombolytic therapy of acute myocardial infarction. Analyses of patient subgroups in the Thrombolysis in Myocardial Infarction (TIMI) Trial, Phase II. *Circulation* 1992;85:1254–1264.
10. Lee KL, Woodlief LH, Topol EJ, et al., for the GUSTO-1 Investigators. Predictors of 30-day mortality in the era of reperfusion for acute myocardial infarction. Results from an international trial of 41,021 patients. *Circulation* 1995;91:1659–1668.
11. Becker RC, Burns M, Gore JM, for the NRMI-2 Investigators. Early assessment and in-hospital management of patients with acute myocardial infarction at increased risk for adverse outcomes: a nationwide perspective of current clinical practice. *Am Heart J* 1998;135:786–796.
12. Hathaway WR, Peterson ED, Wagner GS, for the GUSTO-1 Investigators. Prognostic significance of the initial electrocardiography in patients with acute myocardial infarction. *JAMA* 1998;279:387–391.
13. Ohman EM, Armstrong PW, Christenson RH, for the GUSTO IIA Investigators. Cardiac troponin T levels for risk stratification in acute myocardial ischemia. *N Engl J Med* 1996;335:1333–1341.
14. Morrow DA, Rifan N, Antman EM, et al. Serum amyloid A protein predicts early mortality in acute coronary syndromes: a TIMI 11A substudy. *J Am Coll Cardiol* 2000;35:358–362.
15. Gore JM, Granger CB, Simoons ML, et al., for the GUSTO-1 Investigators. Stroke after thrombolysis. Mortality and functional outcomes in the GUSTO-1 trial. *Circulation* 1995;92:2811–2818.
16. Becker RC, Burns M, Every N, et al., for the National Registry of Myocardial Infarction (NRMI-2) Participants. Early clinical outcomes and routine management of patients with non–ST segment elevation myocardial infarction: a nationwide perspective. *Arch Intern Med* 2000; in press.
17. TIMI Study Group. Comparison of invasive and conservative strategies after treatment with intravenous tissue plasminogen activator in acute myocardial infarction. Results of the Thrombolysis in Myocardial Infarction (TIMI) Phase II Trial. *N Engl J Med* 1989;320:618.
18. Bosch X, Theroux P, Waters DD, et al. Early postinfarction ischemia: clinical, angiographic, and prognostic significance. *Circulation* 1987;5:988–995.
19. Gibson RS, Boden WE, Theroux P, et al. Diltiazem and reinfarction in patients with non–Q-wave myocardial infarction. Results of a double-blind, randomized, multicenter trial. *N Engl J Med* 1986;315:423–429.
20. Schaer DH, Ross AM, Wasserman AG. Reinfarction, recurrent angina and reocclusion after thrombolytic therapy. *Circulation* 1987;76:II–57.
21. ISIS-2 (Second International Study of Infarct Survival) Collaborative Group. Randomized trial of intravenous streptokinase, oral aspirin,

both, or neither among 17,187 cases of suspected acute myocardial infarction: ISIS-2. *Lancet* 1988;2:349.

22. Gruppo Italiano per lo Studio della Streptochinasi nell'Infarto Miocardico (GISSI). Effectiveness of intravenous thrombolytic treatment in acute myocardial infarction. *Lancet* 1986;1:397.

23. Granger CB, Miller JM, Bovill EG, et al. Rebound increase in thrombin generation and activity after cessation of intravenous heparin in patients with acute coronary syndromes. *Circulation* 1995;91:1929–1935.

24. Antman EM, for the TIMI 14 investigators. Abciximab facilitates the rate and extent of thrombolysis: results of the TIMI 14 Trial. *Circulation* 1999;99:2720–2732.

25. Ross AM, Molhoek GP, Knudtson ML, et al. A randomized comparison of low molecular weight heparin and unfractionated heparin adjunctive to tPA thrombolysis and aspirin (HART-II). *Circulation* 2000;102:II-600.

26. TIMI Study Group. Comparison of invasive and conservative strategies after treatment with intravenous tissue plasminogen activator in acute myocardial infarction: results of Thrombolysis in Myocardial Infarction (TIMI) Phase 2 Trial. *N Engl J Med* 1989;320:618–627.

27. Zehender M, Kasper W, Kauder E, et al. Right ventricular infarction as an independent predictor of prognosis after acute inferior myocardial infarction. *N Engl J Med* 1993;328:981–988.

28. Manno BV, Bemis CE, Carver J, et al. Right ventricular infarction complicated by right to left shunt. *J Am Coll Cardiol* 1983;1:554–557.

29. Love JC, Haffajee CI, Gore JM, et al. Reversibility of hypotension and shock by atrial or atrioventricular sequential pacing in patients with right ventricular infarction. *Am Heart J* 1984;108:5–13.

30. Braunwald E, Kloner RA. The stunned myocardium: prolonged post-ischemic ventricular dysfunction. *Circulation* 1982;66:1146.

31. Scott BD, Kerber RE. Clinical and experimental aspects of myocardial stunning. *Prog Cardiovasc Dis* 1992;35:61.

32. Goldberg RJ, Gore JM, Alpert JS, et al. Cardiogenic shock resulting form acute myocardial infarction: a fourteen-year community-wide perspective. *N Engl J Med* 1991;325:1117–1122.

33. Alonso DR, Scheidt S, Post M, et al. Pathophysiology of cardiogenic shock: quantification of myocardial necrosis, clinical, pathologic and electrocardiographic correlations. *Circulation* 1973;48:588–596.

34. Hochman JS, Sleeper LA, Webb JG, et al. Early revascularization in acute myocardial infarction complicated by cardiogenic shock. *N Engl J Med* 1999;341:625–634.

34a. Skillington PD, Davies RH, Luf AJ, et al. Surgical treatment for infarct-related ventricular septal defects: improved early results combined with analysis of late functional status. *J Thorac Cardiovasc Surg* 1990;99:798–808.

35. Becker RC, Charlesworth A, Wilcox RG, et al. Cardiac rupture associated with thrombolytic therapy: impact of time to treatment in the late assessment of thrombolytic efficacy (LATE) study. *J Am Coll Cardiol* 1995;25:1063–1068.

36. Becker RC, Gore JM, Lambrew C, et al. A composite view of cardiac rupture in the United States: National Registry of Myocardial Infarction. *J Am Coll Cardiol* 1996;27:1321–1326.

37. Becker RC, Hochman JS, Cannon CP, et al., and the TIMI 9 Investigators. Fatal cardiac rupture among patients treated with thrombolytic agents and adjunctive thrombin antagonists. *J Am Coll Cardiol* 1999;33:479–487.

38. Tcheng JE, Jackman JD Jr, Nelson CL, et al. Outcome of patients sustaining acute ischemic mitral regurgitation during myocardial infarction. *Ann Intern Med* 1992;117:18–24.

39. Hendren WG, Nemec JJ, Lytle BW, et al. Mitral valve repair for ischemic mitral insufficiency. *Ann Thorac Surg* 1991;52:1246–1251.

40. Hutchins GM, Bulkley BH. Infarct expansion versus extension: two different complications of acute myocardial infarction. *Am J Cardiol* 1978;41:1127.

41. Pfeffer MA, Braunwald E, Moye LA, et al. Effect of captopril on mortality and morbidity in patients with left ventricular dysfunction after myocardial infarction. *N Engl J Med* 1992;327:669.

42. The Acute Infarction Ramipril Efficacy (AIRE) Study Investigators. Effect of ramipril on mortality and morbidity of survivors of acute myocardial infarction with clinical evidence of heart failure. *Lancet* 1993;342:821.

43. Martin RH, Almond CH, Saab S, et al. True and false aneurysms of the left ventricle following myocardial infarction. *Am J Med* 1977;62:418–424.

44. Krainin FM, Flessas AP, Spodick DH. Infarction-associated pericarditis: rarity of diagnostic electrocardiogram. *N Engl J Med* 1984;311:1211–1214.

45. Guillevin L, Valere PE. Pericarditis in acute myocardial infarction. *Lancet* 1976;1:429.

46. Guberman BA, Fowler NO, Engel PJ, et al. Cardiac tamponade in medical patients. *Circulation* 1981;64:633.

47. Miller RR, Lies JE, Carretta RF, et al. Prevention of lower extremity venous thrombus by early mobilization. *Ann Intern Med* 1976;84:700–703.

48. Gueret P, Bubourg O, Ferrier A, et al. Effects of full-dose heparin anticoagulation on the development of left ventricular thrombosis in acute myocardial infarction. *J Am Coll Cardiol* 1986;8:419.

49. Weinreich DJ, Burke JF, Pauletto FJ. Left ventricular mural thrombi complicating acute myocardial infarction: long-term follow-up with serial echocardiography. *Ann Intern Med* 1984;100:789.

50. Keating EC, Gross SA, Schlamowitz RA, et al. Mural thrombi in myocardial infarctions: prospective evaluation by two dimensional echocardiography. *Am J Med* 1983;74:989–995.

CHAPTER 12

Critical Pathway for Unstable Angina

Christopher P. Cannon and Patrick T. O'Gara

A critical pathway for unstable angina and non–ST-segment elevation myocardial infarction (MI) was developed in 1996 at Brigham and Women's Hospital (BWH), Boston, Massachusetts. The first goal was to ensure optimal use of guideline-recommended medications and treatments. In addition, every effort was made to eliminate redundant or unnecessary tests and to reduce the length of hospitalizations. Such measures could reduce costs and allow these resources to be utilized for other beneficial treatments. More recently, as new therapies became available [e.g., low molecular weight heparin (LMWH) or glycoprotein (GP) IIb/IIIa inhibitors for unstable angina], the critical pathway has been used to introduce these agents into the standard of care at BWH and to provide clinicians specific recommendations on which patients should be treated with the new agents.

FIRST TARGET ISSUE

Underutilization of Recommended Medications

A major rationale for the development of a critical pathway for unstable angina was the emerging information from registries showing underutilization of medications such as aspirin. This agent has been shown to be beneficial across the entire spectrum of ischemic coronary syndromes—from primary prevention to unstable angina and acute MI as well as in secondary prevention (1–10). In particular, in unstable angina, aspirin has been shown to reduce death or MI by 50% to 70% (3–6).

However, in the first National Registry of Myocardial Infarction involving 240,989 patients, among those with acute MI not receiving thrombolytic therapy (i.e., largely non–ST-segment elevation MI), only 63% received aspirin (11). In the Thrombolysis in Myocardial Ischemia (TIMI) III Registry of unstable angina or non–ST-segment elevation MI conducted in 1992–1993, 80% of patients received aspirin; and in the Global Unstable Angina Registry and Treatment Evaluation (GUARANTEE) Registry conducted in 1996, 83% of patients received aspirin (12,13).

Similar findings have been observed for beta-blockers and heparin, with heparin being used in only 57% of patients in the TIMI III registry and in 67% of patients in the GUARANTEE registry (12–16). Importantly, recent evidence has suggested that if patients are treated according to the unstable angina guideline recommendations, their adjusted 1-year mortality rate is lower compared with patients who do not receive all guideline-recommended therapies (17). Thus, with these data available nationally, the major focus at BWH was to ensure that all patients received recommended therapies.

More recently, several new classes of drugs have become available for the treatment of unstable angina or non–ST-segment elevation MI. The LMWH agents and the GP IIb/IIIa inhibitors have been shown to be beneficial in reducing death or MI in unstable angina and in non–ST-segment elevation MI (18–24). Accordingly, in early 1999, BWH adapted the pathway to formally incorporate these therapies (see below).

Reducing Other Cardiac Testing

Another area identified at BWH was the potential overutilization of laboratory testing. Patients would often have multiple assessments of their lipid profile during a single hospital stay; or, similarly, full chemistry panels twice daily. It was thought that this might simply be overly cautious house staff ordering tests for completeness. The frequent use of stress testing with radionuclide imaging, for patients who had normal baseline electrocardiograms (ECG) was identified as another area wherein costs savings might be safely achieved.

Reducing Hospital (and Intensive Care Unit) Length of Stay

Reducing the length of hospitalization, which has been the driving force behind the creation of critical pathways, is a relatively easy and efficient way to reduce costs. For the initial critical pathways in cardiac surgical patients, early discharge was the primary outcome variable (25). In unstable angina, hospitalizations were lengthy just 5 years ago. In patients with unstable angina and non–Q-wave MI enrolled in the TIMI IIIB trial, the average length of stay was more than 9 days. In the parallel TIMI 3 registry of patients not entered into the trial, length of stay was also 9 days. Hospitalizations have shortened over recent years—on average 4.4 days in the GUARANTEE registry (26,27). However, opportunities exist to reduce their length further.

Another potential benefit of critical pathways is to improve the triage of patients to the appropriate level of care (28,29). Previously, coronary care unit (CCU) admission was standard. However, in the modern era, CCU admission is generally reserved for ST-segment elevation MI patients and those with hemodynamic compromise or other complications. In the multicenter GUARANTEE registry conducted in the United States in 1996, 62% of patients with non–ST-elevation MI were admitted to the CCU and 36% to a step-down unit (14). Here too, an opportunity exists to reduce admission to the CCU as a means of improving the cost-effectiveness of care.

CRITICAL PATHWAYS DEVELOPMENT

A task force was impaneled to create a critical pathway that would include guidelines for patients with unstable angina and non–Q-wave MI. A draft critical pathway was developed over a 4-month period, which was then distributed to all healthcare professionals who cared for patients with unstable angina, including all physician members of the cardiovascular division, cardiac surgery, cardiovascular nursing, noninvasive testing laboratory, the emergency department (ED), the social service department, case management, and nutrition services. Comments were solicited from all these participants. Their comments were included in the final pathway that was then launched in a pilot fashion in July 1996. The fifth step in the critical pathways development was to collect and monitor data regarding pathway performance. This included evaluating the number of patients for whom the pathway was used, the use of recommended therapies, and length of hospitalizations. The final step was to interpret the initial data and to modify the pathway, as needed. Collectively, the latter three steps consist of the ongoing quality improvement

needed during the implementation of any pathway. In addition, clinical trials are monitored for new therapies that should be added or modified as part of the optimal management of unstable angina.

Goals

The pathway for management of unstable angina or non–ST-segment elevation MI at BWH emphasizes (a) early relief of ischemic pain, a determinant of the development of MI among patients presenting with symptoms of acute ischemia; (b) administration of antithrombotic and antiischemic therapy as outlined above; (c) reminders of eligibility criteria for ongoing clinical trials (e.g., trials of new IIb/IIIa inhibitors or LMWH); (d) a detailed list of suggested blood tests in an effort to reduce unnecessary tests; (e) physician choice of either an early conservative strategy or an early invasive strategy; and (f) early hospital discharge (Fig. 12-1) (29).

Patient Population

Patient eligibility for the pathway was based on clinical criteria for unstable angina (i.e., patients who presented with typical angina at rest or with minimal exertion). It was felt that broad entry criteria were warranted to allow the pathway to potentially benefit as many patients as possible. Because the spectrum of acute coronary syndrome (ACS) is broad, several other pathways were developed in parallel with this unstable angina pathway. For patients in whom the clinical history was less certain for unstable angina, diagnostic chest pain pathways to "rule out MI" were developed (see Chapters 5–7).

Patients were defined as those presenting with ischemic pain occurring either at rest or with minimal exertion and with an accelerating pattern (i.e., Braunwald class 1–3 unstable angina) (30). The ECG provided corroborative information that supported the clinical diagnosis, but was not necessary for inclusion in the pathway. Electrocardiographic changes

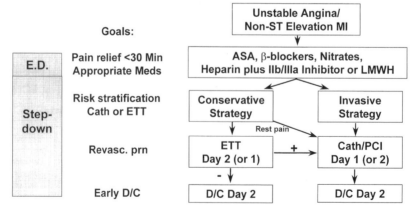

FIG. 12-1. Overview of the Brigham and Women's Hospital critical pathway for unstable angina or non–ST-segment elevation myocardial infarction. ASA, aspirin; Cath, cardiac catheterization; D/C, discharge; ED, Emergency Department; ETT, exercise tolerance test; LMWH, low molecular weight heparin; Meds, medications; MI, myocardial infarction; Min, minutes; PCI, percutaneous coronary intervention.

BWH Critical Pathway: Ischemia (Unstable angina/non-ST elevation MI)   March 1996

	Day 0 Emergency Dept.	Day 0 Stepdown Unit	Conservative Day 1 Stepdown Unit	Conservative Day 2 Stepdown Unit	Invasive Day 1 Stepdown Unit	Invasive Day 2 Stepdown Unit	Post-Discharge
Goals	○ Pain free<30 min ○ Page attending +/or B team fellow ○ Consider TIMI 11		If stable, consider D/C Home with Outpatient ETT	○ ETT ○ If Neg : D/C If Pos: Cath	○ Cath in am ○ If PTCA, sheaths out in pm	○ D/C Home in am ○ Consider enrollment TIMI 12	
Assessment	○ Vitals ○ Cont. ECG monitor ○ Enroll. crit. TIMI 11	○ Vitals q 4h ○ Cont. ECG monitor	○ Vitals q 8h ○ Cont ECG monitor	○ Vitals q 8h ○ D/C Cont. ECG	○ Vitals q 4h ○ Cont. ECG ○ Monitor groin	○ Vitals q 4h ○ monitor groin	
Tests	○ CBC, Chem 20, CK-MB, Troponin I Lipid Profile, PT/PTT ○ ECG	○ CK/MB q 8 x2 ○ PTT 6 h ○ ECG	○ CBC ○ PTT ○ ECG	○ PTT ○ ETT in am	○ AM: CBC, PTT ○ PM: CBC, Chem 7		
Medication	○ ASA ○ IV heparin ○ Metoprolol IV/PO ○ Nitro sl (IV prn)	○ ASA ○ IV heparin ○ Metoprolol ○ Nitrates ○ Ca Antag. prn ○ Lipid low.prn	○ ASA ○ IV heparin ○ Metoprolol ○ Nitrates ○ Ca Antag prn ○ Lipid low.prn	○ ASA ○ IV heparin ○ Beta-blocker ○ Nitrates prn ○ CaAntag prn ○ Lipid low.prn	○ ASA ○ IV heparin pre-cath ○ metoprolol ○ Nitrates ○ Ca Antag prn ○ Lipid low. prn	○ ASA ○ Beta-blocker ○ Nitrates prn ○ CaAntag prn ○ Lipid low. prn	
Treatments	○ O2	○ O2	○ If ischemia: consider cath ○ D/C O2	○ If ischemia: consider cath	○ Cath in am ○ PTCA prn ○ Sheath out in pm		
Activity/Rehab	○ Bedrest	○ Bedrest	○ Ambulate in room	○ Routine activity	○ Bedrest	○ Ambulate	
Diet	○ Heart Healthy Diet	○ Dietary consult	○ Heart Healthy Diet	○ Heart Healthy Diet	○ NPO post MN ○ Heart Healthy in pm	○ Heart Healthy Diet	
Education: Patient and Family	○ Explain Diagnosis /Plan	○ Explain Dx/Plan ○ Cath consent	○ Discuss risk factors, meds	○ D/C instruct.	○ Discuss cath results, risk factors, medications	○ D/C instruct.	
Discharge Planning	○ Admit to Stepdown unit	○ Notify 1° MD ○ Notify Case Manager ○ Soc.Serv. consult prn	○ Call VNA prn ○ Lipid manag. plan (clinic prn) ○ Exercise plan (Card.Rehab prn)	○ If ETT Neg/low risk, D/C home ○ Appt 1° MD ○ Call 1° MD ○ D/C letter	○ Call VNA prn ○ Lipid manag. plan (Appt Lipid clinic prn) ○ Card.Rehab	○ D/C in am ○ Appt 1° MD ○ Call 1° MD ○ D/C letter	○ F/U call Case Manager 24-48h
Variances							

Instructions for the ○: If completed, mark ●. If not done, record a number in the circle, ①, and in the Variances box, record 1: one-two word reason" (Example: if severe COPD, in the Medications section, record ① for metoprolol PO, and in the Variances section: Write "1: Severe COPD")

FIG. 12-2. Initial unstable angina critical pathway—1996.

could include ST-segment depression or transient ST-segment elevation, or new T-wave inversion, although the ST-segment changes are more specific markers of coronary disease and of high risk for adverse outcomes. Of note, ST-segment change of 0.5 mm appears to have equal significance to ST-segment depression of 1 mm or more (13). Because only a third of patients presenting with unstable angina have ECG changes, the admission diagnosis relies predominantly on the history (13).

Medical Management

Initial management, as shown in Figs. 12-1 and 12-2, is with aspirin, heparin, beta-blockers, and nitrates to control ischemic pain. If pain persists despite three sublingual nitroglycerin tablets, intravenous nitroglycerin is used. Calcium antagonists are used if needed to control ischemia after these agents are at optimal therapeutic doses. The heart rate lowering agent diltiazem is generally chosen. However, among patients with bradycardia, long-acting dihydropyridine agents are used.

Because angiotensin converting enzyme (ACE) inhibitors are useful in left ventricular (LV) dysfunction, they are recommended for patients with reduced ejection fraction or symptoms of congestive heart failure. They are not mandatory as initial treatment in the first 24 hours for all patients since the

Gruppo Italiano per lo Studio della Sopravvivenza nell'Infarto Miocardico (GISSI) 3 and International Study of Infarct Survival (ISIS)-4 trials showed no significant benefit in patients with ST-segment depression MI (31,32).

Since the pathway originated, the GP IIb/IIIa inhibitors and LMWH have been added to the pathway. A memorandum was issued updating the pathway recommendations (Fig. 12-3). Below is the brief overview of the new data that were provided to all clinicians to assist them in learning about the new agents and understanding the new pathway recommendations.

Tirofiban

Glycoprotein IIb/IIIa inhibitors bind to the GP IIb/IIIa receptor and prevent the formation (or progression) of a platelet aggregate. Tirofiban is a nonpeptide antagonist of the GP IIb/IIIa receptor. In the Platelet Receptor Inhibition for Ischemic Syndrome Management in Patients Limited by Unstable Signs and Symptoms (PRISM-PLUS) trial (23) involving 1,915 patients with unstable angina and non–ST-segment elevation MI, tirofiban plus heparin and aspirin led to a significantly lower rate of death, MI, or refractory ischemia at 7 days compared with heparin and aspirin (12.9% vs. 17.9%), a 32% risk reduction ($p = 0.004$). This result comprised a 45% reduction in MI and 30% reduction in refractory ischemia. Death or MI at 30 days was reduced by 30%, from 11.9% to 8.7% ($p = 0.03$), and the improvement was consistent across all subgroups and management strategies [i.e., medical therapy (25% reduction), percutaneous transluminal coronary angioplasty (PTCA) (35% reduction), and coronary artery bypass graft (CABG) surgery (30% reduction)]. In the PRISM trial involving 3,232 patients (22), tirofiban reduced the rate of death, MI, or refractory ischemia at 48 hours (3.8% vs. 5.6% for heparin), a 32% reduction ($p = 0.01$). A recent analysis from the PRISM-PLUS trial found that early use of GP IIb/IIIa inhibitors can reduce the size of an evolving non–ST-segment elevation: patients randomized to tirofiban plus heparin had a significantly lower peak troponin (Fig. 12-4) (33). Similar data were observed in the Platelet Glycoprotein IIb/IIIa in Unstable Angina: Receptor Suppression Using

Integrin Therapy (PURSUIT) trial, emphasizing the need to initiate therapy early to reduce the severity of the presenting ischemic episode (33). The cost of tirofiban therapy is approximately $750 per 2-day course.

Eptifibatide

Eptifibatide, a synthetic heptapeptide inhibitor of the GP IIb/IIIa receptor, was studied in the PURSUIT trial involving 10,948 patients. Eptifibatide reduced the rate of death or MI at 30 days by a relative 10% (from 15.7% to 14.2%, $p = 0.042$) (24). A greater benefit was observed in patients who underwent early percutaneous coronary intervention (PCI) on eptifibatide (31% reduction in death or MI at 30 days, 16.7% vs. 11.6%, $p = 0.01$), but no significant benefit (7% reduction,

MEMORANDUM

To:	Cardiovascular Division Staff and Fellows
From:	Christopher Cannon, M.D., Patrick O'Gara, M.D., for the Acute Coronary Syndromes Critical Pathways Committee
Subject:	IIb/IIIa inhibitors and LMWH for the treatment of acute coronary syndromes
Date:	September 7, 2000

As you know, two major advances in the treatment of unstable angina and non-ST elevation MI have recently been approved for use by the Food and Drug Administration: the platelet glycoprotein IIb/IIIa inhibitors, tirofiban (Aggrastat®) and eptifibatide (Integrilin®), and the low molecular weight heparin enoxaparin (Lovenox®). Abciximab (ReoPro®) has already been approved for use during percutaneous coronary intervention (PCI). These new agents have each been shown to afford patients between 10-30% reduction in death or MI at 30 days as compared with aspirin and heparin. We thus feel it is important to incorporate these treatments for appropriate patients in order to offer patients "state-of-the-art" management as summarized below:

Who: High-risk patients as defined by rest pain within the last 24 hours and any one of the following:
- *ECG changes:* ST depression (≥ 0.5 mm), transient ST elevation, or T wave changes
- *Positive serum markers:* Positive CK-MB or Troponin
- *Prior history* of MI, PCI, CABG and a strong clinical history; diabetes and prior aspirin use = high risk
- *Ongoing or recurrent typical ischemic pain* despite IV nitro, aspirin and heparin
- *TIMI Risk Score ≥ 3* .

What: The suggested treatments are based on the strategy chosen (see figure):
> **All patients should get aspirin (325 mg daily)****
- No Cath/PCI planned: Enoxaparin 1 mg/kg subcutaneously bid until hospital discharge
- Cath the same day: Unfractionated heparin and IIb/IIIa inhibitor in cath lab
  (agent selected by Interventional attending)
- Cath the following day: Tirofiban plus unfractionated heparin (APTT 50-70 secs)
  (loading dose 0.4 ug/kg/min x 30 minutes then 0.1 ug/kg/min infusion)

Where:
These agents should be prescribed by the cardiology fellows and staff. Initiation is suggested as soon as possible (e.g. in the Emergency Department) to maximize benefit, as data have recently shown reduction in infarct size and greater reduction in clinical events with earlier initiation. They can also be administered in the CCU and stepdown units.

When:
- These agents should be started during the initial treatment of patients with unstable angina/non-ST elevation MI in the ED or stepdown/CCU or upon transfer to the Brigham of patients who have had recurrent ischemia prior to transfer. The GP IIb/IIIa inhibitors are *continued* during PCI and for 12-24 hours thereafter.
- In patients undergoing PCI who have not already received a IIb/IIIa inhibitor - a IIb/IIIa inhibitor is started just prior to the procedure and continued 12-24 hours thereafter.

FIG. 12-3A. Memorandum to cardiology and other departments describing revised unstable angina critical pathway.

Recommendations – September 2000:

The field of acute coronary syndromes changes rapidly. In particular ongoing trials will address the safety and efficacy of combined use of LMWH and IIb/IIIa inhibitors, and of invasive vs. conservative strategies. At the current time, we recommend the following:

1. **Aggressive Medical Therapy:** Check that aspirin, beta-blockers, etc are actually administered to patients - potentially by using the "Cardiac Checklist" as each patient is admitted
2. **Treatment strategy:** . Thus, for intermediate to high-risk patients, an invasive strategy is recommended. For lower risk patients, either strategy is acceptable
3. **Conservatively managed patients:** Use the LMWH enoxaparin . This is low-cost approach, which may also reduce the *need for* catheterization and revascularization.
4. **Same Day Catheterization / PCI:** Use unfractionated heparin initially, and allow Interventional attending to choose to use IIb/IIIa inhibitor during PCI. (Abciximab has shortest duration of infusion [12 hours], eptifibatide and tirofiban require 18-24 hour infusions but have lower cost)
5. **Catheterization / PCI day after admission:** Begin tirofiban as soon as possible upon admission (ideally in the ED) or at the time of transfer from the other hospital, and continue the infusion during catheterization and PCI and for 12-18 hours post PCI. (We have recommended use of one agent, currently tirofiban, so that the house staff and nursing staff will become familiar with its use, in part to avoid potential dosing errors.)
6. **Combination of LMWH and IIb/IIIa inhibitors** can be considered in high-risk patients. Several pilot studies have shown the combination of LMWH and a IIb/IIIa inhibitor has similar rates of major bleeding as unfractionated heparin and a IIb/IIIa inhibitor.

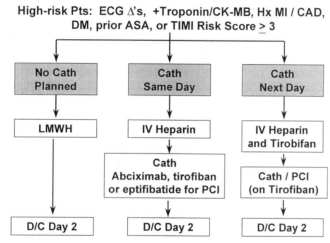

BWH Critical Pathways for Unstable Angina/Non-Q-Wave MI

FIG. 12-3B. Continued.

$p = 0.23$) was seen in those treated medically, with late PCI or CABG. More recently, in the setting of PCI, significant benefit was observed with a double bolus and infusion regimen of eptifibatide (death, MI, or urgent revascularization at 30 days was 10.4% for placebo vs. 6.8% for eptifibatide, $p = 0.004$), with an even greater reduction in the number of patients with ACS (10.5% vs. 5.4%, $p = 0.01$).

Emerging evidence shows an apparent greater benefit of treatment when administered earlier relative to the onset of pain. In the PURSUIT trial, the absolute reduction in death or MI with eptifibatide was 2.8% for patients treated within 6 hours from the onset of pain, 2.3% for those treated between 6 to 12 hours, and 1.7% for those treated 12 to 24 hours following the onset of pain. No benefit was observed in patients treated 24 hours after the onset of pain. Similar data have been observed in PRISM-PLUS (unpublished data),

thus emphasizing the importance of starting therapy as early as possible, ideally in the ED. Cost is approximately $750 per 2-day course of therapy, and approximately $300 for a 12- to 18-hour course of therapy for PCI.

Abciximab

Abciximab, a monoclonal antibody fragment directed at the IIb/IIIa receptor, has been shown in numerous trials to reduce death or MI in patients having PCI (35–38). A long-term mortality benefit has also been observed in one trial, and in a meta-analysis of PCI trials with abciximab (39,40). In patients with unstable angina, benefit was observed in those treated for 24 hours before PCI (38). However, most recently, in the Global Utilization of Strategies to Open Occluded Arteries (GUSTO) IV-ACS trial, in patients not planned for

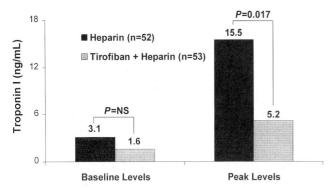

FIG. 12-4. Peak levels of troponin I (TnI) were reduced in patients treated with the glycoprotein IIb/IIIa inhibitor tirofiban compared with aspirin and heparin. These data demonstrate that early treatment (within 12 hours from the onset of chest pain in this study) led to a reduced infarct size among patients with unstable angina and non–ST-segment elevation MI. (Data from Januzzi JL, Hahn SS, Chae CU, et al. Reduction of troponin I levels in patients with acute coronary syndromes by glycoprotein IIb/IIIa inhibition with tirofiban. *Am J Cardiol* 2000;86:713–717).

PCI, no benefit was observed. Cost is approximately $1,400 per 12-hour course of therapy.

Enoxaparin

Low molecular weight heparins are combined factor Xa and thrombin inhibitors. As compared with unfractionated heparin, which has equal antithrombin (factor IIa) and anti-Xa activity, enoxaparin has an increased ratio of anti-Xa to IIa activity of 3:1. The Efficacy and Safety of Subcutaneous Enoxaparin in Non–Q wave Coronary Events (ESSENCE) and TIMI 11B trials compared enoxaparin with unfractionated heparin in unstable angina and non–ST-segment elevation MI in 3,171 and 3,910 patients, respectively. In ESSENCE, death, MI or recurrent ischemia at 14 days was

reduced by a relative 16% (16.6% vs. 19.8%, $p = 0.019$) (19). In addition, the need for cardiac catheterization and PTCA was significantly reduced. In TIMI 11B, death, MI, or urgent revascularization at 14 days was reduced by a relative 15% by enoxaparin (14.2% vs. 16.7% for unfractionated heparin, $p = 0.029$) (21). In the combined meta-analysis, death or MI at 42 days was significantly reduced by 18% ($p = 0.02$) (Fig. 12-5) (20). In the trials, for catheterization and PCI, enoxaparin was usually stopped and unfractionated heparin was used. Cost is approximately $150 for 2-day course of therapy.

TREATMENT STRATEGY

The invasive strategy in the pathway includes the medical management as described above and catheterization within the first 18 hours after admission; thus, for some patients admitted in the morning, the catheterization is performed later in the afternoon. Patients admitted in the afternoon or early evening and who are medically stabilized have catheterization the following morning. Based on the anatomic findings, revascularization is carried out as appropriate. Generally, PCI can be performed immediately. If the patient is referred for CABG, the on-call surgeon is summoned immediately and scheduling is arranged as soon as possible. Patients then follow the CABG pathway (Chapter 14), which targets a 4- to 5-day hospitalization for patients without complications.

The early conservative strategy involves aggressive medical management and clinical monitoring. If the patient has recurrent ischemic pain, an ECG is performed; if the pain is strongly suggestive of ischemia or ECG changes are present, the patient is referred for catheterization that day. In the absence of recurrent ischemia at rest, an exercise test is performed on the morning of day 2; if negative, the patient is discharged home. If ischemia is demonstrated on the stress test, the patient is scheduled for cardiac catheterization that

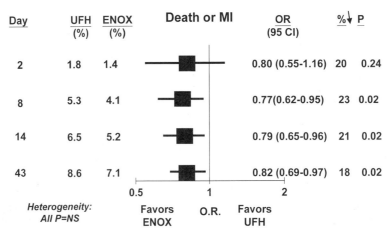

FIG. 12-5. TIMI 11B/ESSENCE metaanalysis. Data from more than 7,000 patients randomized in these two trials show a consistent and significant 20% reduction in the rate of death or myocardial infarction at each of the four time points in patients treated with enoxaparin versus unfractionated heparin. (Adapted from Antman EM, et al. Assessment of the treatment effect of enoxaparin for unstable angina/non–Q-wave myocardial infarction: TIMI 11B-ESSENCE meta-analysis. *Circulation* 1999;100:1602–1608; with permission).

same day. For a patient with abnormal resting ECG (e.g., fixed ST-segment depression, LV hypertrophy with ST-segment depression, or left bundle branch block), a radionuclide stress test is arranged. If the patient is unable to walk, a pharmacologic stress test is arranged—with echocardiography or radionuclide imaging. If the patient has been triaged to the early conservative strategy, non-invasive testing is scheduled within the hours postadmission so that a slot can be reserved for the appropriate day. It should be noted that because unstable angina encompasses such a heterogeneous group of patients and patients at lower risk are managed in the early conservative strategy, exercise testing is sometimes performed on hospital day 1.

Choice of Treatment Strategy

Four randomized trials have compared invasive versus conservative strategies in unstable angina (Fig. 12-6). TIMI IIIB randomized 1,473 patients with unstable angina or non–ST-segment elevation MI. No difference was seen between the two strategies in the primary endpoint (death, MI, or a positive exercise test at 6 weeks): 16.2% vs. 18.1% for the invasive versus conservative strategies ($p =$ NS); or in the endpoint of death or MI at 1 year (10.8% vs. 12.2%, $p =$ NS) (41,42). Similar findings were seen in the much smaller Medicine versus Angioplasty in Thrombolytic Exclusion (MATE) trial (43). The Veterans Affairs Non–Q-Wave Infarction Strategies In-Hospital (VANQWISH) trial, which enrolled 920 patients with non–Q-wave MI, found no significant

difference in death or MI through follow-up (average 23 months): 26.9% in the invasive arm versus 29.9% in the conservative arm ($p = 0.35$) (44). However, significantly more deaths occurred in patients assigned to the invasive compared with the conservative strategy at hospital discharge (4.5% vs. 1.3%, $p = 0.007$), which was sustained at 1 year. This difference was explained in part by a high peri-CABG mortality rate (12.8%) in the invasive group, whereas no adverse outcome was observed in patients treated with PTCA.

More recently, the Fragmin and Fast Revascularization during InStability in Coronary artery disease (FRISC) II trial found a significant reduction in death or MI to 6 months in the invasive group (12.1 vs. 9.4, $p = 0.031$) (45). Subgroup analyses showed that the higher risk groups (e.g., age > 65years, ST-segment depression, or troponin T > 0.01 ng/dl) derived the greatest benefit (46).

The Treat Angina with Aggrastat and determine Cost of Therapy with Invasive vs. Conservative Strategies (TACTICS)–TIMI 18 trial recently showed that for patients at intermediate to high risk, an invasive strategy is superior (46a). For patients at lower risk, either strategy is acceptable.

TESTS ON ADMISSION

The pathway includes three creatine kinase (CK)-MB determinations drawn at baseline, 8 hours, and 16 hours. In addition, a troponin I is drawn at entry to assist in risk stratifying patients. Because serial troponin values have been found to improve the sensitivity of detecting patients at high

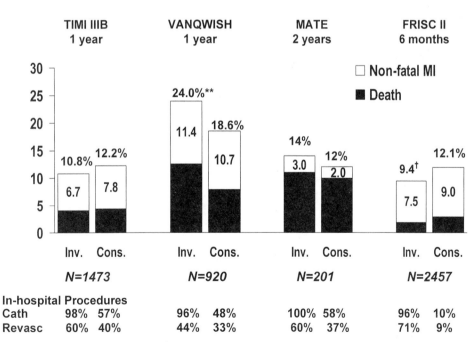

FIG. 12-6. Results from the four randomized trials of invasive versus conservative strategies in unstable angina and non–ST-segment elevation myocardial infarction. The duration of follow-up is shown for each trial at the top, and the number of patients at the bottom. In addition, the rate of cardiac catheterization during the initial hospitalization, as well as the rates of revascularization (revasc) with percutaneous coronary intervention (PCI) or coronary artery bypass graft (CABG). (*p = 0.05; **p = 0.025; +p = 0.031.) (Data from references 42–45).

risk (without ST-segment elevation), serial troponins were recently added to the BWH pathway (47). As will be noted, this is helpful in determining a high-risk group in whom IIb/IIIa inhibitors would have the greatest benefit.

Additional blood work has been limited in the pathway. For example, it has been routine to draw a complete chemistry panel each day that the patient is in the hospital. This has been reduced to one panel on admission, a panel of electrolytes on the second day, and a complete blood count with platelets each day that the patient is on heparin. Because many patients in this population who receive diuretics frequently receive intravenous fluid, both potassium and magnesium are checked on a daily basis for a 2-day period and appropriate replacement given.

Electrocardiograms are performed at baseline, on arrival to the floor, and the following morning to evaluate for any evolution or ST-segment, T-wave, or Q-wave changes. Otherwise, ECGs are performed only for patients with recurrent ischemic pain or other symptoms suggestive of ischemia.

Assessment of LV function, usually with an echo, is recommended for patients with symptoms of congestive heart failure, or for those with evidence of myocardial necrosis.

Cholesterol

Although data are just beginning to emerge from randomized trials to demonstrate an early clinical benefit of starting lipid-lowering therapy in patients with ACS, the early testing and initiation of therapy in the hospital does markedly increase the percentage of appropriate patients who eventually receive therapy. The pathway specifies measurement (within the first 24 hours, because lipid levels will fall over the subsequent days) of total cholesterol, triglycerides, low-density lipoprotein (LDL), and high-density lipoprotein. We do not mandate that this be a fasting level because this infrequently changes the management of the patient and sometimes leads to omission of drawing any cholesterol measurement, thereby missing the opportunity to make the diagnosis.

Length of Stay

The overall goal for length of stay with the pathway is 2 days. This includes patients who have PCI in the early invasive strategy. If patients fail the early conservative strategy and have an angioplasty on day 2, then their target length of stay is 3 days. For patients referred for CABG, the overall target is 7 days, with a 2-day hospitalization for the diagnosis and initial management of unstable angina and 4–5 days for the performance of and recovery from CABG.

SECONDARY PREVENTION AND FOLLOW-UP

Because follow-up is critical, we ensure that both a telephone call and a letter summarizing the hospital events are sent to the primary care physician and all other physicians caring for the patient. This allows continuity of care, and is an opportunity for the cardiologist to provide a rationale for long-term

management of the patient with key medications (e.g., aspirin, beta-blockers, and cholesterol-lowering medications). Given its long-term benefit in secondary prevention, aspirin is recommended at a dose of 81 to 325 mg daily.

Similarly, beta-blockers are recommended for long-term management in all patients without contraindications. Recently, with the results of the Heart Outcomes Prevention Evaluation (HOPE) trial, consideration of ACE inhibitors at discharge has been added for all patients (48). Cholesterol-lowering therapy is a key component of a long-term secondary prevention program and, thus, is recommended (49–51). Follow-up care with the primary care physician to achieve an LDL level less than 100 mg/dl is recommended by the National Cholesterol Education program (52). Finally cardiac rehabilitation is a key component following ACS. For patients with severe limitation of exercise capacity (e.g., the very elderly), transfer to a rehabilitation facility is arranged, especially following CABG, when needed. Patients are approached to participate in a cardiac rehabilitation program, either at our hospital or one near to their home. All patients receive a booklet outlining an exercise program, which is briefly reviewed by the cardiologist and the nurse.

IMPLEMENTATION OF THE CRITICAL PATHWAY

Implementation began with distribution of the pathway, with a cover memorandum that described the goals and contained an overview, to all physicians and nurses caring for patients with unstable angina. In addition, the pathway was presented at both cardiology and medical house staff meetings. An electronic mail message was sent to all physicians, indicating that the pathway was available for use and follow-up reminders were sent by electronic mail each month for the specific physicians on the cardiology service.

Medications:

1.   Aspirin.. ☐
2.   Heparin (or LMWH)................................ ☐
3.   GP IIb/IIIa inhibitor............................... ☐
4.   Beta-blocker .... ☐
5.   Nitrate.. ☐
6.   Heart-rate lowering Ca^{++} blocker .... ☐
7.   ACE inhibitor... ☐

Interventions:

8.   Cath/revascularization for recurrent
   ischemia or in moderate- to
   high-risk patients.. ☐

Secondary prevention:

9.   Cholesterol: check + treat as needed.......... ☐
10.   Treat other risk factors (smoking)............. ☐

FIG. 12-7. Cardiac checklist for unstable angina and non–ST-segment elevation myocardial infarction.

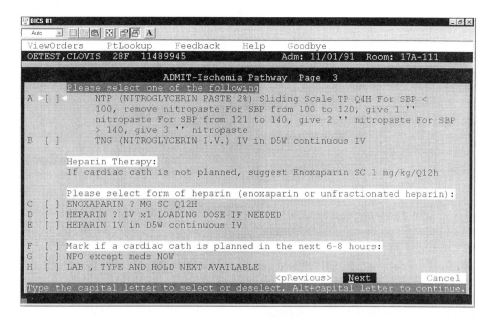

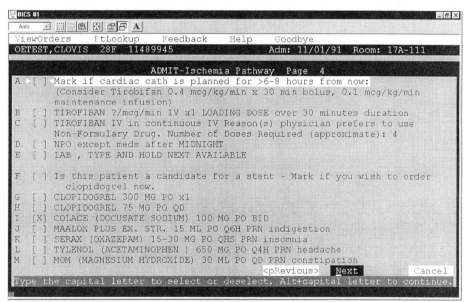

FIG. 12-8. Brigham and Women's Hospital computer order set—pages 3 and 4 of 7 pages. Courtesy of David Morrow, MD.

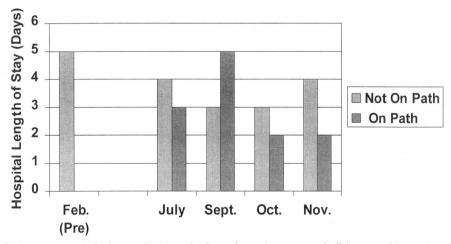

FIG. 12-9. Improvements in the median length of stay for patients on and off the unstable angina pathway.

The second step involved an independent screening of all admissions to the cardiology service for possible inclusion of patients on the pathway. When a patient was identified as eligible—essentially all patients with unstable angina and non–Q-wave MI—a copy of the pathway was placed in the patient's chart and notation left to the team treating the patient. It was quickly noted, however, that the complete pathway document, as shown in Fig. 12-2, took extra time for the physicians to complete and follow, resulting in a low use of the paper pathway (<20% of eligible patients). In keeping with the continuous quality improvement focus, a new approach was developed to have the orders specific to the pathway in a predefined computer-based order set for patients on the pathway, with the orders based on a simple "cardiac checklist" approach (Figs. 12-7 and 12-8).

An alternate approach that some hospitals have used is to have a designated case manager evaluate each patient and ensure that all steps in the pathway are carried out. This approach obviously requires additional resources from the hospital. However, experience with other pathways has shown that it is useful to ensure that patients follow the pathway. We monitored implementation with a designated research assistant.

LENGTH OF STAY RESULTS OF IMPLEMENTATION OF INITIAL PATHWAY

Length of stay, as shown in Fig. 12-9, was reduced after the pathway was instituted. After 1 month of implementation, the target length of stay of 2 days was reached. For patients who did not follow the pathway during the same time period, median length of hospitalization was 3 days. However, in general, length of stay on or off the pathway was reduced, indicating a potential "spill over" effect, whereby general conscientiousness regarding length of stay in patients on the pathway may have translated to similar efforts for patients not formally included on the pathway.

MEDICATION USE

We observed that the use of key medications (e.g., aspirin and heparin), which was already high before institution of the pathway, improved further. Aspirin use in the first 24 hours was 90% before the pathway, and it increased to 100% for patients on the pathway and 95% for those off the pathway during the same period. Heparin use rose from approximately 75% to 80% for patients on the pathway, which may indicate less complete acceptance of the heparin data in the treatment of unstable angina. Use of cholesterol-lowering medications increased from 33% to between 50% and 70%. Further analysis of cholesterol treatment found that of those patients treated medically or with angioplasty, 95% with elevated lipids at entry or who were taking cholesterol-lowering medications at the time of admission were discharged home on a statin medication. In contrast, only 40% of the patients who had CABG were discharged home on a statin.

INITIAL CHANGES TO THE PATHWAY

Based on the above data, one of the first changes was to add criteria for statin medication following CABG. The second change in the pathway was the incorporation of a booklet authored by the nutrition department describing a heart healthy diet and the American Heart Association step I and II diet plans. This booklet became part of the predischarge portfolio. Finally, as noted, new information about LMWH and GP IIb/IIIa inhibitors was added to the pathway.

CONCLUSIONS

The development and implementation of the critical pathway at BWH has evolved over the past 4 years. The goals remain the same: to improve the quality of care by the appropriate use of evidence-based medications, now including the LMWH and IIb/IIIa inhibitors, while improving the cost-efficiency of care by reducing length of stay and unnecessary tests. Initial results have been encouraging, and new data are presently being collected as part of our participation in national registries and as a barometer of our performance. This critical pathway has been beneficial in managing patients, and in providing patients with optimal care.

REFERENCES

1. Willard JE, Lange RA, Hillis LD. The use of aspirin in ischemic heart disease. *N Engl J Med* 1992;327:175–181.
2. Steering Committee of the Physicians' Health Study Research Group. Final report on the aspirin component of the ongoing Physicians' Health Study. *N Engl J Med* 1989;321:129–135.
3. Lewis HD, Davis JW, Archibald DG, et al. Protective effects of aspirin against acute myocardial infarction and death in men with unstable angina. *N Engl J Med* 1983;309:396–403.
4. Cairns JA, Gent M, Singer J, et al. Aspirin, sulfinpyrazone, or both in unstable angina. *N Engl J Med* 1985;313:1369–1375.
5. Theroux P, Ouimet H, McCans J, et al. Aspirin, heparin or both to treat unstable angina. *N Engl J Med* 1988;319:1105–1111.
6. The RISC Group. Risk of myocardial infarction and death during treatment with low dose aspirin and intravenous heparin in men with unstable coronary artery disease. *Lancet* 1990;336:827–830.
7. Roux S, Christeller S, Ludin E. Effects of aspirin on coronary reocclusion and recurrent ischemia after thrombolysis: a meta-analysis. *J Am Coll Cardiol* 1992;19:671–677.
8. ISIS-2 (Second International Study of Infarct Survival) Collaborative Group. Randomised trial of intravenous streptokinase, oral aspirin, both, or neither among 17,187 cases of suspected acute myocardial infarction: ISIS-2. *Lancet* 1988;2:349–360.
9. Klimt CR, Knatterud GL, Stamler J, et al., for the PARIS II Investigator Group. Persantine-Aspirin Reinfarction Study. Part II. Secondary coronary prevention with persantine and aspirin. *J Am Coll Cardiol* 1986;7:251–269.
10. Collaborative overview of randomised trials of antiplatelet therapy. I: Prevention of death, myocardial infarction, and stroke by prolonged antiplatelet therapy in various categories of patients. Antiplatelet Trialists' Collaboration. *BMJ* 1994;308:81–106.
11. Rogers WJ, Bowlby LJ, Chandra NC, et al. Treatment of myocardial infarction in the United States (1990 to 1993). Observations from the National Registry of Myocardial Infarction. *Circulation* 1994;90:2103–2114.
12. Stone PH, Thompson B, Anderson HV, et al. Influence of race, sex, and age on management of unstable angina and non–Q-wave myocardial infarction: the TIMI III Registry. *JAMA* 1996;275:1104–1112.
13. Cannon CP, McCabe CH, Stone PH, et al. The electrocardiogram predicts one-year outcome of patients with unstable angina and non–Q

wave myocardial infarction: results of the TIMI III Registry ECG Ancillary Study. *J Am Coll Cardiol* 1997;30:133–140.

14. Cannon CP, Moliterno DJ, Every N, et al. Implementation of AHCPR guidelines for unstable angina in 1996: unfortunate differences between men and women. Results from the multicenter GUARANTEE registry. *J Am Coll Cardiol* 1997;29[Suppl A]:217A.

15. Alexander KP, Peterson ED, Granger CB, et al. Potential impact of evidence-based medicine in acute coronary syndromes: insights from GUSTO-IIb. *J Am Coll Cardiol* 1998;32:2023–2030.

16. Scirica BM, Moliterno DJ, Every NR, et al. Differences between men and women in the management of unstable angina pectoris (The GUARANTEE Registry). The GUARANTEE Investigators. *Am J Cardiol* 1999;84:1145–1150.

17. Giugliano RP, Lloyd-Jones DM, Camargo CA Jr., et al. Association of unstable angina guideline care with improved survival. *Arch Intern Med* 2000;160:1775–1780.

18. FRagmin during Instability in Coronary Artery Disease (FRISC) Study Group. Low-molecular-weight heparin during instability in coronary artery disease. *Lancet* 1996;347:561–568.

19. Cohen M, Demers C, Gurfinkel EP, et al. A comparison of low-molecular-weight heparin with unfractionated heparin for unstable coronary artery disease. *N Engl J Med* 1997;337:447–452.

20. Antman EM, Cohen M, Radley D, et al. Assessment of the treatment effect of enoxaparin for unstable angina/non–Q-wave myocardial infarction: TIMI 11B-ESSENCE meta-analysis. *Circulation* 1999;100:1602–1608.

21. Antman EM, McCabe CH, Gurfinkel EP, et al. Enoxaparin prevents death and cardiac ischemic events in unstable angina/non–Q-wave myocardial infarction: results of the Thrombolysis in Myocardial Infarction (TIMI) 11B trial. *Circulation* 1999;100:1593–1601.

22. The Platelet Receptor Inhibition for Ischemic Syndrome Management (PRISM) Study Investigators. A Comparison of aspirin plus tirofiban with aspirin plus heparin for unstable angina. *N Engl J Med* 1998;338:1498–1505.

23. The Platelet Receptor Inhibition for Ischemic Syndrome Management in Patients Limited by Unstable Signs and Symptoms (PRISM-PLUS) Trial Investigators. Inhibition of the platelet glycoprotein IIb/IIIa receptor with tirofiban in unstable angina and non–Q-wave myocardial infarction. *N Engl J Med* 1998;338:1488–1497.

24. The PURSUIT Trial Investigators. Inhibition of platelet glycoprotein IIb/IIIa with eptifibatide in patients with acute coronary syndromes. *N Engl J Med* 1998;339:436–443.

25. Nickerson NJ, Murphy SF, Kouchoukos NT, et al. Predictors of early discharge after cardiac surgery and its cost-effectiveness. *J Am Coll Cardiol* 1996;27:264A.

26. Moliterno DJ, Aguirre FV, Cannon CP, et al. The Global Unstable Angina Registry and Treatment Evaluation (GUARANTEE) Study. *Circulation* 1996;94[Suppl I]:I-195.

27. Scirica BM, Moliterno DJ, Every NR, et al. Differences between men and women in the management of unstable angina pectoris (The GUARANTEE Registry). *Am J Cardiol* 1999;84:1145–1150.

28. Cannon CP, Antman EM, Walls R, Braunwald E. Time as an adjunctive agent to thrombolytic therapy. *J Thromb Thrombolysis* 1994;1:27–34.

29. Cannon CP. Optimizing the treatment of unstable angina. *J Thromb Thrombolysis* 1995;2:205–218.

30. Braunwald E. Unstable angina: a classification. *Circulation* 1989;80:410–414.

31. Gruppo Italiano per lo Studio della Sopravvivenza nell' Infarto Miocardico. GISSI-3. Effect of lisinopril and transdermal glyceryl trinitrate singly and together on 6-week mortality and ventricular function after acute myocardial infarction. *Lancet* 1994;343:1115–1122.

32. ISIS-4: randomized factorial trial assessing early oral captopril, oral mononitrate, and intravenous magnesium sulphate in 58,050 patients with suspected acute myocardial infarction. ISIS-4 (Fourth International Study of Infarct Survival) Collaborative Group. *Lancet* 1995;345:669–685.

33. Januzzi JL, Hahn SS, Chae CU, et al. Reduction of troponin I levels in patients with acute coronary syndromes by glycoprotein IIb/IIIa inhibition with tirofiban. *Am J Cardiol* (in press).

34. Alexander JH, Sparapani RA, Mahaffey KW, et al. Eptifibatide reduces the size and incidence of myocardial infarction in patients with non–ST-elevation acute coronary syndromes. *J Am Coll Cardiol* 1999;33[Suppl A]:331A.

35. The EPIC Investigators. Use of a monoclonal antibody directed against the platelet glycoprotein IIb/IIIa receptor in high risk angioplasty. *N Engl J Med* 1994;330:956–961.

36. The EPILOG Investigators. Platelet glycoprotein IIb/IIIa receptor blockade and low-dose heparin during percutaneous coronary revascularization. *N Engl J Med* 1997;336:1689–1696.

37. The EPISTENT Investigators. Randomised placebo-controlled and balloon-angioplasty-controlled trial to assess the safety of coronary stenting with use of platelet glycoprotein-IIb/IIIa blockade. *Lancet* 1998;352:87–92.

38. The CAPTURE Investigators. Randomised placebo-controlled trial of abciximab before and during coronary intervention in refractory unstable angina: the CAPTURE study. *Lancet* 1997;349:1429–1435 [published erratum appears in *Lancet* 1997;350:744].

39. Topol EJ, Mark DB, Lincoff AM, et al. Outcomes at 1 year and economic implications of platelet glycoprotein IIb/IIIa blockade in patients undergoing coronary stenting: results from a multicentre randomised trial. *Lancet* 1999;354:2019–2024.

40. Anderson KM, Fersguon JJ, Stoner GL, et al. Long-term mortality benefit with abciximab in patients undergoing percutaneous coronary intervention (PCI). *Circulation* 1997;96[Suppl I]:I-162.

41. The TIMI IIIB Investigators. Effects of tissue plasminogen activator and a comparison of early invasive and conservative strategies in unstable angina and non–Q-wave myocardial infarction: results of the TIMI IIIB Trial. *Circulation* 1994;89:1545–1556.

42. Anderson HV, Cannon CP, Stone PH, et al. One-year results of the thrombolysis in myocardial infarction (TIMI) IIIB clinical trial. A randomized comparison of tissue-type plasminogen activator versus placebo and early invasive versus early conservative strategies in unstable angina and non–Q-wave myocardial infarction. *J Am Coll Cardiol* 1995;26:1643–1650.

43. McCullough PA, O'Neill WW, Graham M, et al. A prospective randomized trial of triage angiography in acute coronary syndromes ineligible for thrombolytic therapy. Results of the medicine versus angiography in thrombolytic exclusion (MATE) trial. *J Am Coll Cardiol* 1998;32:596–605.

44. Boden WE, O'Rourke RA, Crawford MH, et al. Outcomes in patients with acute non–Q-wave myocardial infarction randomly assigned to an invasive as compared with a conservative strategy. *N Engl J Med* 1998;338:1785–1792.

45. FRagmin and Fast Revascularisation during Instability in Coronary Artery Disease Investigators. Invasive compared with non-invasive treatment in unstable coronary-artery disease: FRISC II prospective randomised multicentre study. *Lancet* 1999;354:708–715.

46. Laqerqvist B, Diderholm E, Lindahl B, et al. An early invasive treatment strategy reduces cardiac events regardless of troponin levels in unstable coronary artery disease (UCAD) with and without troponin-elevation: a FRISC II substudy. *Circulation* 1999;100[Suppl I]:I-497.

46a. Cannon CP. Treat Angina with Aggrastat and determine Cost of Therapy with Invasive vs. Conservative Strategies (TACTICS)–TIMI 18 trial. Presented at the American Heart Association, New Orleans, November, 2000.

47. Newby LK, Christenson RH, Ohman EM, et al. Value of serial troponin T measures for early and late risk stratification in patients with acute coronary syndromes. The GUSTO-IIa Investigators. *Circulation* 1998;98:1853–1859.

48. Heart Outcomes Prevention Evaluation Study Investigators. Effects of ramipril on cardiovascular and microvascular outcomes in people with diabetes mellitus: results of the HOPE study and MICRO-HOPE substudy. *Lancet* 2000;355:253–259.

49. Scandinavian Simvastatin Survival Study Group. Randomised trial of cholesterol lowering in 4444 patients with coronary heart disease: the Scandinavian simvastatin survival study (4S). *Lancet* 1994;344:1383–1389.

50. Sacks RM, Pfeffer MA, Moye LA, et al. The effect of pravastatin on coronary events after myocardial infarction in patients with average cholesterol levels. *N Engl J Med* 1996;335:1001–1009.

51. The Long-Term Intervention with Pravastatin in Ischemic Disease (LIPID) Study Group. Prevention of cardiovascular events and death with pravastatin in patients with coronary heart disease and a broad range of initial cholesterol levels. *N Engl J Med* 1998;339:1349–1357.

52. Summary of the second report of the National Cholesterol Education Program (NCEP) Expert Panel on Detection, Evaluation, and Treatment of High Blood Cholesterol in Adults. *JAMA* 1993;269:3015–3023.

CHAPTER 13

Cardiac Catheterization and Percutaneous Coronary Intervention

Jeffrey J. Popma and Shirley Chan

Coronary arteriography, the "gold standard" for identifying the presence or absence of stenoses caused by coronary artery disease (CAD), provides the most reliable anatomic information needed to determine the appropriateness of medical therapy, percutaneous coronary intervention (PCI), or coronary artery bypass graft (CABG) surgery. Coronary arteriography is performed by directly injecting radiopaque contrast material into the coronary arteries and imaging the coronary anatomy on 35 mm cinefilm, or more recently, digital recordings (1). It is estimated that more than two million patients will have coronary arteriography in the United States this year; of these, more than 700,000 will have PCI, using a variety of devices, including conventional balloon angioplasty, atherectomy, or coronary stents.

The methods used to perform coronary arteriography have evolved substantially over the past few years. A number of factors have contributed to reduced complications and shorter hospitalization periods in patients having cardiac catheterization and PCI. More efficient preprocedural evaluation systems have been established and many diagnostic tests are now performed in the preadmission testing centers, allowing patients "same day" cardiac catheterization within 60 minutes after arrival to the cardiac catheterization laboratory. Smaller (5 to 6 Fr), high-flow injection catheters used during the procedure have replaced larger (8 Fr) thick-walled catheters. The reduced sheath size has allowed coronary arteriography, ambulation, and discharge within 6 to 8 hours following the procedure. The rapid sequence of events that occur today in patients having cardiac catheterization and PCI lends itself to the establishment of "critical pathways" to coordinate the safe and efficient delivery of care in patients with symptomatic CAD. This chapter outlines the indications for cardiac catheterization and PCI and discusses the perioperative management in patients having these procedures.

INDICATIONS FOR CORONARY ANGIOGRAPHY

It is important to make certain that the patient has been referred to the cardiac catheterization suite with a clinical history and physical examination that warrant cardiac catheterization. Although the hemodynamic indications for cardiac catheterization are fairly clear [e.g., valvular heart disease, congestive heart failure (CHF)], indications for coronary arteriography are somewhat more vague. Appropriate guidelines for coronary arteriography have been outlined by a recent consensus statement of the American College of Cardiology (ACC) and American Heart Association (AHA) (1).

The following patients are candidates for coronary angiography:

1. Patients with suspected CAD who have stable angina or asymptomatic ischemia should undergo coronary arteriography if their angina is severe [Canadian Cardiovascular Society (CCS) class III–IV] or if they have "high-risk" criteria for adverse outcome on noninvasive testing.

   High-risk features include severe resting left ventricular (LV) dysfunction [LV ejection fraction (LVEF) <35%], or a standard exercise treadmill test demonstrating hypotension or $\geq$1–2 mm ST-segment depression associated with decreased exercise capacity (2) or an exercise-induced LVEF <35% (1). Stress imaging that demonstrates a large perfusion defect (particularly in the anterior wall), multiple defects, a large fixed perfusion defect with LV dilatation or increased thallium-201 lung uptake, or extensive stress or dobutamine-induced wall motion abnormalities also indicate high-risk for an adverse outcome (1,3).

2. Patients resuscitated from sudden cardiac death, particularly those with residual ventricular arrhythmias are also candidates for coronary arteriography, given the favorable outcomes associated with revascularization in these patients (1).

3. Patients with unstable angina who develop recurrent symptoms despite medical therapy or who are at "intermediate" or "high" risk of subsequent death or myocardial infarction (MI) are also candidates for coronary arteriography (1,4,5). High-risk features include prolonged, ongoing (>20 minutes) chest pain, pulmonary edema or worsening

mitral regurgitation, dynamic ST-segment depression >1 mm, or hypotension (1). Intermediate-risk features include angina at rest (>20 minutes) relieved with rest or sublingual nitroglycerin, angina associated with dynamic electrocardiographic changes, recent onset angina with a high likelihood of CAD, pathologic Q waves or ST-segment depression <1 mm in multiple leads, or age >65 years (1).

4. Patients with Q-wave or non–Q-wave MI who develop spontaneous ischemia or with ischemia at a minimal workload, or when the MI is complicated by CHF, hemodynamic instability, cardiac arrest, mitral regurgitation, or ventricular septal rupture should undergo coronary arteriography. Patients with angina or provocable ischemia after MI should also undergo coronary arteriography (6).

5. Patients presenting with chest pain of unclear cause, particularly those who have high-risk criteria on noninvasive testing, may benefit from coronary arteriography to diagnose or exclude the presence of significant CAD (1). Patients who have undergone prior revascularization should undergo coronary arteriography if suspicion exists of abrupt vessel closure or when recurrent angina develops with high-risk noninvasive criteria in patients who have undergone PCI within the past 9 months.

6. Coronary arteriography should be performed in patients scheduled to undergo noncardiac surgery who develop high-risk criteria on noninvasive testing, have angina unresponsive to medical therapy, develop unstable angina, or have equivocal noninvasive test results and are scheduled to undergo high-risk surgery. Coronary arteriography is also recommended for patients scheduled to undergo surgery for valvular heart disease or congenital heart disease, particularly those with multiple cardiac risk factors and those with infective endocarditis and evidence of coronary embolization (1).

7. Coronary arteriography should be performed annually in patients after cardiac transplantation in the absence of clinical symptoms because of the diffuse and asymptomatic nature of graft atherosclerosis (7). Coronary arteriography is useful in potential donors for cardiac transplantation whose age or cardiac risk profile increases the likelihood of CAD. Coronary arteriography often provides important diagnostic information about the presence of CAD in patients with intractable arrhythmias who are planned to undergo electrophysiologic testing or in patients who present with a dilated cardiomyopathy of unknown cause.

No absolute contraindications are seen for coronary arteriography (1), although cardiac catheterization should be performed with extreme caution in patients with unexplained fever, untreated infection, severe anemia with hemoglobin less than 8 g/dl, severe electrolyte imbalance, severe active bleeding, uncontrolled systemic hypertension, digitalis toxicity, previous contrast allergy but no pretreatment with corticosteroids, or ongoing stroke. Other relative contraindications include acute renal failure, decompensated CHF, severe coagulopathy, and active endocarditis (1).

Risk factors for significant complications after catheterization include advanced age, as well as several general medical, vascular, and cardiac characteristics. Patients with these risk factors should be monitored closely for a minimum of 18 to 24 hours after coronary arteriography, and admission is indicated in patients with severe renal insufficiency (creatinine >2.0 mg/dl) for fluid hydration, uncompensated CHF for diuresis, or advanced age. Coronary arteriography performed under emergency conditions is associated with a higher risk of procedural complications. Careful discussion of the risks and benefits of the procedure, and its alternatives, should be reviewed with the patient and family in all circumstances before coronary arteriography is performed.

INDICATIONS FOR PERCUTANEOUS CORONARY INTERVENTION

The major value of coronary revascularization, whether performed by surgical or percutaneous methods, is the relief of symptoms and signs of ischemic CAD caused by obstructive epicardial disease. A careful assessment of the risks and benefits of coronary revascularization must be reviewed with the patient and family members, if appropriate, before these procedures are performed. The guidelines listed below for the performance of PCI and CABG have been published by the ACC/AHA (8,9).

1. Patients who are asymptomatic or have only mild symptoms are generally best treated with medical therapy, unless one or more significant lesions subtend a large area of viable myocardium that is shown using objective noninvasive testing, the patient prefers to maintain an aggressive lifestyle or has a high risk occupation, and the procedure can be performed with a high chance of success and low likelihood of complications (8).

2. Patients with class II to IV angina, particularly those who are refractory to medical therapy, are suitable candidates for coronary revascularization, provided that the lesion subtends a moderate to large area of viable myocardium by noninvasive testing (8).

3. In selected patients with unstable angina or non–Q-wave MI, PCI may improve prognosis, although it is not clear whether routine PCI is indicated in all patients with acute coronary syndromes (10–12).

4. Cardiac catheterization and selective coronary revascularization in patients who have received thrombolytic therapy is indicated for those with recurrent ischemia, those who present with or develop cardiogenic shock, or those who failed to develop signs of reperfusion after thrombolytic administration (6,13).

PREOPERATIVE EVALUATION

Once the appropriate indications have been established and the risk factors have been determined by the clinician, the patient should be prepared for the catheterization procedure. With the availability of high-resolution playback systems now available with digital angiographic systems, immediate interpretation of the coronary anatomy is available, and PCI is often performed in appropriate patients at the same sitting. As result, patients should be prepared for both coronary angiography and PCI.

Informed Consent

It is incumbent on the physician to fully explain the risks and benefits of the cardiac catheterization and PCI to the patient before the procedure. It is often useful to include family members in this discussion. Major complications (e.g., death, MI) are exceedingly uncommon (<0.3%) after routine coronary arteriography (Table 13-1). In two large registries of patients having femoral artery catheterization, death occurred in 0.10% to 0.14%, MI in 0.06% to 0.07%, cerebral ischemia or neurologic complications in 0.07% to 0.14%, contrast reactions in 0.23%, and local vascular complications in 0.24% to 0.46% (14,15). The incidence of death during coronary arteriography is higher in the presence of left main coronary artery (LMCA) disease (0.55%), LVEF <30% (0.30%), and in patients with New York Heart Association functional class IV (0.29%). More recent registries have identified equivalent complication rates despite increasing age and acuity of illness (16). The risk of clinically significant coronary air embolus during diagnostic coronary arteriography is low, occurring in less than 0.1% of cases. If the syndrome of coronary air embolus and air lock does occur, 100% oxygen by nonrebreathing face mask should be administered, which allows resorption of smaller amounts of air within 2 to 4 minutes. Morphine sulfate can be given for pain relief. Ventricular arrhythmias associated with air embolus can be treated with lidocaine and direct current cardioversion.

The risk factors for PCI are slightly higher than for coronary arteriography alone. Death occurs in less than 0.5% of elective procedures and the frequency of periprocedural Q-wave MI is approximately 1% to 2%. The need for emergency CABG has been reduced substantially in recent years, and is now less than 1% in most centers. Other complications (e.g., groin site bleeding, contrast induced nephropathy, and lesser degrees of myocardial necrosis) occur in an additional 5% of patients after PCI.

TABLE 13-1. *Risk of cardiac catheterization*

Risk factor	SCAI registry (%)
Mortality	0.11
Myocardial infarction	0.05
Cerebrovascular accident	0.07
Arrhythmias	0.38
Vascular complications	0.43
Contrast reaction	0.37
Hemodynamic complications	0.26
Perforation of heart chamber	0.03
Other complications	0.28
Total of major complications	1.70

SCAI, Society for Cardiac Angiography and Intervention.

Preparation of the Patient

Before coronary angiography, comorbid conditions (e.g., CHF, diabetes mellitus, or renal insufficiency) should be stable. A baseline electrocardiogram (ECG), electrolyte and renal function tests, complete blood count, and coagulation parameters should be reviewed before coronary arteriography and PCI. We recommend the following procedural preparations by the patient and clinician:

1. Patients should refrain from eating or drinking after midnight on the evening before the procedure. The patient may take the usual antihypertensive medications and antianginal medication on the morning of the procedure with a small sip of water. A period of fasting (>6 hours) is generally required for conscious sedation in patients having elective coronary arteriography and PCI.
2. Patients who may have PCI immediately following coronary angiography should receive aspirin (100–325 mg) at least 2 hours before the procedure. A few good substitutes for aspirin are available, although pretreatment with ticlopidine or clopidogrel may be used as an alternative in aspirin-sensitive patients. It should be noted that aspirin desensitization can be performed in patients with a history of an allergic reaction to aspirin.
3. Warfarin sodium should be discontinued at least 3 days before elective coronary arteriography and the international normalized ratio should be less than 2.0 before arterial puncture. Patients at increased risk for systemic thromboembolism on withdrawal of warfarin (e.g., those with atrial fibrillation, mitral valve disease, or a history of systemic thromboembolism) can be treated with intravenous unfractionated heparin or subcutaneous low molecular weight heparin (LMWH) in the periprocedural period.
4. After informed consent has been obtained, we recommend that the patients receive diazepam (2.5 to 10 mg) orally, and diphenhydramine, 25 to 50 mg, orally, 1 hour before the procedure. Conscious sedation in the catheterization laboratory can also be performed using intravenous midazolam (0.5–2 mg), and fentanyl (25–50 μg), which are useful agents to provide sedation during the procedure, if oral premedications are not given.
5. Those patients who are receiving intravenous unfractionated heparin should have their infusion discontinued just before the procedure. Patients who are receiving LMWH can safely have coronary angiography, but additional anticoagulation during PCI should be tailored to the timing of the most recent LMWH dose. Although intravenous heparin is no longer required during routine coronary arteriography (17), patients at increased risk for thromboembolic complications, including those with severe aortic stenosis, critical peripheral arterial disease, arterial atheroembolic disease, or those undergoing procedures requiring prolonged (>1–2 minutes) use of guidewires in the central circulation, can be given intravenous heparin (3,000–5,000 U). Patients having brachial or radial artery catheterization may also be given intraarterial unfractionated heparin (2,000–5,000 U). Frequent (every 30–60 seconds) flushing of catheters with contrast medium

or heparinized saline will avoid the formation of micro-thrombi within the catheter tip.

6. In the event that anticoagulation needs to be reversed, the anticoagulant effect of unfractionated heparin can be reversed with protamine (1 mg for every 100 U of heparin). Protamine can cause anaphylaxis or serious hypotensive episodes in approximately 2% of patients. Protamine should not be administered to patients with prior exposure to NPH insulin, because of an increased risk of adverse effects, or in patients with a history of unstable angina, high-risk coronary anatomy, or in those patients who have undergone coronary arteriography via the brachial or radial arteries.

7. After the procedure, femoral sheaths can be removed once the anticoagulant effect of heparin has dissipated [activated clotting time (ACT) <150–180 seconds].

8. Adequate preprocedural fluid hydration is needed in patients at high risk for contrast-induced nephrotoxicity (18), particularly in those patients with prior renal insufficiency, diabetes mellitus, dehydration before the procedure, CHF, larger volumes of contrast, and those with recent (<48 hour) contrast administration (19,20). In patients with baseline renal insufficiency (creatinine >1.5 mg/dl), use of nonionic contrast agents is associated with a lower incidence of contrast nephropathy (21).

9. Patients with a prior history of radiocontrast allergy should also be treated with two doses of prednisone (60 mg, or its equivalent) on the night before and 2 hours before the procedure, based on a randomized study showing that patients given methylprednisolone (32 mg) 12 hours and 2 hours before contrast exposure had a lower (6.4%) incidence of allergic reactions than patients treated with a single dose of methylprednisolone 2 hours before contrast exposure (9.4%) or placebo (9%) ($p < 0.001$) (22). Diphenhydramine (50 mg) and cimetidine (300 mg) should also be given before the procedure (23).

Management of Patients During the Procedure

Patients should be kept modestly sedated during the procedure to reduce their anxiety. When complications do occur, the response should be coordinated with all the catheterization laboratory staff. A few of these complications are discussed below.

Allergic reactions to radiocontrast agents can be classified as mild (grade I: single episode of emesis, nausea, sneezing, or vertigo); moderate (grade II: hives, multiple episodes of emesis, fevers, or chills); or severe (grade III: clinical shock, bronchospasm, laryngospasm or edema, loss of consciousness, hypotension, hypertension, cardiac arrhythmias, angioedema, or pulmonary edema) (22). Although mild or moderate reactions occur in approximately 9% of patients, severe reactions are uncommon (0.15% to 0.7%) (19,20). Contrast reactions can be more difficult to manage in patients receiving beta-blocker therapy. Hives and urticaria can be managed with diphenhydramine (25–50 mg) intravenously, and hypotension can be managed with subcutaneous epinephrine (0.3 ml of a 1:1000 dilution). Shock can be treated with intravenous epinephrine (3 ml of a 1:10,000 solution).

Patients can develop angina during coronary arteriography because of ischemia induced by tachycardia, hypertension, contrast agents, microembolization, coronary spasm or enhanced vasomotor tone, or dynamic platelet aggregation. Sublingual (0.3 mg), intracoronary (50–200 μg) or intravenous (25 μg/minute) nitroglycerin can be given to patients with a systolic blood pressure higher than 100 mm Hg. Patients without contraindications to beta-blockers (e.g., bradycardia, bronchospasm, or LV dysfunction) can be given intravenous metoprolol (2.5–5.0 mg) or propranolol (1–4 mg). Intraaortic balloon counterpulsation is also a useful adjunct in patients with coronary ischemia and left main coronary artery disease, cardiogenic shock, or refractory pulmonary edema.

In patients undergoing PCI who are not given adjunct glycoprotein (GP) IIb/IIIa inhibitors, sufficient intravenous unfractionated heparin should be given to maintain the ACT between 250 to 300 seconds using the Hemochron device (International Technidyne) and 300 to 350 seconds using the Hemochron device. If GP IIb/IIIa inhibitors are given, ACT of more than 200 seconds generally suffices. Based on these studies, GP IIb/IIIa inhibitors should be considered in all patients having coronary intervention, including those having stent implantation. They are particularly beneficial in diabetics, patients with unstable angina with elevated troponins, dynamic ECG changes, or ongoing rest pain, and in those patients with acute MI undergoing primary angioplasty.

Management of the Patient After Cardiac Catheterization and Percutaneous Coronary Intervention

Reduced arterial sheath sizes, reduced anticoagulation, and arterial closure devices have allowed more rapid ambulation in patients undergoing cardiac catheterization and PCI.

Cardiac Catheterization

Most patients can be discharged the same day after diagnostic cardiac catheterization. Following femoral artery catheterization, the 5–6 Fr catheter can be removed manually immediately, and following a period of 6 hours of bedrest with the leg extended, ambulation can be undertaken. Shorter (1–3 hours) periods of bedrest are indicated after the procedure if arterial closure devices [e.g, Angio-Seal (Kensey-Nash Corp., Exton, PA), VasoSeal (Datascope Corp., Montvale, NJ), or Perclose (Abbott Laboratories Co., Redwood City, CA)] are used, but the cost of these devices ($100 to $250) has prevented their widespread clinical use at our institution. No studies have shown a decreased complication rate with new closure devices compared with manual compression.

Because of the administration of radiocontrast agents during coronary angiography, 1 to 2 L of one-half normal saline should be administered intravenously after the procedure. The patient should also be encouraged to drink fluids. In patients with renal insufficiency or CHF, intravenous furosemide (20–80 mg) can be given to initiate a force diuresis and clearance of the radiocontrast agents.

With no signs of bleeding from the arterial puncture site, the patient can be discharged home. Patients undergoing femoral artery catheterization should be counseled to avoid lifting objects weighing more than 10 pounds for the ensuing 48 hours and driving a car for 72 hours. The patient should also be counseled about signs of rebleeding from the access site, and to watch for signs of redness, tenderness, expanding ecchymosis, or extreme tenderness. On occasion, pseudoaneurysms develop after hospital discharge and a low threshold for vascular ultrasound should be undertaken in patients who present with symptoms.

Percutaneous Coronary Intervention

Patients undergoing PCI are generally kept in the hospital overnight, although outpatient PCI has been successfully undertaken at some institutions with extensive follow-up networks. In patients undergoing balloon angioplasty or atherectomy alone, aspirin (80–325 mg daily) is recommended for secondary prevention of coronary events. In those patients receiving a coronary stent, clopidogrel (300 mg) after the procedure, followed by 75 mg daily for 14 to 30 days is given in addition to aspirin to prevent subacute stent thrombosis.

Similar to patients undergoing cardiac catheterization, patients undergoing PCI should also receive 1 to 2 L of one-half normal saline, and patients with renal insufficiency and CHF may also need intravenous furosemide. In the absence of angiographic complications, patients do not require anticoagulation after PCI and the sheaths should be removed when the ACT is less than 150 seconds. Vascular closure devices, which are used more often after PCI, allow ambulation 4 to 6 hours after the procedure. In addition, some clinicians routinely use the radial artery for access, which allows ambulation immediately after the procedure. With no signs of bleeding from the arterial puncture site, the patient can be discharged home the following morning, with the same precautions given those patients undergoing cardiac catheterization.

It is important to emphasize to patients with CAD that atherosclerosis is a ubiquitous disease that manifests clinical symptoms only late in its pathogenic development. Ischemia management in patients with symptomatic CAD should have two major objectives: (a) to relieve the flow-limiting stenosis causing ischemia using stents, balloon catheter, atherectomy devices, or radiation therapy to provide an effective long-term outcome at the site of arterial narrowing, and (b) prevent further episodes of death and MI, which requires aggressive, systemic lipid reduction therapy. Patients, specialists, and primary care physicians each need to take accountability for risk factor modification after coronary revascularization. It should be emphasized to the patient that atherosclerosis is a life-long disease and the measures to improve coronary flow by percutaneous or surgical methods are just palliative—definitive therapy may be too late once symptoms have developed. The objective should be to lower the low-density lipoprotein-cholesterol (LDL-C) to less than 100 mg/dl in all patients and, potentially lower (70–80 mg/dl) in patients with severe comorbid diseases. Once lipid-lowering therapy is begun, regular surveillance according to the National Cholesterol Education Program (NCEP) guidelines should be undertaken to make certain that the treatment goal of LDL-C less than 100 mg/dl is achieved. At the very least, patients with CAD should have a keen awareness of the prognostic implications for maintaining aggressive dietary and pharmacologic approach to lipid-lowering therapy after cardiac catheterization and PCI.

REFERENCES

1. Scanlon P, et al. ACC/AHA guidelines for coronary angiography. *J Am Coll Cardiol* 1999;33:1756–1824.
2. Fletcher GF, et al. Exercise standards: a statement for healthcare professionals from the American Heart Association. *Circulation* 1995;91:580–615.
3. Travin MI, et al. Variables associated with a poor prognosis in patients with an ischemic thallium-201 exercise test. *Am Heart J* 1993;125:335–344.
4. Braunwald E. Unstable angina. A classification. *Circulation* 1989;80(2):410–414.
5. Braunwald E, et al. Diagnosing and managing unstable angina. *Circulation* 1994;90:613–622.
6. Madsen JK, et al. Danish multicenter randomized study of invasive versus conservative treatment in patients with inducible ischemia after thrombolysis in acute myocardial infarction (DANAMI). *Circulation* 1997;96(3):748–755.
7. Fish RD, et al. Responses of coronary arteries of cardiac transplant patients to acetylcholine. *J Clin Invest* 1988;81:21–31.
8. Smith S, Dove J, Jacobs A, et al. ACC/AHA guidelines for percutaneous transluminal coronary angioplasty. *J Am Coll Cardiol* 2000 (in press).
9. Eagle K, et al. ACC/AHA guidelines for coronary artery bypass surgery. *J Am Coll Cardiol* 1999;34:1262–1347.
10. Anderson H, et al. One year results of the thrombolysis in myocardial infarction (TIMI) IIIB clinical trial. *J Am Coll Cardiol* 1995;26:1643–1650.
11. Boden WE, et al. Outcomes in patients with acute non–Q-wave myocardial infarction randomly assigned to an invasive as compared with a conservative management strategy. *N Engl J Med* 1998;338(25):1785–1792.
12. Invasive compared with non-invasive treatment in unstable coronary artery disease: FRISC II prospective randomised multicentre study. *Lancet* 1999;354:708–715.
13. Ryan T, et al. Guidelines for percutaneous transluminal coronary angioplasty: a report of the American College of Cardiology/American Heart Association Task Force on Assessment of Diagnostic and Therapeutic Cardiovascular Procedures. *J Am Coll Cardiol* 1988;12:529–545.
14. Coronary Artery Surgery Study (CASS). A randomized trial of coronary artery bypass surgery: survival data. *Circulation* 1983;68:939–950.
15. Klinke WP, et al. Safety of outpatient catheterizations. *Am J Cardiol* 1985;56:639–641.
16. Johnson LW. Cardiac catheterization 1991. *Cathet Cardiovasc Diagn* 1993;28:219–220.
17. Davis K, Kennedy JW, Kemp HG Jr, et al. Complications of coronary arteriography. *Circulation* 1979;59:1105–1112.
18. Solomon R, et al. Effects of saline, mannitol, and furosemide to prevent acute decreases in renal function induced by radiocontrast agents. *N Engl J Med* 1994;331:1416–1420.
19. Taliercio CP, et al. Nephrotoxicity of nonionic contrast media after cardiac angiography. *Am J Cardiol* 1989;64:815–816.
20. Brogan WC III, et al. Contrast agents for cardiac catheterization: conceptions and misconceptions. *Am Heart J* 1991;122:1129–1135.
21. Hill JA, et al. Multicenter trial of ionic versus nonionic contrast media for cardiac angiography. *Am J Cardiol* 1993;72(11):770–775.
22. Lasser ED, et al. Pretreatment with corticosteroids to alleviate reactions to intravenous contrast material. *N Engl J Med* 1987;317:845–849.
23. Hill J, et al. Radiographic contrast agents. In: Pepine C, Hill J, Lambert C, eds. *Diagnostic and therapeutic cardiac catheterization*. Baltimore: Williams & Wilkins, 1994:182–194.

CHAPTER 14

Pathways for Coronary Artery Bypass Surgery

James D. Rawn, Donna M. Rosborough, and John G. Byrne

BACKGROUND

The development of critical pathways in coronary artery bypass graft (CABG) surgery was initiated primarily in response to cost pressures created by managed care and changes in healthcare reimbursement. These pathways supplemented existing guidelines and practice standards that had evolved over time. CABG surgery was an early target for critical pathways because it is frequently performed and resource intensive, and care processes vary relatively little from patient to patient. It was felt that the implementation of pathways would improve efficiency, decrease costs, and maintain or improve quality. More specific goals include (1):

1. Selecting a "best practice" when practice styles vary unnecessarily.
2. Defining standards for the expected duration of hospital stay and for the use of tests and treatments.
3. Examining the interrelations among the different steps in the care process to find ways to coordinate or decrease the time spent in the rate-limiting steps.
4. Giving all hospital staff a common "game plan" from which to view and understand their various roles in the overall care process.
5. Providing a framework for collecting data on the care process so that providers can learn how often and why patients do not follow an expected course during their hospitalization.
6. Decreasing nursing and physician documentation burdens.
7. Improving patient satisfaction with care by educating patients and their families about the plan of care and involving them more fully in its implementation.

In 1993, an interdisciplinary care improvement team at Brigham and Women's Hospital, Boston, Massachusetts developed critical pathways, with measurable targets and outcomes. Improvement opportunities identified included length of stay, and utilization of laboratory tests, chest x-ray studies, and electrocardiograms (ECG). Consultants reviewed the medical records of 100 patients having coronary bypass surgery. Benchmark data were also reviewed from hospitals with similar cardiac surgery programs. Particular emphasis was placed on six key outcomes (Table 14-1).

The critical pathway contains task categories that include assessment, consult, tests, activity, medications, treatments, diet, education, and discharge. Currently, data entry is computerized and substitutes for nursing documentation. Patient care tasks, expected outcomes, variances, and notes are documented in one of three columns for charting on day, evening, or night shifts. The notes screen enables free text entry for admission, transfer, and discharge. Variances and reasons for variance are documented for patient outcomes that do not meet the expectations of the critical pathway. Analysis of variance provides clinicians with insight into critical steps in the care process and informs them of changes in practice standards.

Implementation of the critical pathway has been one element in a multifactorial approach to improving efficiency and quality and reducing length of stay (2). No controlled trials have demonstrated the benefits of critical pathway implementation, but rapid recovery and early discharge is increasingly becoming the standard of care, and most evidence suggests that outcomes are improved (3). The basic elements of the critical pathway have been incorporated into order sets or into practice guidelines. Our current pathways and guidelines have evolved to reflect our experience as well as nationally accepted standards (4). It should be emphasized that pathways, protocols, and guidelines represent commonly agreed on standards for the care of patients. These practice standards do not always enjoy the support of prospective, randomized trials and remain open to modification. Patients with significant complications or preexisting medical problems are not always candidates for pathways and guidelines. In addition, pathways should never substitute for physician judgment. This chapter summarizes current pathways and guidelines for uncomplicated CABG surgery (guidelines for new onset atrial fibrillation have been included because it occurs so frequently) at Brigham and Women's Hospital.

TABLE 14-1. *CABG critical pathway—key outcomes*

Postoperative day	Outcome
Day of Surgery	Extubation
1	Transfer to intermediate care telemetry unit
2	Tolerating solid foods
3	Removal of pacing wires
4	Tolerating one flight of stairs
5	Discharge from hospital

CABG, coronary artery bypass graft.

PREOPERATIVE PATHWAY

Patients are typically admitted for elective CABG surgery the day of surgery. For patients having more urgent surgery, the basic elements of the pathway are incorporated in the preoperative order set (Fig. 14-1).

A preoperative history and physical examination should be the standard for all patients having a CABG. In addition, standard hematologic and chemistry profiles, urinalysis, ECG, and a chest x-ray study (a lateral film should be included for all reoperations) should be obtained. In addition to coronary angiography, left ventricular function (left ventriculography or echocardiography) is typically assessed. Other studies [e.g., carotid Doppler studies or angiography in patients with transient ischemic attacks (TIA)] can be performed if dictated by the preoperative evaluation.

Several key elements of the preoperative assessment influence perioperative management and determine morbidity and mortality risk. They are discussed below.

History

Factors related to the patient's history include: age; sex; obesity; Stroke or TIA; peripheral vascular disease; diabetes mellitus; renal failure or insufficiency; liver disease; chronic obstructive pulmonary disease; smoking and alcohol history; anginal symptoms; symptoms of congestive heart failure; previous thoracic surgery; recent infection, bleeding, or thrombocytopenia; medications, particularly anticoagulants,

Pre-op for: Tomorrow
Diet: House, NPO after midnight
VS q8h. Please obtain height and weight.
Activity: As tolerated
Allergies: NKDA
IV: heparin lock
EKG
Radiology: Chest PA & Lateral
Laboratory Tests:
        CBC,
        PT, PTT,
        Comprehensive metabolic profile
        U/A, sediment
Cross-match 2 bags PRBC
Cardiac shave & prep chin -> toes. Hibiclens shower.
Keep HOB at 30 degrees.
Face mask: 40% starting on call to OR
NTG 1/150 1 TAB SL x 1 p.r.n. chest pain
Medications:
        (Continue beta-blockers, heparin, TNG)
        Serax 15ñ30 mg PO qhs p.r.n. insomnia
Call HO for T >101, SBP >160, SBP <90, HR >100, RR >30, chest pain

FIG. 14-1. Preoperative order set.

beta-blockers, angiotensin converting enzyme (ACE) inhibitors, diuretics, antiarrhythmics, thyroid medication, insulin and oral hypoglycemics; and allergies.

Physical Examination

The patient should be examined for neurologic deficits; evidence of pulmonary disease; bruits or murmurs; discrepancies in upper extremity blood pressure; signs of peripheral vascular disease; adequacy of peripheral arteries and veins for bypass conduit; and presence of abdominal aortic aneurysm.

Studies and Laboratory Evaluation

The studies and laboratory evaluation are done to uncover any of the following: evidence of renal or hepatic dysfunction; electrolyte abnormalities; coagulation abnormalities, presence of anemia; evidence of infection; presence of left main coronary artery disease; left ventricular ejection fraction; valvular abnormalities; evidence of aortic calcification; evidence of heart failure, pulmonary infiltrates, or congestion.

Two units of packed red blood cells are typically reserved for patients having first time coronary artery surgery and four units are reserved for reoperations. Patients are instructed not to eat or drink after midnight the day before surgery. In general, preoperative antihypertensive, antianginal, and antiarrhythmic medications are continued up until surgery, particularly heparin, nitroglycerin, and beta-blockers. A cephalosporin (e.g., cefazolin) should be provided 30 to 60 minutes prior to incision to maximize its efficacy (5).

Patient and family education is initiated as early as possible and continued throughout the patient's hospitalization. Setting expectations and providing the resources for managing effectively outside of the hospital are critical for safely minimizing the patient's length of stay and ensuring successful outcomes.

POSTOPERATIVE PATHWAY

Day of Surgery

On arrival in the intensive care unit (ICU), surgeons and anesthesiologists communicate the details of the procedure to the nurses and physicians assuming the care of the patient. Hemodynamic, ECG, temperature, and pulse oximetry monitoring are established. Most of the basic elements of the critical pathway are incorporated into the postoperative order set (Fig. 14-2).

Initial Postoperative Assessment

Initial evaluation of the patient following surgery includes the following elements: ECG, chest x-ray study, cardiac output [e.g., thermodilution or Fick method, if a pulmonary artery (PA) catheter is in place; extremity perfusion, urine output, and blood pressure]; assessment of bleeding; laboratory studies [i.e., arterial blood gas; mixed venous blood gas, if a PA catheter is in place; complete blood count; prothrombin time

Admit to Cardiac Surgery Intensive Care Unit
Diagnosis: s/p CABG
Allergies: NKDA
Condition: Stable
Continuous cardiac monitor
Continuous pulse oximetry
Continuous hemodynamic monitoring
Pacemaker wires attached to pacemaker; pacemaker on standby
Vital Signs q15 min
Temperature q1h
CO/CI/SVR/PCWP q4h
NG tube pH, irrigate q8h
I + O q1h
Daily weight
Activity: Soft restraints when intubated
      Elevate the HOB to 30 degrees when hemodynamically stable.
      Turn side to side, reposition q2h
      Elevate vein harvest leg on pillow
      Dangle when extubated
      Dorsiflexion q1h when extubated
      May be out of bed if no pulmonary artery catheter and stable on POD 1
Tubes and drains:
      Foley to gravity
      NGT to continuous suction 60 mmHg
      Chest tube to suction 20 cm H2O
      Begin autotransfusion; total not to exceed 1500cc
Diet: NPO After patient is extubated may have ice chips. Clear liquids up to 60cc/h
      when bowel sounds are present.
Dressings: Dry sterile dressings to sternotomy, leg incisions q.d. starting 24 h post-op
i.v. heparin 3 mL/h in NS (1000U/500mL) continuous i.v.
Medications:
      Cefazolin 1 g IV q8h x 6 doses. D/C when chest tubes are removed, or
         after 6 doses
      Tylenol 650 mg PO/p.r. q6h p.r.n. pain, t >101
      Percocet 1–2 tab PO q3–4h p.r.n. pain
      Morphine 2ñ5 mg i.v. q5min x 3 doses p.r.n. pain
      Propofol 0.05 mL/kg/h in D5W continuous i.v., D/C when patient is
         hemodynamically stable and without significant bleeding
         or ischemia
      Indomethacin 50–100 mg p.r. b.i.d. x 2 doses
      Droperidol 0.625 mg i.v. q20min x 2 doses p.r.n. nausea
      Ketorolac 15—30 mg i.v. q6h x 8 doses p.r.n. pain
      Carafate 1 g pngt/PO q.i.d.
      Hespan 1000–1500 mL total i.v. p.r.n. hypovolemia
      Nitroglycerin 30 mcg/min in D5W (100mg/250cc) continuous i.v., titrate
         to keep SBP <120
      Nitroprusside 0.5 mcg/kg/min in D5W (100mg/500cc) continuous i.v., titrate
         to keep SBP <120
      Dopamine 2.5 mcg/kg/min in D5W (400mg/250cc) continuous i.v.
      Aspirin: 325 mg pngt q.d. Hold if: CT output >50 mL/h starting 6h post-op
      Potassium sliding scale (target K >4.5) i.v. q4h
      Magnesium sliding scale (target Mg > 2.5) i.v. q4h
Ventilator settings mode: SIMV; FiO2: 100%; TV: 800cc; Rate: 10; PEEP: 5 cm H2O;
      Pressure support: 5 cm H2O. Wean ventilator per guidelines.
Ambu, suction q2–4 h p.r.n.
Labs: Ionized-CA, CBC, MG, PT, PTT, basic metabolic (7), VBG
Radiology: Portable chest on arrival in ICU
EKG Stat
Pace for symptomatic bradycardia
Call HO for T >101, SBP >160, SBP <90, HR >100, HR <50, UO <30cc/h

FIG. 14-2. Coronary artery bypass grafting postoperative order set.

1. **Absence of Contraindications**
   Prior to extubation, patients should be:
     • Hemodynamically stable
     • Without evidence of ischemia by 12 lead ECG
     • Bleeding less than 100 cc/h
     • Normothermic (>36°C)
     • Without significant pain.

2. **Adequate Oxygenation**
     • Initial ABG guides subsequent therapy.
     • Trend O2 Sat. while weaning FiO2 to 40%.
     • Target value is O2 Sat. >95%, minimally acceptable pO2 is 75 torr.

3. **Adequate Ventilation**
   Assessment of strength and ability to ventilate
     • Conscious and able to raise head
     • Bilateral hand grasps, leg lifts
     • Gag reflex present
     • Minute ventilation <10–12 L/min
     • Adequate tidal volume by clinical assessment or measurement
        of respiratory mechanics
     • MIF at least −20 cm H2O
     • TV ≥ 5 mL/kg (350 mL for 70 kg)
     • VC ≥ 10 mL/kg (750 mL for 70 kg)
     • RR ≤ 30 breaths/min

   Adequacy of ventilatory drive
     • Initial ABG guides subsequent therapy.
     • Adjust minute ventilation (RR x TV) to maintain target
        pH 7.32–7.45
     • When awake, patients should be able to maintain pH >7.32 during
        weaning of ventilator rate
     • Assess etiology of metabolic acidosis (tissue hypoperfusion,
        renal status) if present

4. **Manageable Secretions**
   Secretions are absent to minimal and easily cleared

FIG. 14-3. Criteria for extubation.

This is facilitated by the use of short-acting anesthetic agents (e.g., propofol). Nonsteroidal antiinflammatory drugs (indomethacin and ketorolac) can provide significant analgesia without sedation and can reduce narcotic requirements (9). Nonsteroidal antiinflammatory drugs should be avoided in patients with renal insufficiency, recent peptic ulcer disease, or significant postoperative bleeding. Patients are ready to be extubated when they have no extrapulmonary contraindications to extubation, and when they have adequate oxygenation and ventilation, and manageable secretions (Fig. 14-3).

POSTOPERATIVE DAY 1

Evaluation of the patient on postoperative day 1 includes the following elements:

1. Vital signs, weight, fluid balance
2. ECG
3. Chest x-ray study
4. Cardiac output: thermodilution or Fick method (if a PA catheter is in place); extremity perfusion, urine output, blood pressure
5. Chest tube output
6. Laboratory studies: arterial blood gas; mixed venous blood gas (if a PA catheter is in place and thermodilution output is marginal); complete blood count, PT, PTT; electrolytes (including magnesium), BUN, creatinine, and glucose

In the absence of contraindications (see "Management Guidelines for Atrial Fibrillation"), all patients are started on beta-blockers. Aspirin is continued. ACE inhibitors are started for patients with low ejection fraction (<40%). Caution is

(PT) and partial thromboplastin time (PTT); electrolytes (including magnesium), blood urea nitrogen (BUN), creatinine, and glucose].

Patients who are cold are actively warmed (6). Laboratory studies are repeated every 8 hours for the first 24 hours, unless clinical circumstances dictate more frequent assessment. Potassium and magnesium levels are determined every 4 hours. Coagulation tests do not need to be repeated, except in cases of significant bleeding. Aspirin is given 6 hours postoperatively except in cases of active bleeding (7). Vasoactive medications are weaned as tolerated. In the absence of complications, early extubation is attempted.

EXTUBATION GUIDELINES

Early extubation can shorten ICU stays, reduce respiratory complications, and lower costs (8). In the absence of complications, patients can be safely extubated within 4 to 6 hours.

exercised in patients with a history of renal insufficiency. Most patients are started on an oral diuretic with potassium replacement. Pain control is assessed.

Pulmonary artery catheters are removed if cardiac output is adequate and the patient is not requiring inotropic medications. Chest tubes are removed if the patient has been mobilized, and if the chest tube output has been <150 ml for the previous 8 hours.

Patients are mobilized from bed to chair. Diet is advanced to clear fluids. In the absence of complications, patients are transferred to an intermediate care, telemetry unit.

POSTOPERATIVE DAYS 2–5

Postoperative evaluation of the patient on days 2 through 5 includes the following elements:

1. Vital signs, weight, fluid balance
2. A chest x-ray study and ECG is obtained the day before discharge
3. Laboratory studies: complete blood count; electrolytes (including magnesium), BUN, creatinine, glucose; potassium and magnesium are determined twice daily.

Beta-blockers, diuretics, ACE inhibitors, and electrolyte replacements are adjusted each morning and as indicated. Patients are mobilized and walk three times daily, advancing to one flight of stairs by postoperative day 4. Diet is advanced to solids by postoperative day 2. Foley catheter and central line are removed on day 2. Pacing wires are removed on postoperative day 3 (Fig. 14-4).

Transfer to step down unit, Cardiac Surgery Service
Diagnosis: s/p CABG POD 1
NKDA
Condition: Stable
Vital signs: q2h on POD 1 and POD 2
Vs q4h on POD 3 and until D/C
Cardiac telemetry
O₂ Sat. q4h on POD 1 and until patient is weaned off oxygen. O₂ Sat. b.i.d. on POD 3 and POD 4.
Titrate FiO₂ to keep O₂ sat >95%
Breath sounds q.i.d. on POD 1–POD 3, breath sounds t.i.d. on POD 4
I+O q4h
Daily weight
Activity:
　　　Dangle x 1, OOB to chair t.i.d., and ambulate x 1 in room with assist on POD 1
　　　Ambulate with assist t.i.d. on POD 2
　　　Ambulate independently q.i.d. on POD 3–POD 4
　　　Climb 1/2 to 1 flight of stairs with assist on POD 4
　　　Limit sitting (with legs down) to meals and bathroom only
Cough and deep-breathe q2h while awake on POD 1 and POD 2
First dressing change 24 h post-op.
Avoid washing front of trunk and leg with incision until post-op day 2
Chest tube site care q.d. POD 1 to POD 4
D/C chest tube site sutures on POD 4
Pacing wire care: Cleanse with NS, apply betadine ointment and occlusive DSD
Tubes and drains:
　　　Chest tube to suction
　　　Foley to gravity. Remove on POD 2.
Anti-embolism—TED stockings. Thigh high for all CABG patients. Remove and reapply each shift
Diet: Advance as tolerated / NAS / low saturated fat; low cholesterol
IV: Heparin lock
Medications:
　　　Metoprolol 12.5 mg PO q.i.d.
　　　Aspirin enteric coated 325 mg PO q.d.
　　　Furosemide 20 mg PO t.i.d.
　　　KCl (potassium chloride) Sliding scale target K >4.5 i.v./PO q12h or MgSO4 (magnesium
　　　　　　　sulfate) sliding scale i.v./PO q.d.
　　　Ranitidine 150 mg PO b.i.d.
　　　Acetaminophen 650 mg PO/p.r. q6h p.r.n. pain, >101. Hold if: concurrently receiving 2 percocet tabs
　　　Droperidol 0.625 mg i.v. q20min x 2 doses p.r.n. nausea
　　　Ibuprofen 200–800 mg PO q4–6h p.r.n. pain. Instructions: do not start until after
　　　　　　　indomethacin x 4 doses is completed. Maximum daily dose = 3200mg. Hold if creatinine >1.5 and
　　　　　　　check with HO.
　　　Percocet 1–2 tab PO q4h p.r.n. pain
　　　Dulcolax (bisacodyl) 10 mg p.r. q.d. p.r.n. constipation
　　　Colace (docusate sodium) 100 mg PO t.i.d. p.r.n. constipation
　　　Lactulose 15 mL PO q6h p.r.n. constipation (until one BM)
　　　MOM (magnesium hydroxide) 30 mL PO q.d. p.r.n. constipation
Laboratory tests:
　　　CBC, Mg, basic metabolic (7) q.d.
　　　K at 4:00 pm POD 1, POD 2
EKG POD 1
CXR POD 1
Care coordination consult

FIG. 14-4. Coronary artery bypass grafting transfer to step down order set.

Need for rehabilitation facility or home resources is identified on postoperative day 1 to 2 and arrangements are facilitated throughout the remainder of the hospital stay.

On day 5, the patient is discharged The overall pathway is shown in Fig 14-6.

MANAGEMENT GUIDELINES FOR ATRIAL FIBRILLATION

Atrial fibrillation is a common complication of chest surgery; it occurs in approximately one third of patients following CABG surgery. Prophylaxis and treatment are controversial, although the use of beta-blockers for prophylaxis is generally accepted (10). The guidelines outlined below are based on the recognition that postoperative atrial fibrillation is generally well tolerated and self-limited and represents one attempt to standardize therapy. Figure 14-5 illustrates a treatment algorithm for postoperative atrial fibrillation.

Prophylaxis

A beta-blocker (metoprolol) should be started or resumed in all patients on postoperative day 1 following cardiac surgery unless specific contraindications exist (11). Patients receiving beta-blockers preoperatively are two times more likely to develop atrial fibrillation postoperatively if the medication is not restarted (12).

Contraindications to beta-blockers include hemodynamic compromise; inotropic support; atrioventricular block (PR interval >0.24, second or third degree block); and known history of beta-blocker–induced bronchospasm.

Metoprolol appears to provide more effective prophylaxis when given four times daily, at a suggested starting dose of 12.5 mg by mouth (po). Patients should be assessed frequently and dosage adjusted to ensure effective beta blockade. If patients do not experience significant atrial arrhythmias they should be transitioned to twice daily dosing or their preoperative beta-blocker by postoperative day 3 or 4.

Initial Assessment

The management of atrial fibrillation should be guided by the answers to the following three questions.

1. Is the patient symptomatic?
   Atrial fibrillation is generally well tolerated, and over-aggressive management can cause significant morbidity. Nonetheless, the first step in the management of atrial fibrillation is an assessment of its hemodynamic significance. Significant symptoms may respond to rate control alone or may require chemical or electrical cardioversion.
   Look for hypotension, changes in mental status, decreased urine output, decreased peripheral perfusion, anginal symptoms, decreased cardiac output, or increased filling pressures.
2. What are the precipitating factors?
   Appropriate management of atrial fibrillation requires identification and treatment of potential risk factors.

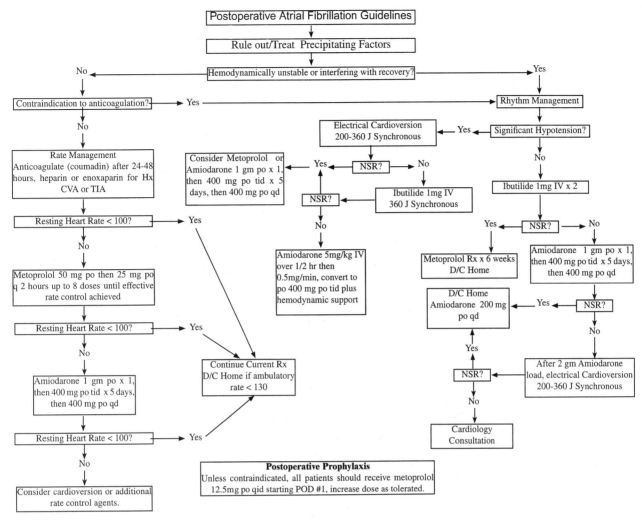

FIG. 14-5.

Atrial fibrillation can result from beta-blocker withdrawal, ischemia, atrial distension, increased sympathetic tone, electrolyte imbalances (particularly, hypokalemia and hypomagnesium, frequently precipitated by diuresis), acid-base disturbances, sympathomimetic medications (inotropes, bronchodilators), pneumonia, atelectasis, and pulmonary embolism.

3. What are the goals of therapy?

Hemodynamic stability is the primary goal. For most patients, rate control is sufficient because 90% of patients with new onset atrial fibrillation following cardiac surgery will be in normal sinus rhythm (NSR) in 6 weeks (13). Evidence of hemodynamic compromise or interference with recovery should prompt chemical or electrical cardioversion.

Drug Therapy

Rate Control Agents

Monodrug therapy is generally better than polydrug therapy.

Beta-blockers, such as metoprolol, should be first-line therapy in most patients. They can be given orally or intravenously. Metoprolol should be titrated to effect with a heart rate goal of <100 beats/minute (bpm) at rest. The suggested treatment for new onset atrial fibrillation is 50 mg po, followed by 25 mg po until NSR or adequate rate control is achieved, up to eight doses. Some patients may require >400 mg/day po.

Of calcium channel blockers, diltiazem is the agent of choice. It can be initiated as a bolus at 0.25 mg/kg intravenously (i.v.), followed by 0.35 mg/kg i.v., followed by a continuous infusion 5–15 mg/hr.

Digoxin can be considered in patients with contraindications to beta-blockers, in particular those with poor ejection fractions. Some evidence suggests that it increases atrial automaticity. It has a half-life of 38 to 48 hours in patients with normal renal function, significant potential toxicity, and a narrow therapeutic range. Levels must be monitored, particularly in patients with renal insufficiency. Many agents, including amiodarone, verapamil, and quinidine, increase its serum level. Digoxin is initially given as a 0.5 mg bolus (i.v. or po) and a total dose of 1 to 1.25 mg is given over a 24-hour period. Maintenance doses are typically 0.125 to 0.25 mg every day.

Following chemical cardioversion, attempts should be made to minimize the number of rate control agents used.

PREOPERATIVE DAY

ASSESSMENT
Vital signs

Weight

Height

CONSULTS
Anesthesia

Cardiology

Social Service/Care Coordination p.r.n.

TESTS
CXR
Profile 20
EKG

Magnesium
UA w/sediment
PT/PTT

CBC
Type and cross 2 units pRBCs

ACTIVITY
Out of bed as tolerated

MEDICATIONS
Cardiac medications as ordered

HS sedation as ordered

TREATMENTS
Hibiclens shower or scrub

DIET
NAS, low fat & low cholesterol diet

NPO after MN

EDUCATION
Provide "Going for Heart Surgery" booklet
View "Going for Heart
  Surgery" video

Review family information pamphlet
Review clinical pathway
Attend preoperative class

Patient states adequate understanding of what
  to expect
Expresses readiness for surgery

DISCHARGE ISSUES
Identify potential date of discharge
Identify preliminary plans for discharge

Identify potential resources for discharge
Care coordination consultation if elderly,

resources are needed, or no family support
Identify potential resources needed for discharge

DAY OF SURGERY

ASSESSMENT
Continuos:
  Hemodynamic monitoring
  ECG monitoring
  Pulse Oximetry
Vital signs q15min
Temps q1h
Breath sounds q4h
Record hemodynamics q4h
CT drainage q1h

Neuro checks q4h
Resting heart rate >60 and <120/min
  With pacemaker
  Without pacemaker
  With antiarrhythmic
  Without antiarrhythmic
Systolic BP >90 and <160 mm Hg
  With vasopressor
  Without vasopressor

CT output <150 cc for previous 8 h
Urine output >30 cc/h
Extubated for 1 h prior to transfer
Resting O₂ sat. >94% on oxygen
Effective cough and airway clearance
Temperature >98° F and <101° F
Bibasilar rales no more than 1/3 of the way up
Moves all extremities
Follows commands

TESTS
ABGs per extubation protocol
VBG if PA line present
CXR on admission to ICU
Profile 7 on admission to ICU

Potassium on admission to ICU and q6h x 3
Ionized Ca on admission to ICU
EKG on admission to ICU
Magnesium on admission to ICU

PT/PTT on admission to ICU
CBC on admission to and q6h x 3
If diabetic: BS q8h

ACTIVITY
Bedrest
Head of bed elevated 30 degrees when
  hemodynamically stable

Turn side to side, reposition q2h
Elevate harvest leg on pillow
Dangle when extubated

Dorsiflexion q1h while awake

MEDICATIONS
As ordered by MD:
  Vasoactive medications
  Antiarrhythmics

Analgesics/sedation
Antibiotics
K, Ca, Mg replacement

Adequate pain control with analgesics

TREATMENTS
ET suction and lavage q4h
Extubation protocol
Auto transfusion per protocol
Pacing wires attached via cable to pacemaker

Pacemaker parameters set
Pacemaker on standby
Soft restraints for hands while intubated
Thigh high TEDS

Coughing/deep breathing q1h after extubated
DC NG tube per HO order
Extubated

DIET
NPO

Ice chips after extubation

EDUCATION
Instruct on:
  Coughing/deep breathing/
    supporting sternotomy incision
  Dorsiflexion

Explain ICU routine to family/significant
  other
Provide ICU number to family/significant
  other

Verify contact person's phone number
Family has adequate understanding of patient's
  condition

POSTOPERATIVE DAY 1 – TRANSFER TO STEP DOWN UNIT

ASSESSMENT
Telemetry
Vital signs q2h
I & O q4h
O₂ sat. q4h while weaning O₂
Breath sounds q6h
Weight

Resting heart rate >60 and < 120/min without
  pacemaker
Systolic BP >90 and <160 mm Hg
Urine output >30 cc/h
Resting O₂ sat. >92% on oxygen
Effective cough and airway clearance

Temperature <101° F
Bibasilar rales no more than 1/3 of the way
  up
Bowel sounds present
Moves all extremities
Alert and oriented x 3

TESTS
CXR
Profile 7
Potassium at 4 pm

EKG
Magnesium
PT/PTT

CBC
If diabetic: BS q8h

ACTIVITY
Dangle when extubated, then out of bed to
  chair t.i.d.
Ambulate in room with assistance

Assist with ADLs
Limit sitting with legs down to meals and BR
  only

Dorsiflexion q1h while awake

MEDICATIONS
As ordered by MD:

Adequate pain control with analgesics

TREATMENT
Heated nebulizer to keep O₂ sat. >92%

Chest PT q.i.d.

Coughing/deep breathing q2h when awake

FIG. 14-6. Brigham and Women's Hospital CABG pathway.

Initial dressing change at 24 h postop
Incision care with DSD q.d.

DIET
Clear fluids

EDUCATION
Provide "Moving Right Along After Heart
  Surgery" booklet
Instruct on dorsiflexion and leg elevation

DISCHARGE ISSUES
Transferred to step down unit within 24 h of
  ICU admission
Identify potential date of discharge
Identify preliminary plans for discharge

DC chest tubes
CT site care q.d.

Patient feels that questions and concerns are
  addressed

Identify potential resources for discharge
Care coordination consultation if elderly,
  resources are needed, or no family support

Thigh high TEDS
Incision without evidence of infection

Family feels that questions and concerns are
  addressed

Identify potential resources needed for
  discharge

POSTOPERATIVE DAY 2 – STEP DOWN UNIT

ASSESSMENT
Telemetry
Vital signs q2h
I & O q8h
O_2 sat. q4h while weaning O_2
Breath sounds q6h
Weight

TESTS
Profile 7
Potassium at 4 pm

ACTIVITY
Ambulate in pod with assistance t.i.d.
Assist with ADLs

MEDICATIONS
As ordered by MD:

TREATMENTS
O_2 via nasal prongs to keep O_2 sat > 95%
Chest PT q.i.d.
Coughing/deep breathing q2h when awake

DIET
Advance to NAS, low fat and low cholesterol diet

EDUCATION
Encourage family to read "Moving Right
  Along After Heart Surgery" booklet
Instruct on dorsiflexion and leg elevation

DISCHARGE ISSUES
Identify potential date of discharge
Identify preliminary plans for discharge
Identify potential resources for discharge

Resting heart rate >60 and <120/min without
  pacemaker
Systolic BP >90 and <160 mm Hg
Resting O_2 sat. >95% on oxygen
Effective cough and airway clearance
Temperature < 101° F

Magnesium
PT if on coumadin

Limit sitting with legs down to meals and BR
  only

Adequate pain control with analgesics

Incision care with DSD q.d.
CT site care q.d.
Thigh high TEDS

Patient feels that questions and concerns are
  addressed

Care coordination consultation if elderly,
  resources are needed, or no family support

Bibasilar rales no more than 1/3 of the way
  up
Alert and oriented x 3

CBC
If diabetic: BS q8h

Dorsiflexion q1h while awake

DC Foley catheter in am, DTV in 8 h
Incision without evidence of infection
Patient voided

Family feels that questions and concerns are
  addressed

Identify potential resources needed for discharge

POSTOPERATIVE DAY 3 – STEP DOWN UNIT

ASSESSMENT
DC telemetry (if no arrhythmias)
Vital signs q4h
I & O q8h
O_2 sat. b.i.d.
Breath sounds q6h

TESTS
Profile 7
Potassium at 4 pm

ACTIVITY
Ambulate in pod with assistance q.i.d.
Assist with ADLs

MEDICATIONS
As ordered by MD:

TREATMENTS
DC O_2
DC pacing wires

DIET
NAS, low fat and low cholesterol diet

EDUCATION
Patient and family to read booklet and view
  video if on coumadin
Diet instruction by dietitian

DISCHARGE ISSUES
Identify potential date of discharge
Identify preliminary plans for discharge
Identify potential resources for discharge

Weight
Resting heart rate > 60 and < 120/min
  without pacemaker
Systolic BP > 90 and < 160 mm Hg
Resting O_2 sat. > 90% on room air

Magnesium
PT if on coumadin

Limit sitting with legs down to meals and BR
  only

Adequate pain control with analgesics

Incision care with DSD q.d.
CT site care q.d.

Medication review
Patient feels that questions and concerns are
  addressed

Care coordination consultation if elderly,
  resources are needed, or no family support
Identify potential resources needed for discharge

Effective cough and airway clearance
Temperature < 101° F
Lungs clear
Alert and oriented x 3

CBC
If diabetic: BS q8h

Able to assist with ADLs
Tolerates independent

Bowel regimen if no BM

Thigh high TEDS
Incision without evidence of infection

Family feels that questions and concerns are
  addressed

Start VNA referral

POSTOPERATIVE DAY 4 – STEP DOWN UNIT

ASSESSMENT
Vital signs q4h
I & O q8h
Breath sounds q t.i.d.
Baseline weight achieved

TESTS
Profile 7
Potassium at 4 pm
Magnesium

ACTIVITY

Resting heart rate > 60 and < 120/min
  without pacemaker
Systolic BP > 90 and < 160 mm Hg
Resting O_2 sat. > 90% on room air

PT if on coumadin
CBC
If diabetic: BS q8h

Effective cough and airway clearance
Temperature < 101° F
Lungs clear
Alert and oriented x 3

CXR
EKG

FIG. 14-6. (*Cont.*)

Ambulate in pod independently q.i.d.	Limit sitting with legs down to meals and BR	Able to assist with ADLs
Assist with ADLs	only	Stairs 1/2 to 1 flight
MEDICATIONS		
As ordered by MD:	Adequate pain control with analgesics	Bowel regimen if no BM
TREATMENTS		
Incision care t.i.d.	Thigh high TEDS	
DC CT sutures	Incision without evidence of infection	
DIET		
NAS, low fat and low cholesterol diet		
EDUCATION		
Instruction on follow-up appointments	Family feels that questions and concerns are	Medication regimen
Medication review	addressed	Diet
Review discharge instruction booklet	Patient and/or family describes:	Warning signs and actions to take
Patient feels that questions and concerns are	Incision care	Plan for follow-up appointments
addressed	Activity progression	Use of TEDs stockings
DISCHARGE ISSUES		
Discuss readiness for discharge	Complete VNA referral	

FIG. 14-6. (*Cont.*)

Antiarrhythmics

Metoprolol (±diltiazem) is also given as an antiarrhythmic. Ibutilide (1 mg) is given as bolus and repeated once if cardioversion fails to occur. Patients need to be monitored for a small but significant incidence of torsade de pointes which may be increased if ibutilide is given in conjunction with amiodarone. Amiodarone can cause myocardial depression and heart block; significant hypotension is most commonly associated with rapid bolus infusion. Significant toxicity is associated with prolonged use of amiodarone, and consideration should be given to discontinuing the drug within 6 weeks of surgery. Adenosine is helpful in the treatment of supraventricular tachycardia. However, it should be avoided in transplant recipients, partially in revascularized patients and in patients with atrial flutter.

Electrical Cardioversion

Electrical cardioversion should be used emergently for the treatment of hemodynamically unstable atrial fibrillation, starting at 200 J (synchronous). Patients should be sedated (e.g., with propofol). In patients with atrial wires who are in atrial flutter, overdrive pacing can be attempted.

Anticoagulation

Patients who remain in atrial fibrillation for more than 24 hours or have multiple sustained episodes over this period should be started on coumadin in the absence of contraindications. Heparin (i.v. or low molecular weight, subcutaneous) should be considered after 48 hours for inpatients with a history of stroke or TIA or a low ejection fraction. Coumadin should not started in patients who may require permanent pacer placement.

REFERENCES

1. Pearson SD, et al. Critical pathways as a strategy for improving care: problems and potential. *Ann Intern Med* 1995;123(12):941–948.
2. Cohn LH, et al. Reducing costs and length of stay and improving efficiency and quality of care in cardiac surgery. *Ann Thorac Surg* 1997;64[Suppl 6]:S58–S60; discussion S80–S82.
3. Cowper PA, et al. Impact of early discharge after coronary artery bypass graft surgery on rates of hospital readmission and death. *J Am Coll Cardiol* 1997;30(4): 908–913.
4. Eagle KA, et al. ACC/AHA guidelines for coronary artery bypass graft surgery. *J Am Coll Cardiol* 1999;34:1262–1346.
5. Kreter B, Woods M. Antibiotic prophylaxis for cardiothoracic operations: meta-analysis of thirty years of clinical trials. *J Thorac Cardiovasc Surg* 1992;104:590–599.
6. Frank SM, et al. Perioperative maintenance of normothermia reduces the incidence of morbid cardiac events. *JAMA* 1997;277:1127–1134.
7. Lorenz RL, et al. Improved aortocoronary bypass patency by low-dose aspirin (100 mg daily): effects on platelet aggregation and thromboxane formation. *Lancet* 1984;1:1261–1264.
8. Lee JH, et al. Cost analysis of early extubation after coronary bypass surgery. *Surgery* 1996;120(4):611–617.
9. Ready LB, et al. Evaluation of intravenous ketorolac administered by bolus or infusion for treatment of postoperative pain. A double-blind, placebo-controlled, multi-center study. *Anesthesiology* 1994;80:1277–1286.
10. Hogue CW, Hyder ML. Atrial fibrillation after cardiac operation: risks, mechanisms, and treatment. *Ann Thorac Surg* 2000;69:300–306.
11. Kowey PR, et al. Meta-analysis of the effectiveness of prophylactic drug therapy in preventing supraventricular arrhythmia early after coronary artery bypass grafting. *Am J Cardiol* 1992;69:963–965.
12. Ali IM, et al. Beta-blocker effects on postoperative atrial fibrillation. *Eur J Cardiothorac Surg* 1997;11:1154–1157.
13. Andres TC, et al. Prevention of supraventricular arrhythmias after coronary artery bypass surgery: meta-analysis of randomized control trials. *Circulation* 1991;84[Suppl III]:236–244.

CHAPTER 15

Aortic Dissection

Michelle A. Albert and Joshua A. Beckman

INTRODUCTION

Acute aortic dissection can be rapidly fatal if assessment and treatment are delayed (1). The natural history of untreated aortic dissection is humbling, with reported mortality reaching 25%, 50%, and 90% by 24 hours, 1 week, and 3 months, respectively. Prompt diagnosis and treatment can significantly improve these results with 5-year survival among patients discharged from the hospital as high as 73% (2–4). More than 200 years after the first comprehensive description by Morgagni, acute aortic dissection remains a diagnostic challenge and is frequently missed by physicians at initial presentation.

EPIDEMIOLOGY

Although the incidence of aortic dissection is unknown, it is estimated that as many as one third of cases are never diagnosed (5). It is the most common acute condition involving the aorta, with an estimated 2,000 new cases per year in the United States (6). Autopsy studies have reported an annual incidence of between 5 to 10 cases per 1 million people (7,8). The incidence of aortic dissection has declined 40% over the last two decades from 3.0/100,000/year to 1.8/100,000/year. Over a 30-year period, Bickerstaff and colleagues studied a white population living in Minnesota, and calculated an incidence of 27 cases per million people per year (9). Blacks have a higher incidence of aortic dissection than their white counterparts, likely because of the higher prevalence of hypertension in the former population (7). In Europe, the incidence is even greater. A recent population-based, longitudinal study from Hungary found an incidence of aortic dissection of 2.95/100,000/year (10). The incidence in Italy was even higher at 4.04/100,000/year (11).

PATHOGENESIS

Classically, aortic dissection begins with a tear within the intima resulting in mural separation and distal propagation of intramural blood driven by the pulsatile surges of ventricular systole (6). The cause of the initiating tear remains unclear. Dissection can also result from spontaneous rupture of the vasa vasorum, with spread of blood into the media and disruption of the aortic wall. This process, which can occur without intimal rupture, is designated an "intramural hematoma" (12). Intramural hematoma can progress to overt dissection or adventitial rupture if left untreated and carries the same prognosis as classic aortic dissection (Fig. 15-1) (13,14). The frequency of intramural hematoma is unclear for a number of reasons. In autopsy series of aortic dissection, the frequency with which an intimal tear is not identified ranges from 0% to 13% (8,15,16). Other variants of aortic dissection include penetrating atherosclerotic ulcers and intimal tears without hematoma (17,18). Penetrating atherosclerotic ulcers disrupt the aortic internal elastic lamina and can present as a localized hematoma, psuedoaneurysm, or frank rupture into the thorax (19). Compared with patients with classic aortic dissection, patients with penetrating atherosclerotic ulcers are usually older, invariably hypertensive, and have severe aortic atherosclerosis.

RISK FACTORS

It is thought that aortic dissection requires the combination of structural weakness in the aortic wall and the presence of luminal shear force to facilitate an intimal tear. Systemic hypertension, the major risk factor for aortic dissection (Table 15-1), is present in an estimated 70% of afflicted individuals (15,20) and more common in individuals with type B aortic dissection (21,22). Other factors associated with aortic dissection include older age (23), male sex (24), aortic valve disease (8), iatrogenic causes, cystic medial necrosis (9,25), cocaine use (26,27), pregnancy (28), and congenital aortic valve disease. Patients with Marfan's syndrome, who are at a markedly increased risk of spontaneous dissection and rupture, will be discussed below (29,30).

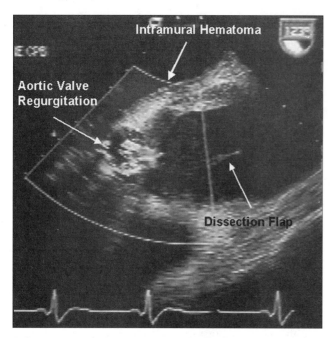

FIG. 15-1. A transesophageal echocardiographic image with evidence of a dissection flap, aortic valvular insufficiency, and intramural hematoma formation superiorly.

CLASSIFICATION AND PROGNOSIS

The Standford system is the most simple and most commonly used classification system for aortic dissection. It divides aortic dissection into those that involve the ascending aorta (type A) and those that do not (type B). This system provides prognostic information which determines proper management. Type A aortic dissections have an extremely high early mortality rate during the first 24 hours, averaging 1% per hour (31). Because this increased mortality occurs despite medical intervention, type A patients are treated surgically. A 6-year series by Wheat (32) demonstrated that type A aortic dissections had a mortality rate of 74% with medical therapy versus 30% when treated surgically. Furthermore, individuals with type A aortic dissections with arch tears fare poorly, possibly reflecting their older age, an increased likelihood of aortic rupture as well as neurologic complications (33), and the technical difficulties of surgical repair.

TABLE 15-1. Risk factors for aortic dissection

Hypertension
Male gender
Older age
Marfan's syndrome
Granulomatous aortitis
Pregnancy
Cocaine use
Congenital aortic valve disease
Cardiac catheterization
Previous aortic or CABG surgery

CABG, coronary artery bypass graft.

Type B dissections are usually managed medically because of the high rates of surgical mortality (26% to 65%) and postoperative paraplegia (10%) (34–37). Medical management of type B dissections is associated with 20% to 30% in-hospital mortality. The high surgical mortality (up to 50%) is predicated, in part, on the fact that surgery is commonly pursued once serious complications have occurred.

SYMPTOMS AND SIGNS

Prompt diagnosis of aortic dissection requires a high index of suspicion and accurate integration of the typical symptoms and signs at presentation (Table 15-2). The sudden onset of a severe sharp or tearing, migratory chest or interscapular pain heralds the presence of an acute aortic dissection in more than 80% of patients (24). Anterior chest and throat pain is more commonly associated with type A dissection, whereas exclusively back pain is more indicative of type B dissection (33). Chest and back pain may reflect other causes such as myocardial infarction or pancreatitis. Renal colic is a common misdiagnosis for type B dissection. Findings such as neck or throat pain, paraplegia, stroke, and syncope are indicative of arch and branch vessel involvement and may reveal the extent of the aortic dissection (38–40). Syncope can be related to cerebrovascular involvement or, more commonly, to aortic rupture into the pericardial space with cardiac tamponade and hemodynamic compromise.

Common physical findings include hypotension, low grade fever, pulse deficits, congestive heart failure, and aortic insufficiency (22,39,41). Aortic insufficiency suggests a proximal (type A) dissection. Myocardial infarction (22) and atrioventricular block (42) are rarely seen. Other unusual manifestations of aortic dissection include superior vena cava syndrome, hematemesis, hemoptysis, Horner's syndrome, and sternoclavicular joint pulsation.

TABLE 15-2. Clinical red flags for aortic dissection

	Study	
	Armstrong (%)	Hagan (%)
Typical symptoms		
−Chest pressure or dull pain	44	
−Sharp chest or back pain	24	64.4
−Migratory pain	16.6	
−Syncope	6	9.4
Typical signs		
−Hypertension	58–90	49
−Pulse deficit	4	15.1
−New aortic insufficiency murmur	31.6	
−Hypotension	8.0	

From Armstrong WF, Bach DS, Carey LM, et al. Clinical and echocardiographic findings in patients with suspected acute aortic dissection. *Am Heart J* 1998;136:1051–1060; and Hagan PG, Nienaber CA, Isselbacher EM, et al. The International Registry of Acute Aortic Dissection (IRAD): new insights into an old disease. *JAMA* 2000;283:897–903; with permission.

LABORATORY FINDINGS

Laboratory findings are usually of limited diagnostic value. Chest radiographic abnormalities are seen in 90% of patients (24). Most patients have an enlarged aortic silhouette. If the aortic knob is calcified, separation (≥1 cm) of the calcium from the soft tissue border of the aorta is suggestive of aortic dissection, but the diagnostic accuracy of chest radiography is low (43). Routine electrocardiography and cardiac enzymes can be helpful to rule out myocardial ischemia or infarction.

DIAGNOSTIC MODALITIES

Currently, transesophageal echocardiography (TEE) and contrast computed tomography (CT) are used most frequently for the rapid diagnosis of an acute aortic dissection. Although TEE, contrast CT, and magnetic resonance imaging (MRI) are all appropriate imaging modalities (44), their use should depend on the clinical scenario and local expertise. Individuals in whom aortic dissection is strongly suggested occasionally have negative diagnostic studies. In these instances, important consideration must be given to unusual types of acute aortic syndromes such as penetrating atherosclerotic ulcer, intramural hematoma, or intimal tear without hematoma. Bansal et al. observed that the primary reason for false-negative findings in aortic dissection was intramural hematoma (45). Table 15-3 details the performance of the various diagnostic modalities.

Echocardiography

Transesophageal echocardiography is an excellent noninvasive method for the rapid diagnosis of acute aortic dissection (46,47). TEE is portable, allows identification of the intimal flap, entry site, true and false lumens, quantification of aortic regurgitation, assessment of coronary ostial involvement, left ventricular function, and pericardial appearance.

Its pitfalls include an inability to image arch vessels and the distal aorta, its relative invasiveness, and the need for sedation.

Transthoracic echocardiography (TTE) can detect some type A dissections that are within 2 to 3 cm of the aortic valve (48) and any associated aortic regurgitation or tamponade. TTE can still fail to identify more than one third of type A dissections and is not recommended as the sole diagnostic test in patients suspected of having aortic dissection.

Contrast-Enhanced Computed Tomography

Contrast CT (49,50), with a diagnostic accuracy of approximately 90%, is able to define the intimal flap and true and false lumens within the aortic wall. Further, it is promptly available and rapid, and allows for patient monitoring during the examination. CT scanning has the disadvantages of the need for ionizing radiation, contrast exposure, poor visualization of secondary and tertiary aortic branch vessels, and failure to show the entry site.

Magnetic Resonance Imaging

Magnetic resonance imaging has 95% or greater sensitivity and specificity and is an excellent modality for long-term follow-up of aortic dissection (51). However, MRI is expensive and time consuming; has limited availability; cannot be used in patients with pacemakers; and does not allow for the monitoring of potentially unstable patients.

Angiography

Angiography has a diagnostic accuracy of approximately 95% (24) and was previously the "gold standard" for the diagnosis of aortic dissection. It is now used only if the coronary anatomy needs to be defined or to confirm negative, noninvasive imaging studies in patients with a high clinical

TABLE 15-3. Diagnostic modalities

Imaging modality	Sensitivity (%)	Specificity (%)	Advantages	Disadvantages
TTE	59–85	63–96	Rapid; provides information regarding LV function, pericardial appearance	Poor diagnostic accuracy
TEE	98–100	90	Safe, rapid, high diagnostic accuracy; can evaluate aortic valve LV function, pericardial appearance	Unable to image arch vessels and distal portion of ascending aorta; sedation required; invasive
Contrast CT scan	83–94	87–100	Readily available and accurate; 3-D reconstruction	Cannot assess aortic valve; i.v. contrast; ionizing radiation
MRI	95–100	95–100	Accurate; high resolution	Expensive; unable to monitor patients
Aortogram	88	95	Previous gold standard—familiar to clinicians	Time consuming; invasive; and insensitive for intramural hematoma

CT, computed tomography; i.v., intravenous; LV, left ventricular; MRI, magnetic resonance imaging; TEE, transesophageal echocardiogram; 3-D, three dimensional; TTE, transthoracic echocardiogram.
Adapted from 44, 51, 64–71.

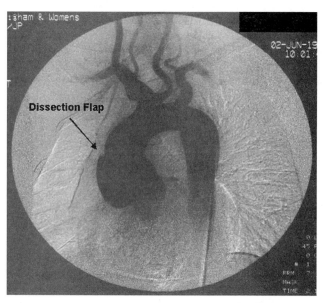

FIG. 15-2. Aortographic image demonstrating a plane of dissection in the ascending aorta.

suspicion of aortic dissection (Fig. 15-2). Drawbacks include its invasiveness, the use of contrast medium, radiation exposure, and time. Additionally, angiography may miss intramural hematoma.

Initial Presentation

Stabilization

1.	Vital signs, Monitor, 2 large bore IVs	☐
2.	ECG	☐
3.	Routine bloods, Type and hold	☐
4.	CXR	☐

Medications

1.	Sodium Nitroprusside IV to maintain SBP 100 - 120 mmHg	☐
2.	Beta-Blocker IV to maintain HR between 60-70 BPM	☐

Diagnostics

1.	Diagnostic test: Contrast CT or TEE	☐
2.	Contact Cardiothoracic surgeon and Cardiologist	☐

Hospital Follow Up

Medications

1)	Beta Blockers	☐
2)	Antihypertensive Therapy	☐

Imaging
Choose and stay with a single modality (CT, MRI, or TEE)

1)	Three Months	☐
2)	Six Months	☐
3)	One Year	☐
4)	Yearly	☐

MANAGEMENT

Patients in whom there is a high clinical suspicion of aortic dissection require urgent institution of medical therapy even before the diagnosis is confirmed (Fig. 15-3). Therapy should consist of agents to decrease blood pressure (e.g., sodium nitroprusside) and its rate of rise (dP/dt), such as a beta-adrenoreceptor blocker. Labetolol, which has alpha- and beta-blocking properties decreases blood pressure as well as dP/dt, combines both aspects of medical therapy, and may be adequate when used alone. In hemodynamically tenuous patients, intravenous esmolol can be used safely for beta-adrenergic blockade because of its ultra-short half-life and rapid titration. Rate-slowing calcium antagonists can be used in patients who are intolerant of beta-blockers (e.g., severe COPD).

In some circumstances, critically ill patients with aortic dissection may present with low blood pressure instead of hypertension. Mechanistically, the cause of the hypotension may be aortic rupture with pericardial tamponade or pseudo-hypotension caused by either an oscillating intimal flapover the origin of a major aortic branch or extension of the dissection into the branch vessel. Patients with a unilateral pulse deficit should have blood pressure titration based on the higher limb.

In the setting of hypotension, norepinephrine or phenylephrine can be useful because they raise blood pressure

FIG. 15-3. Cardiac checklist for acute aortic dissection.

without increasing ventricular contractility or heart rate. During medical stabilization, clinicians should proceed with the appropriate diagnostic test based on the clinical stability of the patient and availability of the appropriate diagnostic imaging study.

The proper management of pericardial tamponade remains unclear. Isselbacher et al. (52) demonstrated a 75% survival rate in patients who were triaged directly to surgery versus 0% survival with initial pericardiocentesis. Because early mortality in this small series was approximately 60% and half of the deaths occurred shortly after pericardiocentesis, emergent surgery without pericardiocentesis is recommended for this subset of patients.

DeBakey revolutionized the surgical treatment of patients with aortic dissection by proposing excision of the intimal tear, obliteration of the false lumen, and placement of a sleeve graft for patients with type A dissection (39). Aortic valve replacement may also be necessary because of aortic valve disruption or regurgitation. Indications for operative intervention in patients with type B dissection include aortic rupture, progression of the dissection despite medical therapy, refractory pain, visceral or extremity end-organ compromise, uncontrolled hypertension, or Marfan's syndrome (35,53). Despite advances in treatment even at leading surgical centers, the in-hospital mortality rate remains approximately 30%.

Risk factors for adverse outcomes in type A dissection include an aortic arch tear or extension of the dissection below the diaphragm. For type B dissections, advanced age, aortic rupture, or complications increase the mortality risk (3). Hospital survival for type B dissection is approximately 80%.

For critically ill patients who are not candidates for complete repair, particularly those with type B dissections or end-organ ischemia, aortic fenestration is sometimes a reasonable alternative. This technique involves transection of the aorta below the renal arteries, excision of a section of the intimal layer from the upper aorta, reapproximation of the intima and adventitia in the distal segment, and reanastomosis of the two aortic segments.

Fenestration, reported to be safe and rapid, had a 62% 5-year survival in one series (37). Recently, percutaneous endovascular stenting and catheter-based fenestration have been applied to increasing numbers of patients at high risk.

CLINICAL FOLLOW-UP OF TREATED PATIENTS

Long-term survival after hospital discharge is estimated at 90%, 80%, and 40% to 60% at 1, 5, and 10 years, respectively (2). Most late deaths are cardiovascular in origin and contribute up to 38% of the fatalities (3). Additionally, rupture of the aorta, more often at the original dissection site than at a remote site, can account for up to 18% of late mortality. Most of these deaths occur within 2 years of the index event

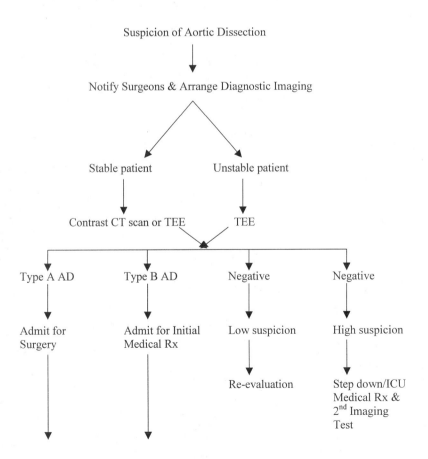

FIG. 15-4. Critical pathway for acute aortic dissection. AD, aortic dissection; Rx, therapy; ICU, intensive care unit; TEE, transesophageal echocardiogram; CT, computed tomography.

(56). Up to 13% and 23% of survivors of aortic dissection need reoperation at 5 and 10 years, respectively (57).

Long-term management of patients must be compulsive. All patients must receive antihypertensive therapy, preferably including beta-blockers. Strict radiographic follow-up should include CT scan or MRI at 3 months, 6 months, 1 year, and then yearly. The same modality should be used after each follow-up visit. Indications for reoperation include branch vessel compromise, aneurysmal dilation or rapid expansion of the aorta, and aortic valve disease. Patients should have an echocardiogram as indicated to assess aortic valve competency.

MARFAN'S SYNDROME

Individuals with Marfan's syndrome and aortic enlargement should be monitored by echocardiography and CT scan every 6 months. Aortic rupture accounts for approximately 60% to 80% of deaths (58). Predictors of poor outcome include patients who have a rapidly dilating aortic root or have first degree relatives with aortic dissection (59). A maximal aortic dissection that exceeds the age-adjusted normal value by 30% or that increases more than 5% per year portends high risk (60). Prophylactic Bentall-deBono surgical repair (resection of the aortic valve, aortic root, and ascending aorta) has a comparatively low mortality rate and should be performed in patients with Marfan's syndrome who are at high risk (29). Unfortunately, many patients with Marfan's syndrome require second surgeries to repair new aneurysms and dissections at other aortic sites, highlighting the pan-aortic pathology in these patients (61). Ultimately, genotypic screening may improve our identification of patients at increased risk of aortic dissection and allow for targeted prophylactic intervention.

CRITICAL PATHWAY FOR EVALUATION OF SUSPECTED AORTIC DISSECTION

Rapid recognition of an aortic dissection is essential to avoid death or serious morbidity. Clinicians must have a high index of suspicion for the condition (Fig. 15-4). In a recent study by Rosman et al., the relationship between the quality of patient history and the diagnosis of aortic dissection was examined (62). The authors performed a retrospective chart review of 83 patients whose diagnosis of aortic dissection was confirmed by autopsy or appropriate imaging modality. Based on the history obtained, the examining physician correctly suspected aortic dissection in only 65% of patients. The report demonstrates that despite technologic advances in diagnostic imaging, clinical judgment is the most important aspect in making the diagnosis. The continued high mortality rate (63) underscores the need for improvement in prevention, diagnosis, and management of acute aortic dissections. We have outlined a critical pathway and checklist for the evaluation of all patients presenting with suspected acute aortic dissection in Figs. 15-3 and 15-4.

REFERENCES

1. Hirst AJ, Johns VJ, Kime SJ. Dissecting aneurysm of the aorta: a review of 505 cases. *Medicine* 1958;37:217.
2. Doroghazi R, Slater E, DeSanctis R, et al. Long-term survival of patients with treated aortic dissection. *J Am Coll Cardiol* 1984;3(4):1026–1034.
3. Glower DD, Speier RH, White WD, et al. Management and long-term outcome of aortic dissection. *Ann Surg* 1991;214(1):31–41.
4. Pokela R, Juvonen T, Satta J, et al. Acute type A aortic dissection—diagnostic aspects and surgical experience. *Scand J Thorac Cardiovasc Surg* 1994;28(2):61–66.
5. Roberts CS, Roberts WC. Aortic dissection with the entrance tear in the descending thoracic aorta. Analysis of 40 necropsy patients. *Ann Surg* 1991;213(4):356–368.
6. Fuster V, Halperin JL. Aortic dissection: a medical perspective. *J Cardiovasc Surg* 1994;9(6):713–728.
7. Lilienfeld DE, Gunderson PD, Sprafka JM, et al. Epidemiology of aortic aneurysms I. Mortality trends in the United States, 1951 to 1981. *Arteriosclerosis* 1987;7(6):637–643.
8. Larson E, Edwards W. Risk factors for aortic dissection: a necropsy study of 161 cases. *Am J Cardiol* 1984;53:849–855.
9. Bickerstaff L, Pairolero P, Hollier L, et al. Thoracic aortic aneurysms: a population-based study. *Surgery* 1982;92(6):1103–1108.
10. Meszaros I, Morocz J, Szlavi J, et al. Epidemiology and clinicopathology of aortic dissection [see comments]. *Chest* 2000;117(5):1271–1278.
11. Giujusa T, Dario C, Risica G, et al. Aortic dissection: an incidence study based on hospital cases. *Cardiologia* 1994;39(2):107–112.
12. Vilacosta I, San Roman JA, Ferreiros J, et al. Natural history and serial morphology of aortic intramural hematoma: a novel variant of aortic dissection. *Am Heart J* 1997;134(3):495–507.
13. Nienaber CA, von Kodolitsch Y, Petersen B, et al. Intramural hemorrhage of the thoracic aorta. Diagnostic and therapeutic implications [see comments]. *Circulation* 1995;92(6):1465–1472.
14. Mohr-Kahaly S, Erbel R, Kearney P, et al. Aortic intramural hemorrhage visualized by transesophageal echocardiography: findings and prognostic implications. *J Am Coll Cardiol* 1994;23(3):658–664.
15. Wilson SK, Hutchins GM. Aortic dissecting aneurysms: causative factors in 204 subjects. *Arch Pathol Lab Med* 1982;106:175–180.
16. Utoh J, Goto H, Hirata T, et al. Acute aortic dissection without intimal tear. *J Cardiovasc Surg (Torino)* 1997;38(4):419–420.
17. Svensson LG, Labib SB, Eisenhauer AC, et al. Intimal tear without hematoma: an important variant of aortic dissection that can elude current imaging techniques. *Circulation* 1999;99(10):1331–1336.
18. O'Gara PT, DeSanctis RW. Acute aortic dissection and its variants. Toward a common diagnostic and therapeutic approach [Editorial] [see comments]. *Circulation* 1995;92(6):1376–1378.
19. Coady MA, Rizzo JA, Elefteriades JA. Pathologic variants of thoracic aortic dissections. Penetrating atherosclerotic ulcers and intramural hematomas. *Cardiol Clin* 1999;17(4):637–657.
20. Lindsay J Jr. Aortic dissection. *Cardiovasc Clin* 1983;13(2):103–119.
21. Chen K, Varon J, Wenker OC, et al. Acute thoracic aortic dissection: the basics. *J Emerg Med* 1997;15(6):859–867.
22. DeSanctis RW, Doroghazi RM, Austen WG, et al. Aortic dissection. *N Engl J Med* 1987;317(17):1060–1067.
23. Pretre R, Von Segesser LK. Aortic dissection. *Lancet* 1997;349(9063):1461–1464.
24. Slater E, DeSanctis R. The clinical recognition of dissecting aortic aneurysm. *Am J Med* 1976;60:625–633.
25. Larson EW, Edwards WD. Risk factors for aortic dissection: a necropsy study of 161 cases. *Am J Cardiol* 1984;53(6):849–855.
26a. Perron AD, Gibbs M. Thoracic aortic dissection secondary to crack cocaine ingestion. *Am J Emerg Med* 1997;15(5):507–509.
26b. Sarasin FP, Louis-Simonet M, Gaspoz JM, et al. Detecting acute thoracic aortic dissection in the emergency department: time constraints and choice of the optimal diagnostic test. *Ann Emerg Med* 1996;28(3):278–288.
27. Rashid J, Eisenberg MJ, Topol EJ. Cocaine-induced aortic dissection. *Am Heart J* 1996;132(6):1301–1304.
28. Nolte JE, Rutherford RB, Nawaz S, et al. Arterial dissections associated with pregnancy. *J Vasc Surg* 1995;21(3):515–520.
29. Gott V, Pyeritz R, Magovern G, et al. Surgical treatment of aneurysms

of the ascending aorta in the Marfan syndrome. *N Engl J Med* 1986;
314(17):1070–1074.

30. Kornbluth M, Schnittger I, Eyngorina I, et al. Clinical outcome in the Marfan syndrome with ascending aortic dilatation followed annually by echocardiography. *Am J Cardiol* 1999;84:753–755.

31. Agnostopoulos C, Prabhakar M, Kittle C. Aortic dissections and dissecting aneurysms. *Am J Cardiol* 1972;30:263–273.

32. Wheat MW Jr. Acute dissecting aneurysms of the aorta: diagnosis and treatment—1979. *Am Heart J* 1980;99(3):373–387.

33. Lansman SL, McCullough JN, Nguyen KH, et al. Subtypes of acute aortic dissection. *Ann Thorac Surg* 1999;67(6):1975–1978; discussion 9–80.

34. Neya K, Omoto R, Kyo S, et al. Outcome of Stanford type B acute aortic dissection. *Circulation* 1992;86[Suppl II]:II-1–II-7.

35. Iguchi A, Tabayashi K. Outcome of medically treated Stanford type B aortic dissection. *Jpn Circ J* 1998;62(2):102–105.

36. Marui A, Mochizuki T, Mitsui N, et al. Toward the best treatment for uncomplicated patients with type B acute aortic dissection: a consideration for sound surgical indication. *Circulation* 1999;100[Suppl 19]:II-275–II-280.

37. Elefteriades JA, Lovoulos CJ, Coady MA, et al. Management of descending aortic dissection. *Ann Thorac Surg* 1999;67(6):2002–2005; discussion 14–19.

38. Crawford ES, Svensson LG, Coselli JS, et al. Aortic dissection and dissecting aortic aneurysms. *Ann Surg* 1988;208(3):254–273.

39. DeBakey ME, McCollum CH, Crawford ES, et al. Dissection and dissection aneurysms of the aorta: twenty-year follow-up of five hundred twenty-seven patients treated surgically. *Surgery* 1982;92:1118–1134.

40. Jex RK, Schaff HV, Piehler JM, et al. Early and late results following repair of dissections of the descending thoracic aorta. *J Vasc Surg* 1986;3(2):226–237.

41. Armstrong WF, Bach DS, Carey LM, et al. Clinical and echocardiographic findings in patients with suspected acute aortic dissection. *Am Heart J* 1998;136(6):1051–1060.

42. Thiene G, Rossi D, Becker A. The atrioventricular conduction system in dissecting aneurysm of the aorta. *Am Heart J* 1979;98(4):447–452.

43. Hartnell GG, Wakeley CJ, Tottle A, et al. Limitations of chest radiography in discriminating between aortic dissection and myocardial infarction: implications for thrombolysis. *J Thorac Imaging* 1993;8(2):152–155.

44. Nienaber C, von Kodolitsch Y, Nicolas V, et al. The diagnosis of thoracic aortic dissection by noninvasive imaging procedures. *N Engl J Med* 1993;328(1):1–9.

45. Bansal RC, Chandrasekaran K, Ayala K, et al. Frequency and explanation of false negative diagnosis of aortic dissection by aortography and transesophageal echocardiography. *J Am Coll Cardiol* 1995;25(6):1393–1401.

46. Vignon P, Gueret P, Vedrinne JM, et al. Role of transesophageal echocardiography in the diagnosis and management of traumatic aortic disruption. *Circulation* 1995;92(10):2959–2968.

47. Kang DH, Song JK, Song MG, et al. Clinical and echocardiographic outcomes of aortic intramural hemorrhage compared with acute aortic dissection. *Am J Cardiol* 1998;81(2):202–206.

48. Sarasin FP, Louis-Simonet M, Gaspoz JM, et al. Detecting acute thoracic aortic dissection in the emergency department: time constraints and choice of the optimal diagnostic test [see comments]. *Ann Emerg Med* 1996;28(3):278–288.

49. Todd GJ, Nowygrod R, Benvenisty A, et al. The accuracy of CT scanning in the diagnosis of abdominal and thoracoabdominal aortic aneurysms. *J Vasc Surg* 1991;13(2):302–310.

50. Sommer T, Fehske W, Holzknecht N, et al. Aortic dissection: a comparative study of diagnosis with spiral CT, multiplanar transesophageal echocardiography, and MR imaging [see comments]. *Radiology* 1996;199(2):347–352.

51. Nienaber CA, Spielmann RP, von Kodolitsch Y, et al. Diagnosis of thoracic aortic dissection. Magnetic resonance imaging versus transesophageal echocardiography. *Circulation* 1992;85(2):434–447.

52. Isselbacher EM, Cigarroa JE, Eagle KA. Cardiac tamponade complicating proximal aortic dissection. Is pericardiocentesis harmful? *Circulation* 1994;90(5):2375–2378.

53. Dailey PO, Trueblood HW, Stinson EB, et al. Management of acute aortic dissections. *Ann Thorac Surg* 1970;10:237.

54. Cachera JP, Vouhe PR, Loisance DY, et al. Surgical management of acute dissections involving the ascending aorta. Early and late results in 38 patients. *J Thorac Cardiovasc Surg* 1981;82(4):576–584.

55. Wolfe WG, Oldham HN, Rankin JS, et al. Surgical treatment of acute ascending aortic dissection. *Ann Surg* 1983;197(6):738–742.

56. Heinemann MK, Ziemer G, Wahlers T, et al. Extraanatomic thoracic aortic bypass grafts: indications, techniques, and results. *Eur J Cardiothorac Surg* 1997;11(1):169–175.

57. Haverich A, Miller DC, Scott WC, et al. Acute and chronic aortic dissections—determinants of long-term outcome for operative survivors. *Circulation* 1985;72(3 Pt 2):II22–II34.

58. Murdoch JL, Walker BA, Halpern BL, et al. Life expectancy and causes of death in the Marfan syndrome. *N Engl J Med* 1972;286(15):804–808.

59. Pyeritz RE, McKusick VA. The Marfan syndrome: diagnosis and management. *N Engl J Med* 1979;300(14):772–777.

60. Legget ME, Unger TA, O'Sullivan CK, et al. Aortic root complications in Marfan's syndrome: identification of a lower risk group. *Heart* 1996;75(4):389–395.

61. Finkbohner R, Johnston D, Crawford ES, et al. Marfan syndrome. Long-term survival and complications after aortic aneurysm repair. *Circulation* 1995;91(3):728–733.

62. Rosman HS, Patel S, Borzak S, et al. Quality of history taking in patients with aortic dissection. *Chest* 1998;114(3):793–795.

63. Hagan PG, Nienaber CA, Isselbacher EM, et al. The International Registry of Acute Aortic Dissection (IRAD): new insights into an old disease. *JAMA* 2000;283(7):897–903.

64. Ballal RS, Nanda NC, Gatewood R, et al. Usefulness of transesophageal echocardiography in assessment of aortic dissection. *Circulation* 1991;84(5):1903–1914.

65. Armstrong WF, Bach DS, Carey L, et al. Spectrum of acute dissection of the ascending aorta: a transesophageal echocardiographic study. *J Am Soc Echocardiogr* 1996;9(5):646–656.

66. Parienty RA, Couffinhal JC, Wellers M, et al. Computed tomography versus aortography in diagnosis of aortic dissection. *Cardiovasc Intervent Radiol* 1982;5(6):285–291.

67. Amparo EG, Hoddick WK, Hricak H, et al. Comparison of magnetic resonance imaging and ultrasonography in the evaluation of abdominal aortic aneurysms. *Radiology* 1985;154(2):451–456.

68. Geisinger MA, Risius B, O'Donnell JA, et al. Thoracic aortic dissections: magnetic resonance imaging. *Radiology* 1985;155(2):407–412.

69. Godwin JD, Herfkens RL, Skioldebrand CG, et al. Evaluation of dissections and aneurysms of the thoracic aorta by conventional and dynamic CT scanning. *Radiology* 1980;136(1):125–133.

70. Hamada S, Takamiya M, Kimura K, et al. Type A aortic dissections: evaluation with ultrafast CT. *Radiology* 1992;183(1):155–158.

71. Thorsen MK, San Dretto MA, Lawson TL, et al. Dissecting aortic aneurysms: accuracy of computed tomographic diagnosis. *Radiology* 1983;148(3):773–777.

CHAPTER 16

Management of Atrial Fibrillation

Leonard I. Ganz

Atrial fibrillation (AF) is the most common sustained arrhythmia encountered in clinical practice. The prevalence of AF increases with age, and occurs more commonly in patients with other cardiovascular diseases. Treatment strategies for AF vary widely among clinicians (1). Clear practice guidelines have not yet emerged; ongoing clinical trials will help shape practice in the future. This chapter outlines strategies for the evaluation and management of patients with AF; it should be emphasized that what follows is the opinion of a single electrophysiologist, rather than an accepted clinical pathway or consensus statement.

The diagnostic evaluation for patients with AF is fairly consistent, independent of whether the patient is encountered in the office, emergency room, or inpatient ward. Conversely, the initial therapeutic approach to the patient with AF depends on the clinical scenario in which the patient is encountered.

DIAGNOSIS

The diagnosis of AF is usually straightforward. Electrocardiographically, AF is characterized by an irregularly, irregular ventricular rhythm, with an absence of discrete P-wave activity. Rather, undulating fibrillatory activity (f waves) are seen on the electrocardiogram between QRS complexes and T waves. Multifocal atrial tachycardia (MAT) also results in an irregularly, irregular ventricular rhythm; MAT, however, inscribes discrete P waves of varying morphologies and axes.

The pattern of AF can be paroxysmal, persistent, or permanent (2). In patients who present with paroxysmal palpitations, ambulatory monitoring can be used to correlate symptoms with a documented dysrhythmia. For patients with infrequent symptoms, event monitoring typically offers a higher yield than continuous Holter monitoring. Once the arrhythmia is recorded electrocardiographically, a diagnosis of AF or some other type of tachyarrhythmia can usually be assigned.

DIAGNOSTIC EVALUATION

Because AF accompanies many cardiovascular and systemic conditions, it is important to look for associated diseases in all patients who present with AF (Table 16-1). Frequently, some other cardiovascular disease process will already be established in patients who present with AF; common examples include hypertension, coronary artery disease, valvular heart disease, and cardiomyopathy. Less commonly, AF will be the initial manifestation of cardiomyopathy or valvular heart disease. Atrial fibrillation that occurs in the absence of associated conditions in patients less than 65 years of age is termed idiopathic or "lone" AF (3).

A small battery of diagnostic tests is recommended in all patients who present with AF (Table 16-2). Thyroid testing will uncover hyperthyroidism, which can precipitate or exacerbate AF. An echocardiogram to assess left ventricular function, atrial size, and valvular function is helpful to define associated conditions, as well as to help predict potential response to various therapies. Although AF can accompany acute pulmonary embolus and acute myocardial infarction (MI), it is extremely rare for AF to be the only presenting sign or symptom of these life-threatening disorders. Thus, assessment for acute pulmonary embolus or MI is recommended only in cases when other symptoms and signs are suggestive of these diagnoses (e.g., dyspnea, chest pain, hemoptysis).

THERAPEUTIC STRATEGIES

Treatment of patients with AF has three components: (a) anticoagulation, (b) control of the ventricular rate, and (c) restoration and maintenance of sinus rhythm. These components of therapy must be considered in all patients with AF. Anticoagulation reduces the risk of thromboembolic complications in patients with AF, whereas rate and rhythm control aim to improve symptomatology. Table 16-3 points out the relative advantages and disadvantages of these strategies.

Anticoagulation

Many clinical studies have established that most patients with AF are at risk for thromboembolic complications, most notably cerebrovascular accident (CVA) and transient ischemic attack (TIA). Moreover, multiple randomized, controlled

163

TABLE 16-1. *Conditions associated with atrial fibrillation*

Cardiovascular
–Hypertension
–Coronary artery disease, chronic or acute
–Cardiomyopathy (e.g., dilated, hypertrophic, infiltrative)
–Valvular heart disease, including rheumatic heart disease
–Cerebrovascular disease
–Pericarditis
–Myocarditis

Pulmonary
–Pulmonary embolus
–Chronic obstructive lung disease

Metabolic
–Hyperthyroidism
–Alcohol intoxication (holiday heart)

Primary dysrhythmic states
–Wolff-Parkinson-White syndrome
–Sick sinus syndrome (bradycardia-tachycardia syndrome)

Miscellaneous
–Postoperative state
 —Coronary artery bypass graft
 —Valve surgery
 —Other thoracotomy

TABLE 16-3. *Rate control vs. rhythm control therapy*

Rate control	Rhythm control
Advantages	
Safe	Symptomatic improvement
Well tolerated	Hemodynamic improvement
Inexpensive	May reduce thromboembolic risk
	May allow discontinuation of anticoagulation
Disadvantages	
Incomplete symptom resolution	Proarrhythmia
Bradycardia	Extracardiac adverse effects
Life-long anticoagulation	Frequently ineffective
Cardiomyopathy, if rate poorly controlled	Expensive

clinical trials have firmly established that in most patient groups, anticoagulation with warfarin to a target international normalized ratio (INR) of 2 to 3 markedly reduces this risk. Table 16-4 reviews guidelines for anticoagulation in patients with AF (4). In short, aspirin is recommended in patients younger than 65 years of age, without risk factors for thromboembolism; patients with idiopathic or "lone" AF have a low risk of stroke (5). Warfarin is typically recommended for patients older than 65 years of age, or with risk factors for thromboembolism. Because anticoagulation is not without risk, particularly in elderly patients, a careful assessment of the potential risks of anticoagulation should be considered in each patient with AF. In patients for whom anticoagulation with warfarin poses excessive risk, aspirin may confer some protection against thromboembolic complications.

All of the long-term clinical trials have evaluated warfarin; few data exist for other anticoagulants and antithrombotics. Unfractionated, intravenous heparin, adjusted to an activated partial thromboplastin time approximately two times control, is frequently used as a bridge until the INR is therapeutic with warfarin. Enoxaparin, a low molecular weight heparin, is used increasingly as a transitional agent at twice

daily doses of 1 mg/kg to bridge chronically anticoagulated patients before and after invasive procedures. No data exist, however, supporting the safety and efficacy of this practice. The ACUTE 2 trial compares subcutaneous enoxaparin with standard unfractionated, intravenous heparin in bridging patients to warfarin following transesophageal echocardiography (TEE)-expedited cardioversion.

Specific guidelines exist regarding anticoagulation related to restoration of sinus rhythm, whether effected electrically or pharmacologically (Table 16-5). In patients with AF known to be of 24 hours duration or less, cardioversion can generally be undertaken without antecedent or subsequent anticoagulation. In all other patients, including those with lone AF in whom chronic anticoagulation is not generally required, one of two approaches should be undertaken. The traditional approach requires therapeutic anticoagulation for at least three continuous weeks before, and for at least four weeks following, cardioversion. Alternatively, the expedited approach

TABLE 16-2. *Diagnostic evaluation of patients with atrial fibrillation*

History and physical examination
Electrocardiogram
Ambulatory monitoring; consider ETT
Thyroid function testing (TSH, free T$_4$)
Transthoracic echocardiogram

ETT, exercise tolerance test; TSH, thyroid-stimulating hormone.

TABLE 16-4. *Guidelines for anticoagulation in patients with atrial fibrillation[a]*

Age (Yr)	Risk factors[b]	Recommendation
<65	Present	Warfarin[c]
	Absent	Aspirin
65–75	Present	Warfarin
	Absent	Warfarin or aspirin
>75		Warfarin

[a]For purposes of anticoagulation, atrial fibrillation and atrial flutter are considered the same, as are paroxysmal and chronic atrial fibrillation.

[b]Clinical risk factors: prior transient ischemic attack or cerebral vascular accident, hypertension, congestive heart failure, coronary artery disease, mitral stenosis, prosthetic heart valve, thyrotoxicosis, hypertrophic cardiomyopathy. Echocardiographic risk factors: left atrial enlargement, left ventricular dysfunction.

[c]Target international normalized ratio 2.5 (range 2.0–3.0).

Adapted from Laupaucis A, Albers G, Dalen J, et al. Antithrombotic therapy in atrial fibrillation. *Chest* 1998; 114:579S–589S, with permission.

TABLE 16-5. *Guidelines for cardioversion of atrial fibrillation*

Duration	Anticoagulation	
	Precardioversion	Postcardioversion
<24–36 h	Not mandatory	Not mandatory
>24–36 h	Three weeks therapeutic INR OR	Four weeks therapeutic INR
	Establish anticoagulation, transesophageal echocardiogram negative for atrial thrombus	Four weeks therapeutic INR

INR, international normalized ratio.

calls for establishment of therapeutic anticoagulation with either warfarin or heparin, and then performance of a TEE. With no evidence of atrial thrombus, cardioversion can be performed. Heparin is continued until the INR is therapeutic, and anticoagulation is continued for at least 4 weeks following cardioversion. In the ACUTE trial, no significant difference was found in the incidence of a cardiovascular accident or TIA in patients randomized to the two strategies. Overall, the risk of cerebrovascular thromboembolism was 0.6% among the 1,222 patients in the study (6).

Because of the high risk of recurrence of AF, warfarin is frequently continued indefinitely in patients with AF. Even when antiarrhythmic drug therapy appears effective in maintaining sinus rhythm, many electrophysiologists favor continuing anticoagulation indefinitely.

Ventricular Rate Control

Pharmacologic therapy to control the ventricular rate has traditionally been prescribed to improve symptoms and hemodynamic parameters in patients with AF (7). In addition, even in asymptomatic patients, chronically elevated ventricular rates can lead to a tachycardia-induced cardiomyopathy. Table 16-6 outlines atrioventricular (AV) nodal blocking agents and dosing information, for both acute and chronic administration.

Few data guide the clinician in assessing adequate rate control. Rate should be assessed both at rest and during exertion, either with a formal exercise test, Holter recording, or informal exercise in the physician's office. As mono-therapy, digoxin is rarely effective in young or active patients. Beta-blockers or rate slowing nondihydropyridine calcium channel blockers tend to be more effective; frequently, combination AV nodal blocking therapy is necessary (8).

Restoration and Maintenance of Sinus Rhythm

Sinus rhythm can be restored spontaneously, pharmacologically, or with direct current cardioversion (DC CV). It should be noted that most short episodes of AF will convert

TABLE 16-6. *Pharmacologic agents used for rate and rhythm control*

Goal	Drug	Dosage
Acute termination	Procainamide (i.v.)	17 mg/kg to 1 g at 20 mg/min
	Ibutilide (i.v.)	1 mg over 10 min (0.01 mg/kg if <60 kg); 2nd. dose if necessary
	Propafenone (po)	600 mg single dose
	Flecainide (po)	300 mg single dose
Acute rate control	Diltiazem (i.v.)	0.25 mg/kg, then 5–15 mg/h
	Verapamil (i.v.)	2.5–10 mg q4h p.r.n.
	Propranolol (i.v.)	1–3 mg q4h p.r.n.
	Metoprolol (i.v.)	5–10 mg q4h p.r.n.
	Esmolol (i.v.)	0.5 mg/kg then 0.05–0.2 mg/kg/min
Chronic rate control	Diltiazem Ext. rel. (po)	120–300 mg q.d.
	Verapamil Ext. rel. (po)	120–240 mg q.d.
	Metoprolol (po)	25–100 mg b.i.d.
	Atenolol (po)	25–200 mg q.d.
	Propranolol Ext. rel. (po)	80–240 mg q.d.
	Digoxin (po)	0.125–0.25 mg q.d.
Sinus rhythm maintenance (suppression of recurrences of atrial fibrillation/flutter)	Quinidine gluconate (po)	324 mg t.i.d.
	Procainamide Ext. rel. (b.i.d.) (po)	1,000–2,000 mg b.i.d.
	Disopyramide Ext. rel. (po)	150–300 mg b.i.d.
	Propafenone (po)	150–300 mg t.i.d.
	Flecainide (po)	50–100 mg b.i.d.
	Sotalol (po)	80–160 mg b.i.d.
	Dofetilide (po)	125–500 μg b.i.d.
	Amiodarone (po)	100–200 mg q.d. (afterload)

b.i.d., twice a day; Ext. rel., extended release formulation which permits once daily dosing; i.v., intravenous; po, oral; prn, as needed; qd, every day; t.i.d., three times a day.

spontaneously to sinus rhythm (9). In patients who are not chronically anticoagulated, it is reasonable to consider cardioversion if AF persists for 12 to 24 hours, so that pericardioversion anticoagulation can be obviated.

Direct current cardioversion has traditionally been effective in restoring sinus rhythm in 80% or more of patients. Recently, biphasic external defibrillators have become available, which markedly increase the success rate of DC CV (10). Pretreatment with ibutilide has also been shown to increase the efficacy of DC CV (11). Predictors of failure of external cardioversion include chronicity of AF, extent of left atrial enlargement, and unfavorable body habitus (e.g., morbid obesity, barrel chest). Internal cardioversion can also be undertaken in refractory patients.

Intravenous procainamide has traditionally been used in efforts to restore sinus rhythm, although data supporting this practice are weak. Newer and more effective dosing regimens for effecting pharmacologic conversion to sinus rhythm are summarized in Table 16-6. Loading doses of the oral IC agents flecainide and propafenone are extremely effective. Patients should be pretreated with a beta-blocker or calcium channel blocker to reduce the risk of atrial flutter with 1:1 AV conduction. These agents are contraindicated in patients with coronary artery disease. Ibutilide is a class III agent available for use intravenously for acute conversion to sinus rhythm. Interestingly, ibutilide is more effective in terminating atrial flutter than AF, and carries with it a risk of inducing polymorphic ventricular tachycardia torsade de pointes (12). Risk factors for torsade de pointes with ibutilide include relative bradycardia, poor ejection fraction, female gender, and history of congestive heart failure. Patients should be monitored for at least 4 hours following ibutilide infusion, or until the QT interval returns to baseline.

Because of the risk of potentially life-threatening proarrhythmia, the precise role of antiarrhythmic therapy in patients with AF remains uncertain. The ongoing Atrial Fibrillation Follow-up Investigation of Rhythm Management (AFFIRM) trial compares the rhythm control and ventricular rate control strategies in patients with AF (13). In patients with symptoms related to AF despite adequate ventricular rate control, antiarrhythmic drug therapy to maintain sinus rhythm is certainly reasonable (14). Table 16-6 summarizes dosing information for the various antiarrhythmic drugs used for AF. Because the likelihood of maintaining sinus rhythm is similar for the different agents, except perhaps for amiodarone, an assessment of the patient's cardiac substrate and potential risk for proarrhythmia should be carefully considered in choosing an antiarrhythmic agent. Complete suppression of AF episodes is rarely achieved; rather, a significant reduction in the frequency, duration, and severity of symptoms with AF episodes should be considered successful therapy. Table 16-7 summarizes reasonable initial choices for antiarrhythmic drug therapy for various patient groups.

Most patients should be hospitalized for continuous telemetry during initiation or dose titration of antiarrhythmic drugs (15). Certainly, patients initiated on QT-prolonging drugs

TABLE 16-7. *Antiarrhythmic drug choice in patients with atrial fibrillation (AF)*

Scenario	First choice	Second choice
Lone AF	Propafenone, flecainide	Sotalol, dofetilide
Coronary artery disease	Sotalol, dofetilide	Amiodarone
Hypertension/left ventricular hypertrophy		
–Uncomplicated	Propafenone, flecainide	Sotalol, dofetilide
–QRS widening and/or strain	Sotalol, dofetilide	Amiodarone
Cardiomyopathy		
–Mild	Sotalol, dofetilide	Amiodarone
–Severe	Amiodarone	Dofetilide
Vagally mediated	Disopyramide	

including quinidine, procainamide, disopyramide, sotalol, and dofetilide should be hospitalized. Patients with structurally normal hearts can frequently have propafenone and flecainide initiated as outpatients. Event monitoring to look for signs of proarrhythmia may facilitate outpatient initiation of these drugs in appropriate patients. These agents should always be used in conjunction with AV nodal blocking agents; exercise testing to exclude exercise-induced proarrhythmia is reasonable once a steady state dose has been achieved. Because the risk of ventricular proarrhythmia with amiodarone is small, this drug can frequently be initiated in outpatients if the risk of significant bradycardia is not felt to be high. Baseline pulmonary, liver, and thyroid function should be assessed before initiating amiodarone therapy.

Patients treated longitudinally with antiarrhythmic drug therapy should be followed carefully, to reduce the risk of proarrhythmia and other potential complications. Table 16-8 lists potential adverse effects of antiarrhythmic drugs, as well as recommended follow-up testing.

APPROACH TO THE PATIENT WITH A FIRST EPISODE OF ATRIAL FIBRILLATION

If a first episode of AF does not revert spontaneously, cardioversion should generally be performed (Fig. 16-1). Beta-blockers can help at promoting conversion by attenuating sympathetic tone, which is frequently elevated at the onset of AF, particularly a first episode. A reasonable practice is to arrange DC CV, after anticoagulation if necessary, and then follow the patient without antiarrhythmic drug therapy to see if AF recurs. It is reasonable to treat with a beta-blocker, verapamil, or diltiazem following cardioversion for two reasons. First, these agents may attenuate the ventricular rate should AF recur. Moreover, intriguing experimental data suggest that these agents can reduce the frequency of recurrent episodes by attenuating atrial electrophysiologic remodeling that accompanies recurrent AF (16). If anticoagulation is

TABLE 16-8. *Potential complications and follow-up of antiarrhythmic drug therapy*

Class	Agent	Toxicity	Follow-up
IA	Procainamide	Blood dyscrasias, GI symptoms, rash, lupus, fever, torsade de pointes	CBC, ANA, QTc, heart rate, Proc/NAPA levels
	Quinidine	GI symptoms, cinchonism, thrombocytopenia, torsade de pointes	QTc, heart rate, quinidine levels
	Disopyramide	Anticholinergic symptoms, torsade de pointes	QTc, heart rate
IC	Flecainide	Atrial flutter with rapid conduction, VT	Exercise test
	Propafenone	Atrial flutter with rapid conduction, VT	Exercise test
III	Sotalol	Bradycardia, torsade de pointes	QTc, heart rate
	Dofetilide	Torsade de pointes	QTc, heart rate
	Amiodarone	Bradycardia, hepatic dysfunction, thyroid dysfunction, pulmonary fibrosis, optic neuritis	Heart rate, LFTs, TFTs, PFTs (with DLCO), ophthalmologic examination

ANA, antinuclear antibodies; CBC, complete blood count; DLCO, diffusing capacity of the lungs for carbon monoxide; GI; gastrointestinal; LFT, liver function test; NAPA, N-acetylprocainamide; PFT, pulmonary function test; QTc, corrected QT interval; TFT, thyroid function test; VT, ventricular tachycardia.

necessary pericardioversion, it is reasonable to continue warfarin for one or more months, with discontinuation of warfarin if sinus rhythm persists.

APPROACH TO THE PATIENT WITH RECURRENT ATRIAL FIBRILLATION

Once AF recurs, it is reasonable to assume that it will continue to recur in the future. The treatment strategy depends on the frequency and duration of AF recurrences, severity of symptoms, and underlying structural heart disease and associated conditions. An overall treatment strategy is presented in Fig. 16-1.

Patients with infrequent, self-limited, minimally symptomatic AF recurrences may be well served with no long-term therapy other than anticoagulation, if indicated. If recurrences are frequent or symptomatic, initial chronic treatment with a rate control agent (beta-blocker or calcium channel blocker) is reasonable. As described, these agents can both reduce the frequency of recurrent episodes and attenuate the symptoms by reducing the ventricular rate. In addition, antithrombotic therapy should be initiated in these patients. For patients with symptomatic AF despite adequate rate control, antiarrhythmic therapy should be considered.

Patients whose primary rhythm disturbance is atrial flutter should be considered for curative catheter ablation relatively early, given the efficacy of this procedure and lack of response to drug therapy (17). The macroreentrant circuit in typical (counterclockwise) atrial flutter includes the tricuspid annulus–inferior vena cava isthmus; ablation to create bidirectional block in this isthmus offers an acute success rate of about 90%, with a recurrence rate of 10%. Patients with both AF and atrial flutter preprocedure may or may not have AF postablation, or may respond better to antiarrhythmic drug therapy (18).

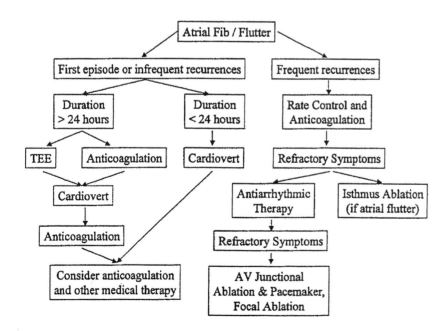

FIG. 16-1. Treatment algorithm for patients with atrial fibrillation.

TABLE 16-9. *Indications for hospital admission in patients with atrial fibrillation (AF)*

Intended therapy	Indications
Rate control	Significant symptoms Extremely rapid rates
Conversion to sinus rhythm	Brief duration AF, to obviate the need for anticoagulation Initiation of antiarrhythmic therapy
Initiation of anticoagulation	Acute CVA or TIA High risk for CVA/TIA (e.g., prior history of CVA or TIA, prosthetic valve, mitral stenosis)
Nonpharmacologic therapy	Refractory symptoms

CVA, cerebrovascular accident; TIA, transient ischemic attack.

INDICATIONS FOR HOSPITAL ADMISSION

Numerous potential reasons are found for hospital admission in patients with AF; these situations are outlined in Table 16-9. Certainly, patients with significant symptoms or signs related to rapid rates should be considered for treatment with intravenous rate control agents. Not all patients with minimally symptomatic AF of uncertain duration require admission for initiation of anticoagulation; patients at high risk for thromboembolic complications should certainly be considered for admission, however. Admission is also reasonable for patients with AF of less than 24 hours to facilitate restoration of sinus rhythm without the need for pericardioversion anticoagulation. As described, antiarrhythmic drug therapy should be initiated in most patients during continuous cardiac monitoring. Certainly, if AF is an epiphenomenon of another acute process (e.g., acute pulmonary embolus, acute myocardial infarction), admission is warranted for the primary problem.

INDICATIONS FOR NONPHARMACOLOGIC THERAPY

Several nonpharmacologic therapies are used with increasing frequency in patients with AF. Catheter ablation of the AV junction with permanent pacemaker implantation should be considered in patients who are refractory to medical therapy, and who remain symptomatic either because of persistently elevated rates or because they are intolerant of the medical therapy to control the ventricular rate (19). Appropriate patients tend to feel much better following the procedure. Because patients are generally pacemaker dependent following the procedure, caution should be exercised in recommending this procedure to relatively young patients. This procedure is palliative, not curative. AF persists in the atria, and chronic anticoagulation remains necessary. Patients with chronic AF receive VVIR pacemakers, whereas a dual chamber pacemaker with automatic mode switching is appropriate in patients with paroxysmal AF.

Maze surgery, as developed by Cox, is extremely effective in preventing recurrent AF (20). At present, this surgery requires a median sternotomy; efforts to develop a less invasive procedure through a limited thoracotomy are underway. Currently, because of the attendant surgical mortality and morbidity, this procedure is best applied to patients with extremely refractory symptoms, or patients who require other cardiac surgical procedures.

Efforts continue to develop a curative catheter ablative approach to AF (21). Current efforts focus on ablation of focal triggers of AF, which seem to arise primarily from the pulmonary venous ostia or from within the veins themselves. This technology is in evolution; important questions include how to select patients likely to benefit from this approach, long-term success rates, and complication rates, including thromboembolism as well as pulmonary vein stenosis.

Device therapy for AF is also evolving (22). Currently, it is commonplace to implant dual chamber pacemakers in patients with tachycardia-bradycardia syndrome to facilitate pharmacologic therapy of the AF. Current efforts focus on more sophisticated pacing algorithms to prevent AF, as well as alternate pacing electrode sites (e.g., atrial septal pacing, multisite atrial pacing). In addition, atrial therapies have been incorporated into some implantable cardioverter defibrillators. In clinical trials, a surprising number of AF episodes have been terminated with high frequency burst pacing. High voltage therapy is also available. It remains unclear what fraction of the AF population will find uncomfortable internal shocks an acceptable therapy for AF.

ATRIAL FIBRILLATION AFTER CARDIAC SURGERY

Atrial fibrillation remains an extremely common complication following cardiac surgery. No consensus exists regarding the optimal management strategy. The incidence appears to be lower in patients who have minimally invasive surgical approaches, but it remains unclear whether this is caused, in part, by differences in patient selection. Beta-blockers are effective in reducing the incidence of AF after cardiac surgery (23). Amiodarone, either administered orally for a week before surgery or intravenously immediately after surgery also reduces the risk of postoperative AF, but has been compared only with placebo, and not with beta-blockers (24,25).

Our usual practice is to initiate beta-blocker therapy postoperatively as soon as patients are extubated, and titrate up the dose as tolerated. If AF develops and persists for more than 24 hours, anticoagulation with heparin and warfarin is initiated. If AF is persistent, DC CV is usually performed after 36 to 48 hours. If AF is paroxysmal, we typically do not cardiovert. Beta-blockers (or calcium channel blockers) are advanced to control the ventricular rate. We tend not to use antiarrhythmic drug therapy unless symptoms persist despite rate control; if antiarrhythmic therapy is necessary, we tend to use amiodarone or sotalol. In most patients, the rate is aggressively controlled, and the patients are discharged when the INR approaches the therapeutic range.

These patients must be followed carefully after cardiac surgery, as they are susceptible to bleeding complications and over-anticoagulation. Patients without a history of AF frequently convert spontaneously to sinus rhythm following discharge from the hospital. If sinus rhythm is present at the 6-week follow-up visit, and there are no symptoms to suggest recurrent AF, antiarrhythmic therapy, if present, can be discontinued. If the patient has not been on antiarrhythmic therapy, warfarin can be discontinued at this time. If the patient has been on an antiarrhythmic agent postoperatively, which is discontinued at the 6-week visit, it is reasonable to continue warfarin for another 4 to 6 weeks to ensure that AF does not recur. If AF persists to the follow-up visit, DC CV is scheduled following verification of adequate anticoagulation.

REFERENCES

1. Prystowsky EN, Benson WD, Fuster V, et al. Management of patients with atrial fibrillation. *Circulation* 1996;93:1262–1277.
2. Gallagher MM, Camm AJ. Classification of atrial fibrillation. *Pacing Clin Electrophysiol* 1997;20:1603–1604.
3. Ganz LI. Idiopathic atrial fibrillation: therapeutic strategies. *Arrhythmia Clinic* 2000;1–12.
4. Laupacis A, Albers G, Dalen J, et al. Antithrombotic therapy in atrial fibrillation. *Chest* 1998;114:579S–589S.
5. Investigators of five studies. Risk factors for stroke and efficacy of antithrombotic therapy in atrial fibrillation. *Ann Intern Med* 1994;154:1449–1457.
6. Klein A. American College of Cardiology Annual Scientific Sessions, 2000.
7. Blitzer M, Costeas C, Kassotis J, et al. Rhythm management in atrial fibrillation-with a primary emphasis on pharmacologic therapy: Part 1. *Pacing Clin Electrophysiol* 1998;21:590–602.
8. Farshi R, Kistner D, Sarma JS, et al. Ventricular rate control in chronic atrial fibrillation during daily activity and programmed exercise: a crossover open-label study of five drug regimens. *J Am Coll Cardiol* 1999;33:304–310.
9. Danias PG, Caulfield TA, Weigner MJ, et al. Likelihood of spontaneous conversion of atrial fibrillation to sinus rhythm. *J Am Coll Cardiol* 1998;31:588–592.
10. Mittal S, Ayati S, Stein KM, et al. Transthoracic cardioversion of atrial fibrillation: comparison of rectilinear biphasic versus damped sine wave monophasic shocks. *Circulation* 2000;101:1282–1287.
11. Oral H, Souza JJ, Michaud GF, et al. Facilitating transthoracic cardioversion of atrial fibrillation with ibutilide pretreatment. *N Engl J Med* 1999;340:1849–1854.
12. Stambler BS, Wood MA, Ellenbogen KA, et al. Efficacy and safety of repeated intravenous doses of ibutilide for rapid conversion of atrial flutter or fibrillation. Ibutilide Repeat Dose Study Investigators. *Circulation* 1996;94:1613–1621.
13. The planning and steering committees of the AFFIRM study for the NHLBI AFFIRM investigators. Atrial fibrillation follow-up investigation of rhythm management—the AFFIRM study design. *Am J Cardiol* 1997;79:1198–1202.
14. Ganz JI, Antman EM. Antiarrhythmic drug therapy in the management of atrial fibrillation. *J Cardiovasc Electrophysiol* 1997;8:1175–1189.
15. Maisel WH, Kuntz KM, Reimold SC, et al. Risk of initiating antiarrhythmic drug therapy for atrial fibrillation in patients admitted to a university hospital. *Ann Intern Med* 1997;127:281–284.
16. Tieleman RG, De Langen C, van Gelder IC, et al. Verapamil reduces tachycardia-induced electrical remodeling of the atria. *Circulation* 1997;95:1945–1953.
17. Cosio FG, Arribas F, Lopez-Gil M, et al. Radiofrequency ablation of atrial flutter. *J Cardiovasc Electrophysiol* 1996;7:60–70.
18. Anselme F, Saoudi N, Poty H, et al. Radiofrequency catheter ablation of common atrial flutter: significance of palpitations and quality of life evaluation in patients with proven isthmus block. *Circulation* 1999;99:534–540.
19. Brignole M, Menozzi C, Gianfranchi L, et al. Assessment of atrioventricular junction ablation and VVIR pacemaker versus pharmacological treatment in patients with heart failure and chronic atrial fibrillation: a randomized, controlled study. *Circulation* 1998;98:953–960.
20. Sundt TM III, Camillo CJ, Cox JL. The maze procedure for cure of atrial fibrillation. *Cardiol Clin* 1997;15:739–748.
21. Chen S-A, Tai C-T, Tsai C-F, et al. Radiofrequency catheter ablation of atrial fibrillation initiated by pulmonary vein ectopic beats. *J Cardiovasc Electrophysiol* 2000;11:218–227.
22. Wellens HJ, Lau CP, Luderitz B, et al. Atrioverter: an implantable device for the treatment of atrial fibrillation. *Circulation* 1998;98:1651–1656.
23. Andrews TC, Reimold SC, Berlin JA, et al. Prevention of supraventricular arrhythmias after coronary artery bypass surgery. A meta-analysis of randomized control trials. *Circulation* 1991;84[Suppl]:III236–III244.
24. Daoud EG, Strickberger SA, Man KC, et al. Preoperative amiodarone as prophylaxis against atrial fibrillation after heart surgery. *N Engl J Med* 1997;337:1785–1791.
25. Guarnieri T, Nolan S, Gottlieb SO, et al. Intravenous amiodarone for the prevention of atrial fibrillation after open heart surgery: the Amiodarone Reduction in Coronary Heart (ARCH) trial. *J Am Coll Cardiol* 1999;34:343–347.

CHAPTER 17

Congestive Heart Failure

Edward F. Philbin, III and Norman W. Lindenmuth

OVERVIEW

Therapies proved to be of benefit for chronic heart failure (HF) can reduce the morbidity and mortality associated with this syndrome. Lifestyle alterations, drug treatments, and surgical therapies, when carefully and correctly applied in the research or clinical setting, reduce symptoms, enhance quality of life, and improve clinical outcomes. Despite these advances, the syndrome of HF is still associated with unacceptably poor clinical outcomes. Death is common (1–5), with 1-year mortality rates exceeding 50% in patients with advanced end-stage disease. HF is the leading cause of hospital admission among patients over the age of 65 years (6,7) and recurrent hospital admissions are common among patients with this disorder (8–10). Why HF remains so morbid a disorder despite powerful treatment options is only partially understood. That existing therapies do not fully attenuate or reverse the relentlessly progressive natural history of HF is one explanation (11). However, imperfect compliance with published treatment guidelines is likely another contributing factor (12). Thus, developing and implementing strategies to measure and improve the quality of care for patients with HF remains a high priority for clinicians and healthcare leaders (13). In fact, compelling evidence indicates that comprehensive, multidisciplinary disease management programs, emphasizing compliance with recommended treatment options, continuing patient education, and careful surveillance, can improve functional status, reduce the risk of hospital readmission, and may lower medical costs for outpatients with HF (14–21). Thus, hope exists that care management strategies for the treatment of hospitalized patients with HF can achieve these same goals.

TREATMENT

Angiotensin converting enzyme (ACE) inhibitors improve symptoms (4,22–25), quality of life (26), and survival, and reduce serious cardiovascular events among patients with symptomatic (4,24,25,27) and asymptomatic (28) left ventricular (LV) systolic dysfunction. These drugs may also be of benefit when used for HF caused by LV diastolic dysfunction (29). The use of ACE inhibitors is a cost-effective strategy (30) and is recommended by expert panels in the United States (1,31,32) and other countries (33). Angiotensin II receptor blockers, which may provide similar benefit to ACE inhibitors, are acceptable alternatives for patients who are intolerant to the latter (34). Other vasodilator strategies (e.g., the combination of hydralazine and isosorbide) have a role as well (27). Digoxin is known to improve symptoms and reduce hospitalizations for patients with HF, without an associated increase in the risk of death (35). Diuretics provide rapid relief of symptoms arising from fluid overload, although their impact on survival is not known (36). Antagonists of the sympathetic nervous system attenuate or partially reverse progression of LV dysfunction and prolong life (37–39). Aldosterone antagonism with spironolactone in class III/IV patients has a favorable impact on survival that is equivalent to, and additive to, beta-adrenergic receptor blockers (40). Potent antiarrhythmia strategies, such as the use of amiodarone (41) and implantable defibrillators (42,43), may also have a beneficial impact on survival among certain subgroups of patients.

Surgical advances, including cardiac transplantation, have improved the quality of life and survival among selected patients (2). Patients with severe coronary artery disease and reduced LV ejection fraction (EF) fare better with coronary bypass surgery than medical treatment (44). Certain patients whose HF is secondary to valvular heart disease, such as those with aortic valve stenosis, also experience better outcomes with surgical treatment (45).

The financial impact of HF is substantial. During 1996, hospital charges for diagnosis related group (DRG) 127 admissions ("congestive heart failure and shock") among Medicare patients alone totaled $6.4 billion. This number grossly underestimates the costs of inpatient care for HF, as DRG 127 would not, by definition, be assigned to patients with HF who had invasive procedures (e.g., cardiac catheterization) or those with HF as a secondary diagnosis. In fact, the care of patients with HF accounts for as much as 5% of the entire national expenditure for healthcare (12). Thus, HF poses a

TABLE 17-1. *Characteristics of outpatients enrolled in seven heart failure care management programs*

Reference	N	Patient characteristics	Mean age (Yr)	Sex (%)	Control or reference group
Fonarow GC, et al. (15)	214	Heart transplant candidates referred to a tertiary hospital	52	19 F 81 M	Patient as own control
Kornowski R, et al. (16)	42	Housebound elderly patients receiving home care in Israel	78	43 F 57 M	Patient as own control
Rich MW, et al. (17)	282	Elderly inpatients at a large, urban teaching hospital	79	63 F 37 M	Random assignment to treatment or control
Shah NB, et al. (18)	27	Outpatient veterans	62	100 M	Patient as own control
Tilney CK, et al. (19)	1,915	Elderly outpatients enrolled in a Medicare-HMO program	74	50 F 50 M	Patient as own control and historical reference
Weinberger M, et al. (20)	1,396	Hospitalized veterans with heart failure (13%), diabetes (35%), chronic lung disease (23%), or >1 diagnoses (28%)	63	1 F 99 M	Random assignment to treatment or control
West JA, et al. (21)	51	Select ambulatory HMO outpatients without serious comorbid illness	66	29 F 71 M	Patient as own control

F, female; HMO, health maintenance organization; M, male.

TABLE 17-2. *Key components of seven care management programs for outpatients with heart failure*

Reference	Duration (mo)	Key programmatic components	Observed changes in medical treatment
Fonarow GC, et al. (15)	6	Transplant cardiologists and nurses focused on medication titration, patient education, lifestyle changes, exercise, and close follow-up	Increased use of ACE inhibitors, diuretics, nitrates, amiodarone, and warfarin; decreased use of type I antiarrhythmic drugs and beta-blockers
Kornowski R, et al. (16)	12	Weekly home visits by internists supported by nurses and therapists	NR
Rich MW, et al. (17)	3	Nurse-managers directing education and surveillance in collaboration with a geriatric cardiologist, dietitian, social worker, and home health professional	NR
Shah NB, et al. (18)	12	Nurse-managers utilizing weekly mailings and phone calls with high-technology home monitoring, supported by primary cardiologist	NR
Tilney CK, et al. (19)	12	Proprietary disease management program (MULTIFIT, Cardiac Solutions, Inc., Sunnydale, CA) which utilized nurse-managers to coordinate care, education, and patient surveillance in collaboration with pharmacists, home care services, and primary physicians	NR
Weinberger M, et al. (20)	6	Intensive outpatient primary care by a dedicated physician/nurse team	NR
West JA, et al. (21)	3.5	MULTIFIT system: Nurse-manager supervised drug titration, patient education and surveillance via telephone	Increased use of ACE inhibitors and vasodilators

ACE, angiotensin converting enzyme; NR, not reported in reference.

TABLE 17-3. *Clinical outcomes of seven care management programs for outpatients with heart failure*

Reference	Clinical outcomes	Resource utilization	%
Fonarow GC, et al. (15)	Improved functional status and aerobic capacity	Reduction in hospital admission rate	85
Kornowski R, et al. (16)	Improved functional status	Reduction in hospital admission rate	62
Rich MW, et al. (17)	Improved quality of life measures	Reduction in hospital admission rate	56
Shah NB, et al. (18)	NR	Reduction in hospital admission rate	50
Tilney CK, et al. (19)	A 20% reduction in daily dietary salt intake Improved functional status	Reduction in hospital admission rate	60
Weinberger M, et al. (20)	No change in quality of life measures Improved patient satisfaction scores	Increase in general medical visit rate Reduction in subspecialty clinic visit rate Increase in hospital readmission rate	68 5 36
West JA, et al. (21)	Improved symptoms and functional status A 38% reduction in daily dietary salt intake	Reduction in general medical visit rate Reduction in cardiology visit rate Reduction in emergency room visit rate Reduction in hospital admission rate	23 31 53 74

NR, not reported in reference.

significant societal burden in terms of medical care costs, as well as loss of life and productivity (7,12). As the population continues to age, it is likely that HF will become even more prevalent, likely affecting more than 5,000,000 Americans by the year 2030 (7).

RATIONALE FOR MANAGING THE CARE OF PATIENTS

Physician and management team adherence to evidence-based recommendation for care remains suboptimal. For example, only 51% of patients hospitalized for HF in the community setting were discharged on ACE inhibitors (46). Although the use of ACE inhibitors has increased (47), improper prescribing habits continue to limit the full potential of these drugs. Furthermore, we found low rates of compliance with other recommended practices, such as documentation of LV systolic function (48), proper dietary counseling (48), and the use of beta-adrenergic receptor blockers (49). Poor clinical practices, if highly prevalent, are meaningful, as process of care has been linked to clinical outcomes in HF (50,51). Thus, developing and implementing strategies to measure and improve the quality of care for HF remains a high priority for clinicians and health care leaders (13). Care management programs, practice guidelines, and critical care pathways for the treatment of patients with HF hold promise to achieve this goal.

EXPERIENCE WITH HEART FAILURE CARE MANAGEMENT IN THE OUTPATIENT DOMAIN

In recent years, care management programs for HF have become increasingly common. Some of these initiatives have focused on finite goals (e.g., reducing length of stay for hospitalized patients) (13,52). Others have been broader in scope and have extended to outpatient practice. We performed a systematic evaluation of the impact of comprehensive, multidisciplinary disease management programs for HF on process of care, resource utilization, healthcare costs, and clinical outcomes across the longer-term continuum of this disorder (14). A total of seven articles met the search criteria for inclusion in this systematic review (15–21). The characteristics of the patients enrolled are summarized in Table 17-1. The key clinical components of the management programs tested in these studies are summarized in Table 17-2. The effects of the multidisciplinary programs on drug use are also summarized in Table 17-2. The impact of the multidisciplinary

TABLE 17-4. *Economic utility of seven care management programs for outpatients with heart failure*

Reference	Difference in charges or costs ($/patient)	Costs of intervention ($/patient)	Net economic impact ($/patient/mo)
Fonarow GC, et al. (15)	−$15,894[a]	$6,350[b]	−$1,591[a]
Kornowski R, et al. (16)	NR	NR	NR
Rich MW, et al. (17)	−$1,058[a]	$552	−$153[a]
Shah NB, et al. (18)	NR	NR	NR
Tilney CK, et al. (19)	−55%[c]	NR	NR
Weinberger M, et al. (20)	NR	NR	NR
West JA, et al. (21)	NR	NR	NR

NR, not reported in reference.
[a]These values essentially reflect changes in hospital charges, as total healthcare costs were not reported.
[b]Includes charge for initial hospitalization, averaging $6,050 per patient, plus $300 cost of postdischarge nursing care.
[c]Reported as percentage only, actual value not given.

TABLE 17-5. *Common causes of exacerbation of heart failure symptoms necessitating hospital admission in patients previously treated for heart failure*

Cause	Mechanisms
Noncompliance with medications	Habitual noncompliance, inadequate patient education, poor understanding of medication regimen, complexity of the medication regimen, excessive cost, perceived lack of efficacy, social factors (e.g., inflexibility of work schedule)
Noncompliance with dietary recommendations	Habitual noncompliance, inadequate patient education, poor understanding of dietary regimen, complexity of the dietary regimen (e.g., simultaneous recommendations for weight-reducing, low cholesterol, "diabetic" or "renal" diets), inadequate family participation, excessive cost, perceived lack of efficacy, social factors (e.g., inflexibility of work schedule)
Inadequate diuretic program	Progression of underlying cardiac dysfunction, diminished absorption of medications, development of diuretic resistance
Increased cardiac demand	Excessive activity or exercise, intercurrent illness
Intercurrent illness	Pain, fever, infection, pulmonary illness, anemia, gastrointestinal bleeding, renal insufficiency, nephrotic syndrome, thyroid disease, other endocrine abnormalities
New cardiac event	Myocardial ischemia, valvular regurgitation, cardiac arrhythmia (atrial or ventricular)
Use of a new medication	Nonsteroidal antiinflammatory agents, corticosteroids, calcium channel blockers, beta-blockers

TABLE 17-6. *Targets for education of patient and family regarding management of heart failure*

Domain	Subtopics and recommendations
Readiness for learning	Consider formal or informal testing to assess patient's readiness for learning, including assessment of denial response, capacity for comprehension, language skills, and prior fund of knowledge
Pathophysiology	Causes of heart failure, role of abnormalities in cardiac contraction and relaxation
Prognosis	Potential for progression of underlying cardiac dysfunction; significance of worsening heart failure, palpitations, syncope or chest pain
Medication use	Names (generic and brand), basic mechanisms of action, duration of action, side effects, drug interactions, contraindicated medications
Self-management	Daily weights, sliding scale diuretics (optional for selected patients)
Dietary restrictions	Low-salt, calorie restriction (for obese patients)
Lifestyle modification	Cessation of alcohol consumption and tobacco use
Exercise and activities	Low-level aerobic exercise is recommended for all compensated patients (functional class $\geq$III); consider referral to formal cardiac rehabilitation, when feasible; address timing of return to work in employed patients
Sexual habits	Intercourse is considered safe for all compensated patients (functional class $\geq$III)
Follow-up program	Confirm arrangements for first postdischarge office visit, establish frequency of future office visits, discuss future considerations regarding medication changes and medical procedures
Accessing healthcare	Strategies for when and whom to notify for worsening symptoms, new events, or questions
Comprehension	Consider formal or informal testing to assess patient's comprehension and retention of information

programs on clinical outcomes and resource utilization is summarized in Table 17-3. Finally, the economic utility of these programs is summarized in Table 17-4.

Strong emphasis on general treatment principles, such as aggressive patient education and close clinical follow-up, considered markers of high quality care have been proposed (1,13). From the pharmacologic standpoint, the two studies that emphasized proper drug titration demonstrated success in these efforts (15,21). The uniformity of the direction and magnitude of the effect of these programs on the risk of hospital admission across the studies was compelling: six of the seven studies demonstrated a 50% to 85% reduction in hospital admissions. This association between "better care" and "better outcomes" is comforting because it is intuitive and compatible with the results of large clinical trials.

The demographic and clinical characteristics of patients enrolled in the care management programs were broad and varied, spanning the diffuse spectrum of individuals likely to be encountered in typical clinical practice. Unfortunately, none of the studies reported subgroup analyses to detect classes of patients more likely to be "responders." However, in the absence of evidence to the contrary, it would seem reasonable that most patients with chronic HF would be candidates for HF care management programs. No evidence suggests this is a "niche technology" only appropriate for selected patients. From the public health perspective, these are highly relevant observations, as the essential manpower and technology required to initiate and sustain these programs should be available in most clinical settings. Moreover, these studies provide proof-of-concept that aggressive management of HF within the confines of a structured system of care is feasible, and offer hope that similar strategies executed in the in-hospital environment will yield similar benefits.

CLINICAL GOALS DURING HOSPITALIZATION FOR DECOMPENSATED HEART FAILURE

Surveillance for Signs of Poor Short-Term Outcome

The mortality rate associated with hospitalization for decompensated HF is high. In a statewide sample of patients with HF hospitalized in New York during 1995, the in-hospital mortality rate was 7% (3,106 of 44,926 patients) (53). Among a smaller cohort of 2,906 patients with HF treated in community hospitals, 157 (5%) died during the index hospitalization (5). In this same study, 568 of 2,508 patients (23%) followed during the acute hospitalization and for 6 months after discharge died during the period of observation. Most deaths were attributed to progressive pump failure or sudden cardiac death. Thus, an acute hospitalization for HF identifies a group with poor short- and intermediate-term outcome.

Controversy surrounds the notion that specific preventative steps will reduce the risk of death during an individual episode of hospital treatment for decompensated HF. Park et al. argue that hospital mortality for HF is more related to severity of illness on hospital admission (not modifiable by the treating clinician) than to process of care (54). Conversely, certain characteristics of the hospital environment may be associated with lower risk of death (55). However, which component(s) of the hospital environment or process of care explains these differences in hospital mortality has not been elucidated. Although providing high quality medical care for all inpatients with HF is rational and should be the goal in every clinical setting, no compelling evidence indicates that any single component of the process of care alters the immediate risk of death during an individual episode of hospitalization for HF. As HF is a chronic and largely irreversible disorder managed over a much longer continuum than any single hospital episode, clinicians should address the issue of a patient's prognosis from this perspective. Thus, hospitalization for HF provides the opportunity to identify patients who are at high risk of death during both the hospitalization and the months following discharge. Markers of particularly high risk include low LV EF (31,56–59); complex ventricular arrhythmias (57,58); advanced HF symptoms and abnormal hemodynamics, especially when refractory to

TABLE 17-7. *Goals of the first clinical encounter following discharge from the hospital after treatment for heart failure*

Domain	Goals or recommendations
Clinical status	Assess the presence and severity of heart failure, other cardiac conditions (e.g., ischemia, arrhythmia, and valvular regurgitation), and comorbid medical diseases.
Medication program	Add, discontinue, or titrate medications as indicated.
Lifestyle modification	Address comprehension and compliance with lifestyle modification program, including diet, weight reduction, exercise, and alcohol and tobacco abstention.
Patient education	Assess patient's comprehension and retention of information taught in the hospital; initiate, repeat, or supplement teaching, as needed.
Review hospitalization	Review the adequacy of diagnostic and therapeutic maneuvers performed in the hospital; schedule or perform additional tests, treatments, or consultations, as indicated.
Follow-up treatment plan	Confirm arrangements for next office visit; establish frequency of future office visits; discuss future considerations regarding medication changes and medical procedures.
Return to work	Address timing of return to work in employed patients.
Patient or family questions	Provide the patient or family ample opportunity to ask questions relative to heart failure or other medical problems.
Communication	Communicate with other physicians who share in the patient's care regarding current status, treatment changes, and future plans.

medical therapy (58–60); ischemic heart disease (61), hyponatremia (58), and evidence of end-organ hypoperfusion, such as renal insufficiency (59,62).

Relieving Symptoms of Fluid Overload

Symptoms and signs of fluid overload are the most common presenting complaints among patients hospitalized for decompensated HF. Thus, a frequent and immediate goal in managing hospitalized patients with HF is the initiation of steps to return the patient toward the euvolemic state.

The restriction of dietary salt is an important therapeutic maneuver in the management of acute and chronic HF (1,31,32). Salt restriction alone restores and maintains euvolemia in only a few hospitalized patients with HF. It is an important adjunct to drug therapy, however, and generally is considered good clinical practice (13). Fluid restriction is also used by many clinicians as an adjunct to salt restriction

CONGESTIVE HEART FAILURE CLINICAL PATHWAY TREATMENT GUIDELINES

CHECK PHYSICIAN ORDERS DAILY BEFORE INITIATING

CATEGORIES	DAY ONE	DAY TWO	DAY THREE	DAY FOUR	DAY FIVE	DAY SIX
ASSESSMENT and MONITORING	VS q4h----------------> Lung Assess TID & prn Skin Assessment q8h---> ✓ Perip edema 1-4+ prn---> Weigh daily---------------> TC & DB TID & PRN--> Sputum assess, color, consistency, amount prn Foley/ voiding Q8H----> Bowel Sound Q shift- --> Check for BM--------- ---> HOB Elevated------- Psychosocial--------------	VS q Shift-------> ----------------> ----------------> ----------------> ----------------> ----------------> ----------------> Foley Out?-----> ----------------> ----------------> ---------------->	----------------> ----------------> ----------------> ----------------> ----------------> ----------------> ----------------> voiding qs Laxative per order	----------------> ----------------> ----------------> ----------------> ----------------> ----------------> ----------------> Check for BM----	----------------> ----------------> ----------------> ----------------> ----------------> ----------------> ---------------->	VITAL SIGNS LUNG ASSESSMENT SKIN ASSESSMENT CHECK EDEMA WEIGHT SPUTUM ASSESSMENT CHECK VOIDING CHECK BOWEL SOUNDS CHECK FOR BM
DIET	2 Gm Sodium Diet----------> Fluid Restriction ?	Dietitian to screen ---------------->	----------------> ---------------->	----------------> ---------------->	----------------> ---------------->	
MOBILITY ACTIVITY/ SAFETY	Bedrest OOB/chair/Commode BRP with Assist------> ROM Exercises	OOB/Chair 30 min.TID ----------------> ----------------> ---------------->	----------------> Eval ADLs Q8h Ambulate 2 min TID Activity in Room ad lib	----------------> Amb 3 to 4 mins TID (see Consult)	Amb 4 to 5 mins TID	
DIAGNOSTICS	CXR, EKG, CBC, Chem-7 Chem-13 Consider: ABGs or oximetry Mg++ Digoxin Level, PT, PTT Thyroid elevation Cardiac Enzymes Telemetry as needed	Consider: Echocardiogram Cardiac Enzymes Chem-7	Consider repeat: CXR Chem 7, Chem 13 ABG's / oximetry on room air, if poss. Digoxin level D/C Telemetry	Oximetry	Consider repeat: Chem 7, Chem 13 Digoxin Level Oximetry on room air	
CONSULT		Cardiac Rehab ?		If not Ambulating, PT/OT Respiratory Therapy Cardiac Rehab ?		
TREATMENTS	O₂, per order------------> Diuretic per order-------> Saline Lock---------------> Consider: (per order) K+ supplement----------> Nitrates----------------- ACE inhibitor----------> Digoxin---------------> Consider Sub-Q heparin	----------------> Evaluate dose-------> ----------------> ----------------> ----------------> ---------------->	Evaluate need O₂ Evaluate dose------> ----------------> Evaluate dose-----> ----------------> ----------------> Evaluate dose----->	Consider D/C O₂ Select QD dose------> Consider D/C saline lock ----------------> ----------------> ----------------> ---------------->	Home O₂: if on room air PO₂ <55, SAT <88 Evaluate medications for discharge------------------>	
PATIENT/FAMILY EDUCATION	Review Patient Map Initiate teaching tool	Per teaching tool	Per teaching tool	Per teaching tool	Review discharge instructions	
DISCHARGE PLAN	Discharge planning assessment by Nursing and Plan initiated Needs identified	---------------->	---------------->	---------------->	Review discharge plan, sign 24 hr notice	

MR 500 11/96 5/29/97chf/chfguide

FIG. 17-1. Heart Failure Guide, a critical care pathway for heart failure in the format of a time-task matrix or Gantt chart.

and diuresis, although its safety and utility have not been well studied in prospective clinical trials.

In most cases, the intravenous administration of loop diuretics is the most appropriate pharmacologic strategy to induce rapid and predictable naturesis and relieve symptoms of fluid overload. Using intravenous rather than oral diuretics obviates concerns regarding the limited and unpredictable bioavailability of oral preparations that is common in patients with decompensated HF (63,64). The loop diuretic torsemide boasts 100% bioavailability even in the decompensated state, making it appropriate for some patients, particularly those without intravenous access or those with only mild volume overload (64,65). In some patients, administration of a continuous drip of a loop diuretic by the intravenous route is preferred (64). In patients refractory to loop diuretics alone, a second diuretic (e.g., a thiazide or metolazone) may be required (63,64). In patients with moderate or severe renal insufficiency, diuretics—even at high dose—may be ineffective, necessitating the use of renal dialysis or hemofiltration.

Returning the patient to the euvolemic state is the goal of salt restriction and diuresis in decompensated HF. Careful patient monitoring during diuresis (i.e., recording of the daily body weight and measuring intake and output) may obviate side effects or complications such as hypotension and renal insufficiency. In fact, the frequency with which the daily weight is recorded in the medical chart is considered by some to be a process marker of quality of care (13). In most patients with normal resting cardiac output and no intrinsic renal parenchymal or vascular disease, a reduction of 1 kg of body weight or net urinary output of 1 L/day will preserve intravascular volume to the extent that hypotension and renal insufficiency are less likely to develop. Other common complications of diuresis that warrant monitoring include electrolyte disturbances (e.g., hyponatremia, hypokalemia, and hypomagnesemia). The use of diuretic agents is not proved of benefit in reducing the mortality rate in acute or chronic HF (36) and they clearly activate neurohormonal systems that are known to promote progression of this syndrome (66). Thus, diuretics should be used as needed, but with caution, toward the goal of restoring euvolemia. They have not proved to have a role in patients who are euvolemic without them.

Use of intravenous inotropes and vasodilators is increasingly common in hospitalized patients with decompensated HF. Use of these drugs is associated with prompt

CHF PATIENT LANGUAGE MAP

Each person is unique, and this plan may vary to best suit your individual needs!

	DAY 1	DAY 2	DAY 3	DAY 4	DAY 5	DAY 6 DISCHARGE
GOALS AND OUTCOMES	Breathe easier	Breathe easier while out of bed	Breathe easier with increased activity Understand diet	Breathe easier and tolerate an increase in activity	Breathe easier with activity Demonstrate understanding of diet, medications and activity	Know all your discharge instructions
NURSING CARE AND TREATMENTS	Vital signs every 4 hrs Lung sounds every 4 hrs Weigh in AM If needed: Oxygen Heart monitor Blood work Measure oxygen level Chest X-ray	Vital signs every 8 hrs Lung sounds every 8 hrs Weigh in AM If needed: Oxygen Heart monitor Blood work Echocardiogram	Vital signs every 8 hrs Lung sounds every 8 hrs Weigh in AM If needed: Oxygen Stop heart monitor Blood work Chest X-ray	Vital signs every 8 hrs Lung sounds every 8 hrs Weigh in AM If needed: Stop oxygen Measure oxygen level every 8 hrs	Vital signs every 8 hrs Lung sounds every 8 hrs Weigh in AM If needed: Blood work Measure oxygen level	Vital signs Lung sounds Weigh in AM
DIET	Low salt diet Fluids restricted	Low salt diet	Dietitian to visit	Low salt diet	Any questions? Call Dietitian	Review Discharge Instructions
ACTIVITY (As Tolerated)	Walk to bathroom with assist	Sit up in chair for 30 min. Walk to bathroom with assist	Be as independent as possible with bathing and dressing	Increase walking distance Strive for continued independence	Increase distance Be as independent as possible	
MEDICATIONS	IV Medications	IV/Oral Medications	IV/Oral Medications	Oral Medications	Oral Medications	If you have any questions about your medications, ask your Nurse!
DISCHARGE PLANNING/ TEACHING	The nurse will ask questions about your home situation to see if you qualify for help at home.	------------------>	If you have concerns about going home, tell your nurse	Social Work will visit to see if you need equipment or more help at home.	Review discharge instructions. Sign 24 hr discharge notice	

FIG. 17-2. Heart Failure Patient Map, a language map for patients with heart failure, linked to the critical care pathway.

improvement or normalization of resting hemodynamics, rapid diuresis, and shorter hospitalizations. The hospital environment provides the setting for monitoring of the common side effects of the use of intravenous agents, including hypotension, myocardial ischemia, and cardiac arrhythmias. However, the safety and efficacy of this approach (compared with conventional therapy) has not been studied in large randomized trials. Perhaps, the results of the Outcomes of a Prospective Trial of Intravenous Milrinone for Exacerbations (OPTIME) study will provide more insight in this regard.

Identifying the Immediate Cause of Worsening Heart Failure

Among patients previously treated for HF, clinical exacerbations leading to hospitalization frequently occur because of readily identifiable and remediable causes (1,67). In fact, it has been estimated that as many as 50% of hospitalizations for worsening HF can be prevented. Frequently, these culprits can be identified with simple and low technology maneuvers, such as careful interview of the patient and family. The common causes of HF exacerbation are listed in Table 17-5. When a preventable cause of HF exacerbation is identified, corrective action should be taken, if possible.

Establishing the Primary Cause of Heart Failure

Heart failure is not a single disease, but rather a syndrome that occurs when a pathologic process impairs the contraction or relaxation properties of the heart. The primary causes of HF are numerous and a complete iteration of them is beyond the scope of this chapter. In Western cultures such as the United States, however, as many as 70% of patients with HF will have coexistent coronary atherosclerosis, whereas in 50% of patients, coronary artery disease appears to be the primary cause (68). Most patients with HF will also have hypertension (69), although it is implicated as the primary cause of HF in a smaller percentage. Other causes of HF include valvular heart disease and various toxic exposures and systemic disorders. Even with thorough clinical investigation, the cause is idiopathic in 10% or more of patients (5).

The cause of HF has important implications for the management of this syndrome. Prognosis is related to cause: patients with ischemic cardiomyopathy have a worse prognosis than some others (61). Conversely, some causes of HF (e.g., acute myocarditis, alcoholism, and hypothyroidism) have significant potential for improvement with proper medical management. The cause of HF is also relevant to treatment choices. For example, patients with ischemic or valvular causes may be candidates for revascularization or valve

INTERDISCIPLINARY TEACHING TOOL

Congestive Heart Failure Clinical Pathway

To Whom Taught: _____

Directions: Assess knowledge/abilities, provide education
if needed, indicate method of instruction and response,
date and initial where indicated.

Survival Skills Criteria to be assessed / taught		METHOD USED			PATIENT / SO RESPONSE			TEACHING DONE (by whom and date)		

Date / Initials
_____/___
_____/___
_____/___
_____/___
	View "Understanding CHF"
	  Channel 50 (9 AM & 4 PM)
	Given CHF teaching materials
	Given Patient Language Map
	other:
		D = Demonstration
		P = Pamphlet
		TV = Video/TV
		V = Verbal Inst. 1:1
		W = Written instruction
		N/A = Not Applicable
					Demo/verbalize material.
					NR = Needs
					      Reinforcement
					G = Goal Met
					N/A = Not Applicable
								With Patient or S.O.
								Date and Initial each
								teaching session
								(up to 3x)		

TOPICS	**GOALS**	1st	2nd	3rd	1st	2nd	3rd	1st	2nd	3rd
General Facts	Describes CHF	___	___	___	___	___	___	___	___	___
Medications	Understands drug name, dose, purpose, schedule, of following: Diuretic: _____ Ace Inhibitor: _____ Digoxin: _____ Beta Blocker: _____ Relates importance of taking medications as directed Given med teaching sheets *list*: _____ _____ Relates significant side effects and drug-food interactions	___ ___ ___ ___ ___ ___ ___ ___ ___ ___	___ ___ ___ ___ ___ ___ ___ ___ ___ ___	___ ___ ___ ___ ___ ___ ___ ___ ___ ___	___ ___ ___ ___ ___ ___ ___ ___ ___ ___	___ ___ ___ ___ ___ ___ ___ ___ ___ ___	___ ___ ___ ___ ___ ___ ___ ___ ___ ___	___ ___ ___ ___ ___ ___ ___ ___ ___ ___	___ ___ ___ ___ ___ ___ ___ ___ ___ ___	___ ___ ___ ___ ___ ___ ___ ___ ___ ___

Nutrition	Knowledgeable regarding:
	  Low sodium diet and
	  Importance of weight loss
		___	___	___	___	___	___	___	___	___

Activities	Understands the importance
	  of regular exercise
	Relates ways to improve
	  exercise / activity tolerance
		___
		___
			___
			___
				___
				___
					___
					___
						___
						___
							___
							___
								___
								___
									___
									___
										___
										___

Precautions	Relates home care plan and
	  MD follow-up
	Relates symptoms to report to
	doctor:
	1-SOB at night/unable to lie flat.
	2-Increased difficulty breathing
	  with the same activity.
	3-Weight gain >2 lb/day
	4-Swelling of legs or feet
	5-Very slow or very rapid pulse.
	6-Increased/unusual dizziness
	7-Chest pain
	Smoking Cessation
		___
		___
		___
		___
		___
		___
		___
		___
		___
			___
			___
			___
			___
			___
			___
			___
			___
			___
				___
				___
				___
				___
				___
				___
				___
				___
				___
					___
					___
					___
					___
					___
					___
					___
					___
					___
						___
						___
						___
						___
						___
						___
						___
						___
						___
							___
							___
							___
							___
							___
							___
							___
							___
							___
								___
								___
								___
								___
								___
								___
								___
								___
								___
									___
									___
									___
									___
									___
									___
									___
									___
									___
										___
										___
										___
										___
										___
										___
										___
										___
										___

FIG. 17-3.A. The Heart Failure Patient Education Document, a tool that assists with documentation of the patient education process for heart failure.

surgery (44,45). Patients with severe HF secondary to causes that are unlikely to improve or perhaps progress despite good care may be candidates for cardiac transplantation (2). Thus, proper management of patients with HF requires identifying its primary cause. A complete discussion of the diagnostic evaluation of HF is beyond the scope of this chapter. However, the clinical history, physical examination, and basic laboratory tests often provide clues to the cause (1,31). The clinician should carefully select diagnostic studies based on evidence and suspicion arising from the initial clinical assessment. Invasive or noninvasive laboratory tests should be performed only when clinical suspicion is justified by the patient's history, physical examination, and basic diagnostic studies (31). No expectation exists that laboratory test results will exclude all potential causes of HF in all patients. Conversely, the label "idiopathic cardiomyopathy" should be reserved for patients

INTERDISCIPLINARY TEACHING TOOL

Congestive Heart Failure	The heart is unable to pump enough blood to consistently meet all the body's needs, especially increased activity. This usually occurs because of weakness, fatigue or stiffness of the heart muscle. In any event, not enough blood is pumped out of the heart to keep up with the body's needs. The result is symptoms of chest pain, shortness of breath, fatigue, swelling, palpitations and passing out. As a rule, CHF gets worse over time, particularly if not treated in the correct fashion.

Medications
 	
Medication Precautions
	Diuretic: Takes excess sodium out of body and thereby "pulls" out excess fluid. Too much fluid overwhelms the weak or stiff heart muscle.
	ACE inhibitor: Decreases the work load of the heart.
	Digoxin: Improves the contraction of the heart muscle.
	    (Nurse FYI: Especially helpful in patients with systolic dysfunction or atrial fibrillation. May not be helpful in hypertrophic cardiomyopathy.)
	Beta blocker: Most patients benefit from beta blockers. They prevent disease progression by antagonizing the effects of catecholamines on the failing heart.
	Importance of taking the medications: These medications help to control the problem but do not cure it. If you stop the medications, the symptoms will likely recur.
	
	NSAIDS: Are pain relievers that can cause sodium retention (e.g., Advil, Nuprin).
	    (Nurse FYI: Aspirin and acetaminophen are generally well tolerated.)
	Antacids: Some antacids can cause sodium retention. Ask your doctor what to use.
	Decongestants: Ask your doctor which decongestant to use.

Diet	**Sodium reduction** is the key. Excess sodium makes your body retain fluid which, in turn, overwhelms the weak heart muscle. Grams (gm) and milligrams (mg) are units of measure *(like ounces and pounds)*. Read food labels. Avoid salt in foods. Limit your sodium to 2,000 milligrams (mg) per day. *(Nurse: Review what gm and mg mean and how to read food labels for sodium content.)* Review common foods to avoid (e.g., fast foods). Fruits and vegetables are generally okay. **Diuretics** also take potassium out of your body. Foods rich in potassium *(e.g., bananas)* are generally helpful. *(Nurse FYI: Caution regarding renal failure and ACE inhibitors.)* **Losing weight** makes less work for the heart. *A small pump (heart) in a big machine (a large body) has to work harder to run the machine.*
Activity	The heart, like any muscle, becomes weaker if not exercised. **Regular exercise as tolerated is important.** Modifications to exercise, such as pacing activity may make getting enough exercise easier and not worsen your symptoms. **Alternate activity and rest**. For example, sit down and rest after bathing and dressing. **Walking is generally a safe form of exercise.** Start slowly, 2-5 minutes a day for a week, then 5-10 minutes a day for a week, depending on your tolerance. **Short exercise periods spaced throughout the day are as effective as one long exercise session.** Talk with your doctor about planning safe activity.

Precautions	Call your doctor if you experience these symptoms which might indicate worsening CHF
	  1. Awakening with shortness of breath at night and/or inability to lie flat.
	  2. Increased difficulty breathing with activity previously easy to do.
	  3. Weight gain of more than 2 lb per day for 2 days. (Weigh yourself daily at same time of day wearing the same amount of clothes. Note your weight on a calendar.)
	  4. Increased swelling of your legs or feet.
	  5. Very slow or very rapid pulse.
	  6. Increased or unusual dizziness.
	  7. Chest pain.
	Smoking Cessation Very important to overall health. Many benefits are apparent immediately. Ask your doctor about the best methods to help you quit smoking.

FIG. 17-3.B. Continued.

who have had a thoughtful and appropriate diagnostic evaluation with all studies being negative.

In our experience in the community hospital setting, 36% of all hospital admissions for HF are the first episode of medical care for HF for that individual (5). A patient's presentation to the hospital with newly diagnosed HF provides the opportunity to initiate the diagnostic evaluation. Certainly, a thorough history, physical examination, and basic laboratory studies including blood chemistries, complete blood count, urinalysis, electrocardiogram, and chest radiograph should be performed on hospital admission in all patients with acute cardiac disorders. The clinician should critically analyze and synthesize these data to allow a succinct differential diagnosis of HF. From there, deciding which if any diagnostic studies to pursue in the hospital would be guided by the level of clinical suspicion, the availability of diagnostic services, the degree of the patient's medical stability, patient preferences, and so forth.

Most hospital admissions for HF are not the first for that patient; many patients, therefore, will have had the cause of

Congestive Heart Failure
Clinical Pathway

Day of Admission   Date:_____

Patient Stamp

Check Physician Orders Daily Before Initiating		2400-0700	0700-1500	1500-2400
Neurological	Alert & oriented x 3			
Comfort	Patient comfortable			
Respiratory	Lung assessment WNL			
	TC DB			
	O₂ Therapy (Type/Liter)			
	Oximetery (document on O₂ Sat Report)			
	No cough			
Circulatory	VS stable			
	Assess edema			
	Telemetry			
GI/GU	ABD assessment WNL			
	Continent of (A) urine (B) stool			
	Voiding QS *or* Foley patent (choose criteria for Foley) (A) Relieve obstruction (B) Neurogenic bladder (C) Accurate I & O (D) Urologic or adjacent surgery			
	Foley patent _____ cc 24 hr			
	Date of last BM			
	Weight per protocol			
Diet	Type	B L D		
	Percent eaten	B ____ % L ____ % D ____ %		
	Feeds (A) self (B) w/assist (C) total			
	Fluid restriction			
Skin	Skin WNL			
	Braden Scale Score (frequency per standard)			
Hygiene	Per standard (A) Self (B) Partial (C) Complete			
Mobility	Bedrest			
Activity	(A) Commode (B) BR *w/assist of* (C) 1 (D) 2			
	(A) Chair *w/assist of* (B) 1 (C) 2 (D) Lift			
	ROM exercises (Nursing)			
Safety	Siderails up #	#	#	#
	Call bell within reach			
	Fall Prevention Protocol reassess daily			
	(A) Restraints (see Flowsheet) (B) Alternatives to restraints used			
	IV rounds q 1hr			
Psychosocial	(A) Anxiety controlled (B) Pt/SO concerns verbalized			
Teaching	Initiate Interdisciplinary teaching tool			
	Per _____ tool			
D/C Planning	Admission Assessment complete day 1			
Plan of Care	(A) Reviewed (B) Revised			
Consult				
Other				

FIG. 17-4.A. Heart Failure Days, a tool that incorporates the nursing care plan and nursing documentation. The form becomes part of the patient's permanent medical record at our institution. A. Admission, day 1. B. Day 2. C. Day 3. D. Day 4. E. Day 5. F. Day 6 (discharge).

their HF previously diagnosed and documented. However, in our experience in the community setting, more than 20% of patients with one or more previous hospitalizations for HF will not have a presumed or established cause of HF documented in their medical chart (48). Moreover, errors occur in assigning a cause of HF. Therefore, the clinician should critically analyze all relevant data, including the patient's previous medical records, toward the goal of documenting the most reasonable cause of HF.

Evaluating Left Ventricular Systolic Function

Left ventricular contractile function is abnormal in most patients with chronic HF, but normal or nearly normal in

Congestive Heart Failure

Clinical Pathway

Day 2   DATE:_____

Patient Stamp

CHECK PHYSICIAN ORDERS DAILY BEFORE INITIATING		2400-0700	0700-1500	1500-2400
Neurological	Alert & Oriented x 3			
Comfort	Patient comfortable			
Respiratory	Lung assessment WNL			
	TC DB			
	O₂ Therapy (Type/Liter)			
	Oximetery (document on O₂ Sat Report)			
	No cough			
Circulatory	VS stable			
	Assess Edema			
	Telemetry			
GI/GU	ABD assessment WNL			
	Continent of (A) urine (B) stool			
	Voiding QS *or* Foley patent (choose criteria for Foley) (A) Relieve obstruction (B) Neurogenic bladder (C) Accurate I & O (D) Urologic or adjacent surgery			
	Foley D/C voiding qs			
	Date of last BM			
	Weight per protocol			
Diet	Type	B_____	L_____	D_____
	Percent eaten	B_____ %	L_____ %	D_____ %
	Feeds (A) self (B) w/assist (C) total			
	Fluid restriction			
Skin	Skin WNL			
	Braden Scale Score (frequency per standard)			
Hygiene	Per standard A)Self B)Partial C)Complete			
Mobility	OOB to chair x 30 minutes TID			
Activity	(A) Commode (B) BR *w/assist of* (C) 1 (D) 2			
	(A) Chair *w/assist of* (B) 1 (C) 2 (D) Lift			
	ROM exercises (Nursing)			
Safety	Siderails up #	#	#	#
	Call bell within reach			
	Fall Prevention Protocol (reassess daily)			
	(A) Restraints (see Flowsheet) (B) Alternatives to restraints used			
	IV rounds q 1 hr			
Psychosocial	(A) Anxiety controlled (B) Pt / SO concerns verbalized			
Teaching	Per Interdisciplinary Teaching Tool			
	Per _____ tool			
Plan of Care	(A) Reviewed (B) Revised			
Consult				
Other				

FIG. 17-4.B. Continued.

as many as 40% to 45% of this population (29,70–72). Measures of contractile function, including EF, are highly relevant to diagnosis (31,70,73,74), prognosis (31,56–59, 74–77), and treatment (29,31,46,47,56,70,73,74,77) of HF. Ejection fraction, which is inversely related to mortality (31,56–59,74–77), is perhaps the best prognostic index for HF. On this basis, experts recommend that systolic function be assessed at least once in all cases of suspected HF (1,31–33).

Certain factors (e.g., older age, female sex, hypertension, and normal cardiothoracic ratio on chest radiograph) often exist when HF occurs in the presence of normal EF, or so-called "diastolic failure" (29,59,71,72,74,78–81). In evaluating a patient with HF, the presence of one or more of these factors may promote a false sense that EF can be estimated on clinical grounds, and that measurement is not necessary. In our experience in the community hospital setting, 25% of patients with documented HF are managed without assessment

Congestive Heart Failure

CLINICAL PATHWAY

Day 3　　　　DATE:_____

Patient Stamp

CHECK PHYSICIAN ORDERS DAILY BEFORE INITIATING		2400-0700	0700-1500	1500-2400
Neurologic	Alert & oriented x 3			
Comfort	Patient comfortable			
Respiratory	Lung assessment WNL			
	TC & DB			
	O$_2$ Therapy (Type/Liter)			
	Oximetery (document on O$_2$ Sat Report)			
	No cough			
Circulatory	VS stable			
	Assess Edema			
	Telemetry D/C			
GI/GU	ABD assessment WNL			
	Continent of (A) urine (B) stool			
	Voiding QS *or* Foley patent (choose criteria for Foley) (A) Relieve obstruction (B) Neurogenic bladder (C) Accurate I & O (D) Urologic or adjacent surgery			
	Date of last BM			
	Weight per protocol			
Diet	Type	B_____ L:_____	D:_____	
	Feeds (A) self (B) w/assist (C) total	B_____ %L:_____	%D:_____ %	
	Fluid restriction			
Skin	Skin WNL			
	Braden Scale Score (frequency per standard)			
Hygiene	Per Standard (A)Self (B)Partial (C)Complete			
Mobility	Ambulate in room TID *w/assist of* (A) 1 (B) 2			
Activity	Distance			
	(A) Commode (B) BR *w/assist of* (C) 1 (D) 2			
	(A) Chair *w/assist of* (B) 1 (C) 2 (D) Lift			
	ROM exercises (Nursing)			
Safety	Side rails up #	#	#	#
	Call bell within reach			
	(A) Restraints (see Flowsheet) (B) Alternatives to restraints used			
	IV rounds q 1 hr			
	Fall Prevention Protocol reassess qd			
Psychosocial	(A) Anxiety controlled (B) Patient/SO concerns verbalized			
Teaching	Per Interdisciplinary teaching tool			
	Per _____ tool			
Plan of Care	(A) Reviewed (B) Revised			
Consult				
Other				

FIG. 17-4.C. Continued.

of systolic function (48). In point of fact, we have shown that the cardiothoracic ratio does not reliably predict EF for individuals with HF, even after accounting for the cause of HF, presence of right ventricular failure, and method of EF measurement (82). In a more comprehensive analysis of the utility of clinical estimation of EF, we examined data from 7,534 patients with HF enrolled in the Digitalis Investigators'

Group (DIG) trial (83). We attempted to derive a prediction rule for EF using multiple regression analyses and more than 80 predictor variables from the clinical history, physical examination, and basic laboratory tests. Among the 38% of patients who had the lowest values of predicted EF, measured EF was frequently less than 0.45. However, among the remaining 62% of patients, this method did not reliably distinguish

Congestive Heart Failure

CLINICAL PATHWAY

Day 4   DATE:_____

Patient Stamp

CHECK PHYSICIAN ORDERS DAILY BEFORE INITIATING		2400-0700	0700-1500	1500-2400
Neurologic	Alert & oriented x 3			
Comfort	Patient comfortable			
Respiratory	Lung assessment WNL			
	TC & DB			
	O$_2$ Therapy (Type/Liter)			
	Oximetery (document on O$_2$ Sat Report)			
	No cough			
Circulatory	VS stable			
	Assess Edema			
GI/GU	ABD assessment WNL			
	Voiding QS *or* Foley patent (choose criteria for Foley) (A) Relieve obstruction (B) Neurogenic bladder (C) Accurate I & O (D) Urologic or adjacent surgery			
	Continent of (A) urine (B) stool			
	Date of Last BM			
	Weigh daily per protocol			
Diet	Type	B_____ L_____ D_____		
	Percent eaten	B_____ % L_____ % D_____ %		
	Feeds (A) self (B) w/assist (C) total			
	Fluid restriction			
Skin	Skin WNL			
	Braden Scale Score (frequency per standard)			
Hygiene	Per standard (A) Self (B) Partial (C) Complete			
Mobility	Tolerating increased activity			
Activity	Ambulate in hall TID *w/assist of* (A) 1 (B) 2			
	ROM exercises (Nursing)			
Safety	Siderails up #	#	#	#
	Call bell within reach			
	(A) Restraints (see Flowsheet) (B) Alternatives to restraints used			
	Fall Prevention Protocol reassess qd			
Psychosocial	(A) Anxiety controlled (B)Pt/SO concerns verbalized			
Teaching	Per Interdisciplinary Teaching Tool			
	Per _____ Tool			
Plan of Care	(A) Reviewed (B) Revised			
Consult				
Other				

FIG. 17-4.D. Continued.

those with normal from low EF. Pending further refinement of clinical prediction rules which might prove them to be both valid and convenient for bedside use, our results support expert recommendations that objective testing be used to assess systolic function in all patients suspected of having HF (1,13,31–33). Assessment of LV systolic function in hospitalized patients with newly diagnosed HF, or previously treated patients without prior assessment, is a preferred practice. The utility of repeated assessment of systolic function (at regular intervals in the outpatient clinic, with each hospitalization for HF, or both) is an unproved strategy, the utility of which has never been assessed in a rigorous scientific

manner. To our knowledge, no experts recommend such a practice. Pragmatic considerations include the following:

1. Once HF has been documented as "systolic" or "diastolic," changes in EF within the abnormal or normal range, respectively, although they may occur, have limited implications for most decisions regarding therapy of HF.
2. Patients with previously documented diastolic failure uncommonly have a significant fall in EF in association with hospital admission for decompensated HF.
3. Among patients with previously documented systolic HF, repeat assessment of LV function at the time of worsening

Congestive Heart Failure

CLINICAL PATHWAY

Day 5   DATE:_____

Patient Stamp

CHECK PHYSICIAN ORDERS DAILY BEFORE INITIATING		2400-0700	0700-1500	1500-2400
Neurologic	Alert & oriented x 3			
Comfort	Patient comfortable			
Respiratory	Lung assessment WNL			
	TC & DB			
	O$_2$ Therapy (Type/Liter)			
	Oximetery (document on O$_2$ Sat Report)			
	No cough			
Circulatory	VS stable			
	Assess Edema			
GI/GU	ABD assessment WNL			
	Voiding QS *or* Foley patent (choose criteria for Foley) (A) Relieve obstruction (B) Neurogenic bladder (C) Accurate I & O (D) Urologic or adjacent surgery			
	Continent of (A) urine (B) stool			
	BM			
	Weight daily per protocol			
Diet	Type	B_____ L_____ D_____		
	Percent eaten	B_____% L_____% D_____%		
	Feeds (A) self (B) w/assist (C) total			
	Fluid restriction			
Skin	Skin WNL			
	Braden Scale Score (frequency per standard)			
Hygiene	Per standard (A) Self (B) Partial (C) Complete			
Mobility	Tolerating increased activity			
Activity	Ambulate in hall TID with assist of (A) 1 (B) 2			
	Distance			
	ROM exercises			
Safety	Siderails up #	#	#	#
	Call bell within reach			
	(A) Restraints (see Flowsheet) (B) Alternatives to restraints used			
	Fall Prevention Protocol reassess qd			
Psychosocial	(A) Anxiety controlled (B) Pt/SO concerns verbalized			
Teaching	Per Interdisciplinary Teaching Tool			
	Per _____ Tool			
Discharge Plan	Initiate discharge paperwork			
	Sign 24 hr Notice			
Plan of Care	(A) Reviewed (B) Revised			
Consult				
Other				

FIG. 17-4.E. Continued.

symptoms or hospitalization usually does not give much valuable or unique information regarding the cause of exacerbation.

In summary, a recommended clinical practice is to differentiate systolic from diastolic HF, usually by measuring EF, using objective tests such as echocardiography. In patients with newly diagnosed HF, or those previously treated without prior assessment, this is often done during an acute hospitalization. In most cases, patients who have had prior documentation of systolic or diastolic HF usually do not require routine repeat measurement of EF to be managed effectively.

Initiating or Adjusting "Maintenance" Pharmacologic Therapy

Hospitalization provides a valuable opportunity to critique and potentially modify the treatment regimen of patients with newly diagnosed or previously treated HF. For new patients,

Congestive Heart Failure

CLINICAL PATHWAY

Day 6 Discharge DATE:_____

Patient Stamp

CHECK PHYSICIAN ORDERS BEFORE INITIATING		2400-0700	0700-1500	1500-2400
Neurologic	Alert & oriented x 3			
Comfort	Patient comfortable			
Respiratory	Lung assessment WNL			
	TC & DB			
	O₂ Therapy (Type/Liter)			
	Oximetry (document on O₂ Sat Report)			
	No cough			
Circulatory	VS stable			
	No peripheral edema			
GI/GU	ABD assessment WNL			
	Voiding QS *or* Foley patent (choose criteria for Foley) (A) Relieve obstruction (B) Neurogenic bladder (C) Accurate I & O (D) Urologic or adjacent surgery			
	Continent of (A) urine (B) stool			
	BM			
	Weight per protocol			
Diet	Type	B_____ L_____ D_____		
	Percent eaten	B_____ % L_____ % D_____ %		
	Feeds (A) self (B) w/assist (C) total			
	Fluid restriction			
Skin	Skin WNL			
	Braden Scale Score (frequency per standard)			
Hygiene	Per standard (A) Self (B) Partial (C) Complete			
Mobility	Ambulates (A) ad lib, *w/assist of* (B) 1 (C) 2			
Activity	Distance			
	Tolerating ADL's			
	ROM WNL (Nursing)			
Safety	Siderails up #	#	#	#
	Call bell within reach			
	(A) Restraints (see Flowsheet) (B) Alternatives to restraints used			
	Fall Prevention Protocol (reassess daily)			
Psychosocial	(A) Anxiety controlled (B) Pt/SO concerns verbalized			
Teaching	Reviewed D/C instructions			
	Per Interdisciplinary Teaching Tool			
	Per _____ Tool			
Discharge Plan	Finalized			
Plan of Care	Goals met			
Consult				
Other				

FIG. 17-4.F. Continued.

initiation of carefully chosen drugs in the hospital setting provides the opportunity for careful monitoring of efficacy and side effects. For patients who have had prior treatment for HF, most clinicians view a hospitalization itself as a marker of failure of the previous regimen and an indication to advance the treatment program. However, special conditions and circumstances need to be considered.

As presented earlier in this chapter, noncompliance with the previously prescribed medical regimen is a frequent cause of HF exacerbation. Reasons for low compliance are listed in Table 17-5. In many cases, a simple discussion with the patient or family will uncover the presence and cause(s) of inadequate compliance. Sometimes, serum assays (e.g., of digitalis) will reveal undetectable levels that are a clue. In cases of inadequate compliance, recommendation of more or higher doses of medications may be ineffective, unnecessary, or inappropriate. Rather, facilitating compliance with previously recommended treatments, perhaps in association with a reduction in the complexity of the treatment regimen, may be all that is indicated.

The use of ACE inhibitors is a proved and accepted strategy in the treatment of HF. In the Cooperative North Scandinavian Enalapril Survival Study (CONSENSUS), patients with advanced HF (New York Heart Association functional class IV) who were treated with enalapril experienced a significant reduction in mortality during 1 year of follow-up compared with those randomized to placebo (4). In this study, the mortality curves showed significant separation within a few months after randomization favoring the enalapril-treated group. Therefore, the early use of ACE inhibitors in hospitalized patients with HF is rational. However, the timing of drug initiation and up-titration requires caution. Patient who are receiving aggressive diuresis are particularly susceptible to the renal toxicities of ACE inhibition (84). Consequently, withholding ACE inhibitors until patients have achieved a euvolemic state is sometimes prudent. Further up-titration of ACE inhibitors toward the chosen dose can then be achieved during the subacute period following hospitalization.

Beta-adrenergic blocker use in stable, ambulatory outpatients with HF is well tolerated and reduces disease progression and mortality (37–39). Therefore, their use is recommended in such circumstances. However, the use of beta-blockers in sicker patients with class IV HF is associated with a higher incidence of side effects (85), and perhaps, less efficacy (38). Therefore, the use of such drugs in hospitalized patients poses more challenges. As none of the major, large randomized trials of beta-blockers enrolled hospitalized patients (in fact, excluded them), we cannot recommend routine initiation of these drugs for inpatients with HF, particularly severe HF. However, the simultaneous use of a phosphodiesterase inhibitor is a promising, albeit unproved, strategy for facilitating the initiation and up-titration of beta-blockers during a hospitalization for decompensated HF (86). Among patients previously treated with beta-blockers who experience worsening HF, increasing the concomitant therapy (e.g., diuretics) but continuing the beta-blocker is a rational first step (32). For patients refractory to this maneuver, reducing the dose of beta-blockers, or slowly weaning them, is then acceptable. For patients who require beta-receptor agonists (e.g., dobutamine), weaning or discontinuation of beta-blockers is preferred.

Compared with placebo, the use of digoxin is associated with improved symptoms of HF and lower risk for hospitalization, with a negligible impact on mortality (35). Thus, it is rational to use digoxin in patients who remain symptomatic on ACE inhibitors and diuretics (±beta-blockers) with a goal of improving symptoms and quality of life while reducing the risk for rehospitalization. As such, initiation of digoxin in the hospital is an acceptable if not preferred practice. When used properly, the incidence of side effects will be low; routine surveillance with assays for serum digoxin level is usually unnecessary.

In the Randomized Aldactone Evaluation (RALES) study, when spironolactone (12.5 to 25 mg/day) was added to background therapy of ACE inhibitors, digitalis, and diuretics (±beta-blockers) among patients with chronic HF, a 30%

reduction in the risk of death was observed (40). As these findings were published in late 1999, they are too recent to be reflected in any of the published authoritative HF treatment guidelines available today. Anecdotally, we have witnessed an abrupt rise in the use of spironolactone following publication of the RALES results, and we use the drug liberally in our own practice. When employing it in euvolemic patients (or nearly euvolemic patients) for the reasons it was used in the RALES study, we use the study dose (12.5–25 mg/day). Also, we generally restrict its use to sicker (class III and IV) patients, such as those enrolled in RALES. This strategy would include most patients who are hospitalized for HF. As spironolactone can cause a rise in blood potassium level, careful monitoring is appropriate.

Educating the Patient and Family

Whether educating patients and families regarding clinical issues surrounding HF alone improves clinical outcomes has not been studied in prospective, randomized trials (13). However, patient and family education is a core component of all successful HF disease management programs (14–21). It is considered good practice in general and is recommended by most expert panels (1,31,32). In fact, patient and family education is considered by some to be a process marker of quality of care for HF (13). The educational process should not be limited to verbal teaching, but rather, supplemented by written or visual aids. The educational process should be tailored to the literacy level, language preference, and ethnic and cultural habits of the patient and family. The key topics to be covered in the educational process are listed in Table 17-6.

Planning for Timely and Appropriate Hospital Discharge and Postdischarge Care

Patients with HF who are unstable at the time of discharge are at higher risk for hospital readmission (50). Even patients who receive excellent medical care are at significant risk of ongoing morbidity, recurrent hospitalization, and death during the intermediate-term period after hospital discharge. Therefore, planning for proper postdischarge care is an important component of the hospital-based management of this disorder. Some or many patients benefit from referral to specialized HF care management programs or HF clinics (14–21). Others may benefit from enrollment in a home care program. Most experts recommend an outpatient office or home visit by a skilled clinician within 1 week after discharge (1). The goals of this clinical encounter are listed in Table 17-7.

A CRITICAL PATHWAY FOR MANAGEMENT OF PATIENTS WITH HEART FAILURE

Having established the goals and processes that we consider proper in the hospital-based management of HF, we now present a template critical care pathway (Fig. 17-1 to 17-4).

The Heart Failure Guide (Fig. 17-1) is organized as a time-task matrix or Gantt chart. It is the backbone of the pathway process. The document itself is placed in the front of the patient's medical chart to serve as a resource for all staff. It is not part of the permanent medical record and is discarded when the patient is discharged from the hospital.

The Heart Failure Patient Map (Fig. 17-2), a simplified version of the "Heart Failure Guide," is designed for use by the patient and family to familiarize them with the process of care for HF at our institution. It is organized in a fashion similar to the "Heart Failure Guide" (Fig. 17-1). It is placed at the patient's bedside and is not a part of the permanent medical record.

The Heart Failure Patient Education Document (Fig. 17-3) is a tool that assists the patient's nurse with documentation of the educational process. It ensures consistent education and documentation across patients and providers. It is a permanent part of the medical record.

Heart Failure Days 1 through 6 (Fig. 17-4) are also nursing documentation tools that incorporate the nursing care plan and allow the patient's nurse to document by exception. The presumption is that all activities on the document have occurred as planned unless otherwise noted. If the activity occurs as planned, the nurse simply initials the block. In cases of variance, the nurse places an asterisk in the box and writes a note to document the alternative action that was taken and the reason for it.

When a patient with HF is admitted to our hospital, all of the materials for the HF pathway process are placed in the patient's chart. This includes a preprinted order sheet containing a standard set of admission orders for HF. The admitting physician simply checks all of the orders to be implemented for that patient and then adds supplemental orders, as appropriate, for HF or other concurrent medical problems. Among other things, the preprinted orders are designed to focus the admitting physician on the need to initiate diuresis early after hospital admission (51). In addition, the preprinted orders draw attention to the importance of assessing LV systolic function and prescribing ACE inhibitors. Printed educational materials are available on all medical wards where patients with HF are treated. Their use ensures that care providers, in particular the patient's nurse, address prespecified key issues (e.g., diet and medications) and compliance with them. In addition, the day-by-day care plan helps physicians and nurses focus on other key management principles such as the need for accurate intake and output records and daily weights. Nutritional counseling and physical therapy are also initiated by the patient's nurse.

Outcome measures defined by the "Heart Failure Guide" for each day help all care providers stay focused on the goals for the hospitalization. Each outcome is tracked and profiled, stratified by attending physician. We have found it important that all physicians have an opportunity to review proposed outcome measures before tracking and profiling are initiated. Periodic reports of pathway compliance by outcome per physician encourage outlying physicians to comply with the treatment guidelines, and provide opportunities for our performance improvement team to address areas where compliance might be improved.

The pathways and outcome tracking become an integral part of the organization's performance improvement process. The PDCA (Plan-Do-Check-Act) cycle is complete. The pathway (PLAN) is developed with multidisciplinary input. It is then implemented (DO) with defined outcome measures (CHECK). Variances from expected outcomes are identified and changes made in the pathway (ACT). In our institution, the PDCA process is repeated every 3 to 6 months.

At our institution, more than 70% of patients with the primary diagnosis of HF are treated "on the pathway." Use of this pathway process has resulted in excellent compliance (>80%) with recommended management strategies that are considered key process markers of quality, such as proper dietary counseling, measurement of LV systolic function, and use of ACE inhibitors.

REFERENCES

1. Konstam MA, Dracup K, Bottoroff MB, et al. Quick reference guide for clinicians No. 11. Heart failure: management of patients with left ventricular systolic dysfunction. Rockville, MD: Agency for Health Care Policy and Research, Public Health Service, United States Department of Health and Human Services, AHCPR Publication No. 94-0613, 1994.
2. Costanzo MR, Augustine S, Bourge R, et al. Selection and treatment of candidates for heart transplantation. A statement for health professionals from the Committee on Heart Failure and Cardiac Transplantation of the Council on Clinical Cardiology, American Heart Association. *Circulation* 1995;92:3593–3612.
3. Domanski MJ, Garg R, Yusuf S. Prognosis in congestive heart failure. In: Hosenpud JD, Greenberg BH, eds. *Congestive heart failure: pathophysiology, diagnosis and comprehensive approach to management.* New York: Springer-Verlag, 1994:622–627.
4. The CONSENSUS Trial Study Group. Effects of enalapril on mortality in severe congestive heart failure: results of the Cooperative North Scandinavian Enalapril Survival Study. *N Engl J Med* 1987;316:1429–1435.
5. Philbin EF, Rocco TA, Lindenmuth NW, et al. Clinical outcomes in heart failure: report from a community hospital–based registry. *Am J Med* 1999;107:549–555.
6. Parmley W. Pathophysiology and current treatment of congestive heart failure. *J Am Coll Cardiol* 1989;13:771–785.
7. Cardiology Preeminence Roundtable. Beyond four walls. Cost-effective management of chronic congestive heart failure. Washington, DC: The Advisory Board Company; 1994:39–47.
8. Krumholz HM, Parent EM, Tu N, et al. Readmission after hospitalization for congestive heart failure among Medicare beneficiaries. *Arch Intern Med* 1997;157:99–104.
9. Philbin EF, DiSalvo TG. The influence of race and gender on process of care, resource utilization, and hospital-based outcomes in congestive heart failure. *Am J Cardiol* 1998;82:76–81.
10. Philbin EF, DiSalvo TG. Prediction of hospital readmission for heart failure: development of a simple risk score based on administrative data. *J Am Coll Cardiol* 1999;33:1560–1566.
11. Mann DL. Mechanisms and models in heart failure. A combinatorial approach. *Circulation* 1999;100:999–1008.
12. O'Connell JB, Bristow MR. Economic impact of heart failure in the United States: time for a different approach. *J Heart Lung Transplant* 1994;13:S107–S112.
13. Krumholz HM, Baker DW, Ashton CM, et al. Evaluating quality of care for patients with heart failure. *Circulation* 2000;101:e122–e140.
14. Philbin EF. Comprehensive multidisciplinary programs for management of patients with congestive heart failure. *J Gen Intern Med* 1999;14:130–135.
15. Fonarow GC, Stevenson LW, Walden JA, et al. Impact of a comprehensive heart failure management program on hospital readmission and

functional status of patients with advanced heart failure. *J Am Coll Cardiol* 1997;30:725–732.

16. Kornowski R, Zeeli D, Averbuch M, et al. Intensive home-care surveillance prevents hospitalization and improves morbidity among elderly patients with severe congestive heart failure. *Am Heart J* 1995;129:762–766.

17. Rich MW, Beckman V, Wittenberg C, et al. A multidisciplinary intervention to prevent the readmission of elderly patients with congestive heart failure. *N Engl J Med* 1995;333:1190–1195.

18. Shah NB, Der E, Ruggerio C, et al. Prevention of hospitalizations for heart failure with an interactive home monitoring program. *Am Heart J* 1998;135:373–378.

19. Tilney CK, Whiting SB, Horrar JL, et al. Improved clinical and financial outcomes associated with a comprehensive congestive heart failure program. *Disease Management* 1998;1:175–183.

20. Weinberger M, Oddone EZ, Henderson WG. Does increased access to primary care reduce hospital readmissions? *N Engl J Med* 1996;334:1441–1447.

21. West JA, Miller NH, Parker KM, et al. A comprehensive management system for heart failure improves clinical outcomes and reduces medical resource utilization. *Am J Cardiol* 1997;79:58–63.

22. Captopril Multicenter Research Group. A placebo-controlled trial of refractory chronic congestive heart failure. *J Am Coll Cardiol* 1983;2:755–763.

23. Packer M, Lee WH, Yushak M, et al. Comparison of captopril and enalapril in patients with severe chronic heart failure. *N Engl J Med* 1986;315:847–853.

24. Kjekshus J, Swedberg K. Tolerability of enalapril in congestive heart failure. *Am J Cardiol* 1988;62:67A–72A.

25. The SOLVD Investigators. Effect of enalapril on survival in patients with reduced left ventricular ejection fractions and congestive heart failure. *N Engl J Med* 1991;325:293–302.

26. Rogers WJ, Johnstone DE, Yusuf S, et al. Quality of life among 5,025 patients with left ventricular dysfunction randomized between placebo and enalapril: the studies of left ventricular dysfunction. *J Am Coll Cardiol* 1994;23:393–400.

27. Cohn JN, Johnson G, Zieshe S, et al. A comparison of enalapril with hydralazine-isosorbide in the treatment of chronic congestive heart failure. *N Engl J Med* 1991;325:303–310.

28. Pfeffer MA, Braunwald E, Moye LA, et al. Effect of captopril on mortality and morbidity in patients with left ventricular dysfunction after myocardial infarction. *N Engl J Med* 1992;327:669–677.

29. Philbin EF, Rocco TA. The utility of angiotensin-converting enzyme inhibitors in heart failure with preserved systolic function. *Am Heart J* 1997;134:188–195.

30. Paul SD, Kuntz KM, Eagle KA, et al. Costs and effectiveness of angiotensin converting enzyme inhibition in patients with congestive heart failure. *Arch Intern Med* 1994;154:1143–1149.

31. Williams JF, Bristow MR, Fowler MB, et al. Guidelines for the evaluation and management of heart failure. Report of the American College of Cardiology/American Heart Association Task Force on Practice Guidelines (Committee on Evaluation and Management of Heart Failure). *Circulation* 1995;92:2764–2784.

32. Advisory Council to Improve Outcomes Nationwide in Heart Failure. Consensus recommendations for the management of chronic heart failure. *Am J Cardiol* 1999;83[Suppl 2A]:1A–38A.

33. Johnstone DE, Abdulla A, Arnold JMO, et al. Diagnosis and management of heart failure. *Can J Cardiol* 1994;10:613–631.

34. Pitt B, Segal R, Martinez FA, et al. Randomised trial of losartan versus captopril in patients over 65 with heart failure (Evaluation of Losartan in the Elderly Study, ELITE). *Lancet* 1997;349:747–752.

35. The Digitalis Investigation Group. The effect of digoxin on mortality and morbidity in patients with heart failure. *N Engl J Med* 1997;336:525–533.

36. Philbin EF, Rocco TA, Cotto M, et al. Association between attenuated diuretic response and death in acute heart failure. *Am J Cardiol* 1997;80:519–522.

37. Packer M, Bristow MR, Cohn JN, et al. The effect of carvedilol on morbidity and mortality in patients with chronic heart failure. *N Engl J Med* 1996;334:1349–1355.

38. MERIT-HF Study Group. Effect of metoprolol CR/XL in chronic heart failure: metoprolol CR/XL Randomized Intervention Trial in Congestive Heart Failure (MERIT-HF). *Lancet* 1999;353:2001–2007.

39. CIBIS-II Investigators and Committees. The Cardiac Insufficiency Bisoprolol Study II (CIBIS-II): a randomised trial. *Lancet* 1999;353:9–13.

40. Pitt B, Zannand F, Remme WJ, et al. The effect of spironolactone on morbidity and mortality in patients with severe heart failure. *N Engl J Med* 1999;341:709–717.

41. Doval HC, Nul DR, Vancelli HO, et al. Randomized trial of low-dose amiodarone in severe congestive heart failure. *Lancet* 1994;344:493–498.

42. Buxton AE, Lee KL, Fisher JD, et al. A randomized study of the prevention of sudden death in patients with coronary artery disease. *N Engl J Med* 1999;341:1882–1890.

43. Moss AJ, Hall WJ, Cannom DS, et al. Improved survival with an implanted defibrillator in patients with coronary disease at high risk for ventricular arrhythmia. *N Engl J Med* 1996;335:1933–1940.

44. Killip T, Passamani E, Davis K. Coronary artery surgery study (CASS): a randomized trial of coronary bypass surgery. Eight years follow-up and survival in patients with reduced ejection fraction. *Circulation* 1985;72[Suppl V]:V102–V109.

45. Smith W, McAnulty JH, Rahimtoola SH. Severe aortic stenosis with impaired left ventricular function and clinical heart failure: results of valve replacement. *Circulation* 1978;58:258–264.

46. Philbin EF, Andreou C, Rocco TA, et al. Patterns of angiotensin-converting enzyme inhibitor use in congestive heart failure in two community hospitals. *Am J Cardiol* 1996;77:832–838.

47. Philbin EF. Factors determining angiotensin-converting enzyme inhibitor use in heart failure in the community setting. *Clin Cardiol* 1998;21:103–108.

48. Philbin EF, Lynch LJ, Rocco TA, et al. Does quality improvement work? The Management to Improve Survival in Congestive Heart Failure (MISCHF) Study. *Jt Comm J Qual Improv* 1996;22:721–733.

49. Philbin EF, Rocco TA, Jenkins PL. β-blocker use in heart failure: which patient characteristics determine physician use of β-blockers in community practice? *J Am Coll Cardiol* 2000;35[Suppl A]:217A(abst).

50. Ashton CM, Kuykendall DH, Johnson ML, et al. The association between the quality of inpatient care and early readmission. *Ann Intern Med* 1995;122:415–421.

51. Philbin EF, Rocco TA, Lynch LJ, et al. Predictors and determinants of hospital length of stay in congestive heart failure in ten community hospitals. *J Heart Lung Transplant* 1997;16:548–555.

52. Weingarten S, Riedinger M, Conner L, et al. Reducing lengths of stay in the coronary care unit with a practice guideline for patients with congestive heart failure: insights from a controlled clinical trial. *Med Care* 1994;32:1232–1243.

53. Philbin EF, Jenkins PL. Differences between heart failure patients treated by cardiologists, internists, family physicians and other physicians: analysis of a large, statewide database. *Am Heart J* 2000;139:491–496.

54. Park RE, Brook RH, Kosecoff J, et al. Explaining variations in hospital death rates. *JAMA* 1990;264:484–490.

55. Rosenthal G, Harper D, Quinn L, Cooper G. Severity-adjusted mortality and length of stay in teaching and non-teaching hospitals. *JAMA* 1997;278:485–490.

56. Cintron G, Johnson G, Francis G, et al. Prognostic significance of serial changes in left ventricular ejection fraction in patients with congestive heart failure. *Circulation* 1993;87[Suppl VI]:VI-17–VI-23.

57. Cohn JN, Johnson GR, Shabetai R, et al. Ejection fraction, peak exercise oxygen consumption, cardiothoracic ratio, ventricular arrhythmias and plasma norepinephrine as determinants of prognosis in heart failure. *Circulation* 1993;87[Suppl VI]:VI-5–VI-16.

58. Gradman A, Deedwania P, Cody R, et al. Predictors of total mortality and sudden death in mild to moderate heart failure. *J Am Coll Cardiol* 1989;14:564–570.

59. Franciosa JA. Why patients with heart failure die: hemodynamic and functional determinants of survival. *Circulation* 1987;75[Suppl IV]:IV-20–IV-27.

60. Stevenson LW, Tillisch JH, Hamilton M, et al. Importance of hemodynamic response to therapy in predicting survival with ejction fraction less than or equal to 20% secondary to ischemic or nonischemic dilated cardiomyopathy. *Am J Cardiol* 1990;66:1348–1354.

61. Felker GM, Thompson RE, Hare JM, et al. Underlying causes and long-term survival in patients with initially unexplained cardiomyopathy. *N Engl J Med* 2000;342:1077–1084.

62. Philbin EF, Santella RN, Rocco TA. Angiotensin-converting enzyme inhibitor use in heart failure complicated by renal impairment. *J Am Geriatr Soc* 1999;47:302–308.

63. Brater DC. The use of diuretics in congestive heart failure. *Semin Nephrol* 1994;14:479–484.

64. Brater DC. Diuretic therapy. *N Engl J Med* 1998;339:387–395.

65. Vargo DL, Kramer WG, Black PK, et al. Bioavailability, pharmacokinetics, and pharmacodynamics of torsemide and furosemide in patients with congestive heart failure. *Clin Pharmacol Ther* 1995;57:601–609.

66. Bayliss J, Norell M, Canepa-Anson R, et al. Untreated heart failure: clinical and neuroendocrine effects of introducing diuretics. *Br Heart J* 1987;57:17–22.

67. Ghali JK, Kadakia S, Cooper R, et al. Precipitating factors leading to decompensation of heart failure: traits among urban blacks. *Arch Intern Med* 1988;148:2013–2016.

68. Gheorghiade M, Bonow RO. Chronic heart failure in the United States: a manifestation of coronary artery disease. *Circulation* 1998;97:282–289.

69. Ho KK, Pinsky JL, Kannel WB, et al. The epidemiology of heart failure: the Framingham Study. *J Am Coll Cardiol* 1993;22[Suppl A]:6A–13A.

70. Bonow RO, Udelson JE. Left ventricular diastolic dysfunction as a cause of congestive heart failure: mechanisms and management. *Ann Intern Med* 1992;117:502–510.

71. Vasan RS, Benjamin EJ, Levy D. Prevalence, clinical features and prognosis of diastolic heart failure. *J Am Coll Cardiol* 1995;26:1565–1574.

72. Senni M, Tribouilloy CM, Rodeheffer RJ, et al. Congestive heart failure in the community. A study of all incident cases in Olmstead County, Minnesota, in 1991. *Circulation* 1998;98:2282–2289.

73. Aguirre FV, Pearson AC, Lewen MK, et al. Usefulness of Doppler echocardiography in the diagnosis of congestive heart failure. *Am J Cardiol* 1989;63:1098–1102.

74. Goldsmith SR, Dick C. Differentiating systolic from diastolic heart failure: pathophysiologic and therapeutic considerations. *Am J Med* 1993;95:645–655.

75. Cohn JN, Rector TS. Prognosis of congestive heart failure and predictors of mortality. *Am J Cardiol* 1988;62[Suppl A]:25A–30A.

76. Keogh AM, Baron DW, Hickie JB. Prognostic guides in patients with idiopathic or ischemic dilated cardiomyopathy assessed for cardiac transplantation. *Am J Cardiol* 1990;65:903–908.

77. Cohn JN, Archibald DG, Francis GS, et al. Veterans Administration cooperative study on vasodilator therapy of heart failure: influence of prerandomization variables on the reduction of mortality by treatment with hydralazine and isosorbide dinitrate. *Circulation* 1987;75[Suppl IV]:IV-49–IV-54.

78. McDermott MM, Feinglass J, Sy J, et al. Hospitalized congestive heart failure patients with preserved versus abnormal left ventricular systolic function: clinical characteristics and drug therapy. *Am J Med* 1995;99:629–635.

79. Pernenkil R, Vinson JM, Shah AS, et al. Course and prognosis in patients >70 years of age with congestive heart failure and normal versus abnormal left ventricular ejection fraction. *Am J Cardiol* 1997;70:216–219.

80. Wong WF, Gold S, Fukuyama O, et al. Diastolic dysfunction in elderly patients with congestive heart failure. *Am J Cardiol* 1989;63:1526–1528.

81. Ghali JK, Kadakia S, Cooper RS, et al. Bedside diagnosis of preserved versus impaired left ventricular systolic function in heart failure. *Am J Cardiol* 1991;67:1002–1006.

82. Philbin EF, Garg R, Danisa K, et al. The relationship between cardiothoracic ratio and left ventricular ejection fraction in congestive heart failure. *Arch Intern Med* 1998;158:501–506.

83. Philbin EF, Hunsberger S, Garg R, et al. Did clinical features distinguish low from normal ejection fraction in chronic heart failure in the DIG Trial? *J Am Coll Cardiol* 1998;31[Suppl A]:116A(abst).

84. Packer M, Lee WH, Medina N, et al. Functional renal insufficiency during long-term therapy with captopril and enalapril in severe chronic heart failure. *Ann Intern Med* 1987;106:346–354.

85. Macdonald PS, Keogh AM, Aboyoun CL, et al. Tolerability and efficacy of carvedilol in patients with New York Heart Association class IV heart failure. *J Am Coll Cardiol* 1999;33:924–931.

86. Shakar SF, Abraham WT, Gilbert EM, et al. Combined oral positive inotropic and beta-blocker therapy for treatment of refractory class IV heart failure. *J Am Coll Cardiol* 1998;31:1336–1340.

CHAPTER 18

Deep Venous Thrombosis

Samuel Z. Goldhaber

The diagnosis and management of deep venous thrombosis (DVT) can be standardized and adapted to a critical pathway. Although patients with DVT are generally managed by internists, cardiologists need to be adept in detecting DVT among their patients and in managing complicated cases that require catheter-directed thrombolysis, mechanical thrombectomy, or placement of an inferior vena caval filter. Furthermore, cardiologists should set the standard for recommending and implementing prophylaxis among their hospitalized patients and among patients for whom they consult preoperatively.

EPIDEMIOLOGY

Deep venous thrombosis is underdiagnosed because about half the time it is completely asymptomatic. Often, the best clue to the possibility of DVT is based on an assessment of predisposing risk factors, including prior venous thromboembolism (1–3), cancer, surgery, trauma, bedrest, or immobilization, which are beyond control of the patient; and "environmental factors" such as obesity, cigarette smoking, hypertension, oral contraceptives, pregnancy, and hormone replacement therapy.

Deep venous thrombosis is problematic because it predisposes patients to pulmonary embolism (PE), which is potentially life threatening, as well as to venous insufficiency, which impairs the quality of life because of chronic leg swelling, pain, and occasional ulceration. Venous insufficiency is surprisingly common. It can develop in as many as one third of patients who have DVT. Often, it develops as a late complication, years after the thrombotic event.

DIAGNOSIS

The most common history is a cramp or "charley horse" in the lower calf that does not abate and gradually worsens after several days. Discomfort, at first intermittent, becomes persistent. Swelling may then ensue. Sudden, excruciating calf discomfort is most likely caused by a ruptured Baker's cyst.

Fever and chills usually suggest cellulitis rather than DVT, although DVT may be present concomitantly.

When detected early after onset, the physical findings may be minimal, consisting of mild palpation discomfort in the lower calf. If the DVT propagates proximally because it is not recognized at an early stage, massive thigh swelling and marked tenderness might be found when palpating the inguinal area over the course of the femoral vein. Such patients often have difficulty walking and may need to use a cane, crutches, or walker. If a patient has upper extremity venous thrombosis, asymmetry may be seen in the supraclavicular fossae or in the girth of the upper arms. A prominent superficial venous pattern may also be seen over the anterior chest wall.

Erythema usually suggests concomitant superficial venous phlebitis with saphenous vein involvement or coexisting cellulitis. If the leg is diffusely edematous, DVT is unlikely. Much more common is an acute exacerbation of venous insufficiency caused by a postphlebitic syndrome.

Once suspected, DVT is diagnosed in a relatively straightforward manner because it relies on the venous ultrasound examination (Fig. 18-1). In an attempt to use the ultrasound most effectively, a formal scoring system was developed in Canada to assess the pretest probability of DVT (6). Although simple, this system has never gained enough popularity to be used routinely in clinical decision-making. The scoring system, as with all diagnostic algorithms, relies on the principle of integrating risk factors, symptoms, and signs to assess likelihood (7).

At Brigham and Women's Hospital (BWH), Boston, Massachusetts, we begin our diagnostic workup with the venous ultrasound (8,9), which we believe is especially reliable in symptomatic patients. The sensitivity of the venous ultrasound decreases among patients who are asymptomatic and having routine screening (10). Of particular importance is the proper interpretation of the ultrasound report. Unfortunately, the distal portion of the deep femoral vein is called the "superficial femoral vein." Even though superficial is part of the name of this vein, it is a deep vein and patients with superficial femoral vein thrombosis should be treated for

191

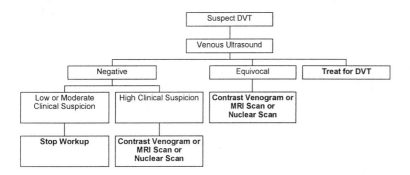

FIG. 18-1. Deep venous thrombosis diagnosis.

DVT. They should not be discharged home with the misdiagnosis of superficial thrombophlebitis (11).

Usually, the venous ultrasound examination is definitive in detecting or excluding DVT in the large upper extremity veins as well as the deep veins from the common femoral proximally to the calf veins distally. Occasionally, the imaging test is equivocal because of the patient's body habitus, recent leg trauma or surgery, or profound edema that limits compression of vascular structures. Under these circumstances, other imaging tests can be considered, specifically contrast venography, magnetic resonance imaging (MRI), or nuclear scanning (Fig. 18-1). Of these alternatives, contrast venography has been the traditional "gold standard," even though the trend is moving toward MRI. At BWH, we have found nuclear imaging difficult and not always reliable.

Magnetic resonance imaging can provide surprisingly precise, detailed information about the venous system. MRI is especially useful in assessing suspected pelvic vein thrombosis and in defining the extent of upper extremity vein thrombosis. MRI can also help estimate the age of the thrombus, based on various "spin" characteristics of the image.

In 1998, the US Food and Drug Administration (FDA) approved technetium-99m-apcitide (AcuTect; Diatide, Inc.; Londonderry, NH) for the diagnosis of acute leg DVT. A complex of the synthetic peptide, apcitide, and the radionuclide, technetium, binds preferentially to the glycoprotein IIb/IIIa receptors found on activated platelets. This diagnostic modality can complement ultrasonography and provide information on pelvic vein thrombosis (not ordinarily imaged by ultrasound), acute superimposed on chronic DVT (not well differentiated by ultrasound), and acute DVT when the interpretation of the ultrasound examination is limited by

body habitus or ambiguous findings. However, broad clinical experience with this technique is not yet available.

TREATMENT

The treatment of DVT has changed dramatically during the past several years. The low molecular weight heparin (LMWH), enoxaparin, is now the preferred anticoagulant to manage DVT. Enoxaparin has received FDA approval for outpatient (12,13) DVT treatment, as a "bridge" to warfarin, because of its superior efficacy (14) and safety as well as cost-effectiveness (15) compared with unfractionated heparin. It is administered as a fixed dose according to weight (1 mg/kg twice daily) and is cost-effective because no routine laboratory testing is required. Low molecular weight heparin has become the foundation of anticoagulation treatment of DVT patients (Fig. 18-2) and can facilitate complete outpatient treatment of this disease among properly selected patients. Over the past few years, an increasing proportion of DVT patients are being treated entirely on an outpatient basis (16), based on landmark trials by Canadian and Dutch investigators (17–19).

The popularity of LMWH reflects the difficulty in achieving effective doses of continuous intravenous unfractionated heparin, despite the proliferation of weight-based nomograms (20). Although a robotic dosing system has been successfully tested (21), the need for traditional heparin appears to be limited to patients who are massively obese or in renal failure or who have an abhorrence of injections.

Even those patients who require hospitalization (Fig. 18-3) can usually be managed with LMWH until they achieve a stable and therapeutic level of warfarin, based on

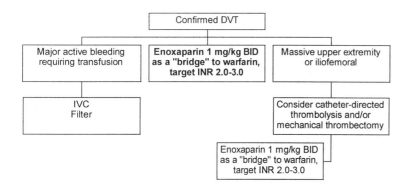

FIG. 18-2. Deep venous thrombosis treatment.

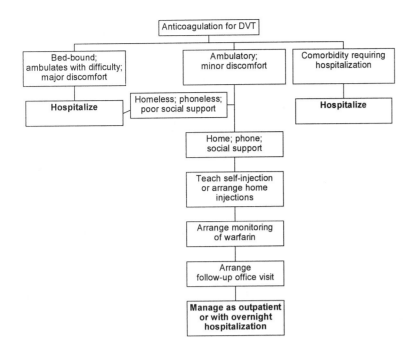

FIG. 18-3. Deep venous thrombosis: patient triage and disposition.

a target international normalized ratio (INR) of 2.0–3.0. The success of an anticoagulation critical pathway depends on reliable dosing and monitoring of warfarin.

The optimal duration of anticoagulation remains one of the most controversial areas within the field of DVT management (22). Currently, the standard duration of anticoagulation is 3 months for upper extremity or isolated calf DVT. For proximal leg DVT, our critical pathway recommends 6 months of therapy.

Patients who suffer idiopathic DVT outside the setting of cancer, surgery, or trauma may benefit from prolonged anticoagulation, possibly with a less intensive target INR than the usual 2.0–3.0. To test this hypothesis, the ongoing Prevention of Recurrent Venous Thromboembolism (PREVENT) trial, sponsored by the National Institutes of Health, is recruiting such patients at about 30 hospitals across the United States and 6 to 8 in Canada. After the standard duration of anticoagulation has been completed, patients are counseled about the trial and are encouraged to enroll. Those who participate are randomized in a double blind manner to either low intensity warfarin (target INR of 1.5 to 2.0) or to its control. They are followed for the ensuing 3 to 4 years for clinical evidence of venous thromboembolism or hemorrhage (23).

At BWH, the PREVENT trial has an important role at the end of our critical pathway for DVT treatment. We have recruited more than 70 patients into this study. For possible enrollment in PREVENT at one of the trial centers in the United States or Canada, telephone (617-732-7566) or E-mail me (sgoldhaber@partners.org) to discuss any patients with idiopathic DVT in whom the optimal duration of anticoagulation is uncertain.

Certain principles have recently been elucidated to improve anticoagulation with warfarin. First, it is preferable to initiate warfarin in a dose of 5 mg daily rather than the traditional higher dose of 10 mg daily (24). Second, be aware that

1% to 3% of patients have a genetic mutation that predisposes them to warfarin sensitivity. They have difficulty metabolizing the S-racemer of warfarin and, therefore, become fully anticoagulated with tiny doses of warfarin, in the range of 1.0 to 1.5 mg daily (25). Third, for patients requiring indefinite anticoagulation with warfarin, effective therapy can often be better achieved with self-monitoring at home with a finger-stick machine rather than traditional phlebotomy performed in a laboratory (26,27).

At BWH, we established an anticoagulation service in our cardiac center 4 years ago. A specially trained nurse and hospital pharmacist under the supervision of a cardiologist (S.Z.G.) runs this service day-to-day. It has become indispensable in the successful implementation of critical pathways that depend on successful management of anticoagulated patients and optimization of their therapy. This centralized resource facilitates the outpatient management of patients with DVT who require close telephone follow-up, and helps ensure that they are improving clinically.

With respect to safety, drugs such as acetaminophen, that were traditionally thought to have no interaction with warfarin, actually potentiate its effect (28). If a patient does become excessively anticoagulated, small doses of oral vitamin K appear effective (29–31) and are preferable to large doses of parenteral vitamin K, which often preclude resumption of adequate therapy for several weeks.

Beyond Anticoagulation

The indications for DVT thrombolysis are uncertain. Theoretically, DVT thrombolysis should restore venous valve patency and function, thereby preventing the development of venous insufficiency and the postthrombotic syndrome. However, this hypothesis has not been proved. In addition, DVT thrombolysis may be especially useful in patients who have developed an upper extremity thrombosis because of a long-term indwelling central venous catheter that must remain in place, if possible, to complete additional courses of chemotherapy or to provide nutritional supplementation. At BWH, we advise DVT catheter-directed thrombolysis for young, otherwise healthy patients who have massive iliofemoral DVT with marked leg swelling, leg tenderness, and difficulty walking. The usual dosing regimen is a bolus of approximately 10 mg of tissue plasminogen activator (tPA) injected directly into the thrombus, followed by an 8- to 12-hour infusion of 1 to 2 mg/hour. For patients with large DVT who require intervention in addition to anticoagulation, a combination of catheter-directed thrombolysis and catheter-assisted thrombectomy is usually used.

Inferior vena caval filters are mechanical devices that are ordinarily placed below the renal veins to prevent embolization of thrombus from the pelvic or deep leg veins to the pulmonary arteries. The principal two indications for filter placement are (a) active bleeding (e.g., gastrointestinal hemorrhage requiring transfusion) that precludes anticoagulation; and (b) well-documented occurrence of a new PE despite several days of therapeutic levels of anticoagulation. Other indications for PE are "soft" but might include unusual situations such as preoperative insertion in a patient with recent PE who must have emergency hip fracture surgery.

Filters are almost always effective in preventing PE, but they do nothing whatsoever to halt the thrombotic process. Furthermore, in long-term follow-up, the filters appear to be thrombogenic (32). Therefore, in general, once a bleeding problem has been brought under control, anticoagulation should be initiated.

Aside from anticoagulation, thrombolysis, and mechanical interventions, important adjunctive measures for DVT management should not be overlooked (Table 18-1). Whether to proceed with a hypercoagulable workup is controversial, and this issue is not addressed in our critical pathways. However, providing vascular compression stockings to avoid subsequent venous insufficiency is considered mandatory (4). We emphasize the importance of providing emotional support as well as intensive education about DVT and anticoagulation. To this end, we created a Web site in which we respond to "frequently asked questions" (http://web.mit.edu/karen/www/faq.html).

TABLE 18-1. *Adjunctive measures for deep venous thrombosis management*

Obtain family history and consider hypercoagulable workup.
Prescribe below knee vascular compression stockings, 20–30 or 30–40 mm Hg, to prevent venous insufficiency.
Provide emotional support.
Educate regarding low molecular weight heparin and warfarin.
Offer Web addresses of educational sites.
Explain controversy concerning optimal duration of anticoagulation.

TABLE 18-2. *Venous thromboembolism prevention*

Condition	Consider following prophylactic regimen
Orthopedic surgery	Enoxaparin 30 mg s.c., b.i.d., or Enoxaparin 40 mg q.d., or Dalteparin 5,000 U q.d., or Warfarin, target INR 2.0–2.5
General surgery	Enoxaparin 40 mg q.d., or Dalteparin 2,500 or 5,000 U q.d., or Heparin 5,000 U b.i.d. or t.i.d., or Intermittent pneumatic compression devices
Medical patients	Enoxaparin 40 mg q.d., or Heparin 5,000 U b.i.d. or t.i.d., or Intermittent pneumatic compression devices

b.i.d., twice daily; INR, international normalized ratio; qd, every day; s.c., subcutaneously; t.i.d., three times daily.

PREVENTION

Prevention of DVT is of paramount importance. Both mechanical (32a,33) and pharmacologic modalities are available. Mechanical methods include vascular compression stockings, intermittent pneumatic compression boots, and inferior vena caval filters. Pharmacologic prevention involves anticoagulation with minidose unfractionated heparin (5,000 U twice or three times daily); LMWH (e.g., enoxaparin 40 mg daily or dalteparin 5,000 U daily); or warfarin, with a target INR of 2.0 to 3.0. Recently, a megatrial of 13,356 patients with hip fracture indicated that 160 mg of aspirin daily for 5 weeks can reduce by one third the risk of venous thromboembolism (34).

Among surgical patients, especially those having hip or knee replacement, it has become apparent that the risk of developing DVT persists for weeks after the operation and long after hospital discharge (35). Therefore, most critical pathways for DVT prevention provide for prolonged prophylaxis that continues when patients at high risk for venous thromboembolism are transferred to a skilled nursing facility or are discharged home.

Medical patients (36), especially those in medical intensive care units (37,38), have an especially high rate of asymptomatic but clinically important DVT. LMWH use seems to be especially safe in these patients and possibly causes fewer bleeding complications than minidose unfractionated heparin (39). Recently, enoxaparin (40 mg) once daily was compared with placebo in medical patients at moderate risk for DVT. Those prophylaxed with enoxaparin enjoyed a two-third reduction in DVT rate, including proximal DVT (40).

CONCLUSIONS

Diagnosis, management, and prevention of DVT is a field that lends itself well to the development and implementation of critical pathways. The adverse endpoints, recurrent thrombosis and hemorrhage, are well defined. Diagnosis can usually be established or excluded quickly if a skilled technologist is available. Management is increasingly undertaken as a complete outpatient program with enoxaparin as a bridge to warfarin. Finally, all potentially preventable DVT should be prophylaxed to avoid the inconvenience and possible morbidity associated with the diagnosis and treatment of this disease.

REFERENCES

1. Hansson PO, Sörbo J, Eriksson H. Recurrent venous thromboembolism after deep vein thrombosis: incidence and risk factors. *Arch Intern Med* 2000;160:769–774.
2. Heit JA, Mohr DN, Silverstein MD, et al. Predictors of recurrence after deep vein thrombosis and pulmonary embolism: a population-based cohort study. *Arch Intern Med* 2000;160:761–768.
3. Heit JA, Silverstein MD, Mohr DN, et al. Risk factors for deep vein thrombosis and pulmonary embolism: a population-based case-control study. *Arch Intern Med* 2000;160:809–815.
4. Brandjes DP, Büller HR, Heijboer H, et al. Randomised trial of effect of compression stockings in patients with symptomatic proximal-vein thrombosis. *Lancet* 1997;349:759–762.
5. Ibrahim S, MacPherson DR, Goldhaber SZ. Chronic venous insufficiency: mechanisms and management. *Am Heart J* 1996;132:856–860.
6. Wells PS, Anderson DR, Bormanis J, et al. Value of assessment of pretest probability of deep-vein thrombosis in clinical management. *Lancet* 1997;350:1795–1798.
7. Kahn SR. The clinical diagnosis of deep venous thrombosis. Integrating incidence, risk factors, and symptoms and signs. *Arch Intern Med* 1998;158:2315–2323.
8. Cogo A, Lensing AWA, Koopman MMW, et al. Compression ultrasonography for diagnostic management of patients with clinically suspected deep vein thrombosis: prospective cohort study. *BMJ* 1998;316:17–20.
9. Cornuz J, Pearson SD, Polak JF. Deep venous thrombosis: complete lower extremity venous US evaluation in patients with known risk factors—outcome study. *Radiology* 1999;211:637–641.
10. Jongbloets LMM, Lensing AWA, Koopman MMW, et al. Limitations of compression ultrasound for the detection of symptomless postoperative deep vein thrombosis. *Lancet* 1994;343:1142–1144.
11. Bundens WP, Bergan JJ, Halasz NA, et al. The superficial femoral vein. A potentially lethal misnomer. *JAMA* 1995;274:1296–1298.
12. Baron RM, Goldhaber SZ. Deep venous thrombosis: outpatient management is now FDA approved. *J Thromb Thrombolysis* 1999;7:113–122.
13. Dunn AS, Coller B. Outpatient treatment of deep vein thrombosis: translating clinical trials into practice. *Am J Med* 1999;106:660–669.
14. Gould MK, Dembitzer AD, Doyle RL, et al. Low-molecular-weight heparins compared with unfractionated heparin for treatment of acute deep venous thrombosis. A meta-analysis of randomized, controlled trials. *Ann Intern Med* 1999;130:800–809.
15. Gould MK, Dembitzer AD, Sanders GD, et al. Low-molecular-weight heparins compared with unfractionated heparin for treatment of acute deep venous thrombosis: a cost-effectiveness analysis. *Ann Intern Med* 1999;130:789–799.
16. Harrison L, McGinnis J, Crowther M, et al. Assessment of outpatient treatment of deep-vein thrombosis with low-molecular-weight heparin. *Arch Intern Med* 1998;158:2001–2003.
17. Koopman MMW, Prandoni P, Piovella F, et al., for the Tasman Study Group. Treatment of venous thrombosis with intravenous unfractionated heparin administered in the hospital as compared with subcutaneous low-molecular-weight heparin administered at home. The Tasman Study Group. *N Engl J Med* 1996;334:682–687.
18. Levine M, Gent M, Hirsh J, et al. A comparison of low-molecular-weight heparin administered primarily at home with unfractionated heparin administered in the hospital for proximal deep-vein thrombosis. *N Engl J Med* 1996;334:677–681.
19. The Columbus Investigators. Low-molecular-weight heparin in the treatment of patients with venous thromboembolism. *N Engl J Med* 1997;337:657–662.
20. Raschke RA, Reilly BM, Guidry JR, et al. The weight-based heparin dosing nomogram compared with a "standard care" nomogram. A randomized controlled trial. *Ann Intern Med* 1993;119:874–881.
21. Cannon CP, Dingemanse J, Kleinbloesem CH, et al. Automated heparin-delivery system to control activated partial thromboplastin time: evaluation in normal volunteers. *Circulation* 1999;99:751–756.
22. Kearon C, Gent M, Hirsh J, et al. A comparison of three months of anticoagulation with extended anticoagulation for a first episode of idiopathic venous thromboembolism. *N Engl J Med* 1999;340:901–907.
23. Ridker PM, for the PREVENT Investigators. Long-term low-dose warfarin among venous thrombosis patients with and without factor V Leiden mutation: rationale and design for the Prevention of Recurrent Venous Thromboembolism (PREVENT) trial. *Vasc Med Rev* 1998;3:67–73.
24. Harrison L, Johnston M, Massicotte MP, et al. Comparison of 5-mg and 10-mg loading doses in initiation of warfarin therapy. *Ann Intern Med* 1997;126:133–136.
25. Aithal GP, Day CP, Kesteven PJL, et al. Association of polymorphisms in the cytochrome P450 CYP2C9 with warfarin dose requirement and risk of bleeding complications. *Lancet* 1999;353:717–719.
26. Ansell JE. Empowering patients to monitor and manage oral anticoagulation therapy. *JAMA* 1999;281:182–183.
27. Sawicki PT. A structured teaching and self-management program for patients receiving oral anticoagulation: a randomized controlled trial. *JAMA* 1999;281:145–149.
28. Hylek EM, Heiman H, Skates SJ, et al. Acetaminophen and other risk factors for excessive warfarin anticoagulation. *JAMA* 1998;279:657–662.
29. Hirsh J. Reversal of the anticoagulant effects of warfarin by vitamin K_1. *Chest* 1998;114:1505–1508.
30. Weibert RT, Le DT, Kayser SR, et al. Correction of excessive anticoagulation with low-dose oral vitamin K1. *Ann Intern Med* 1997;126:959–962.
31. Wentzien TH, O'Reilly RA, Kearns PJ. Prospective evaluation of anticoagulant reversal with oral vitamin K1 while continuing warfarin therapy unchanged. *Chest* 1998;114:1546–1550.
32. Decousus H, Leizorovicz A, Parent F, et al. A clinical trial of vena caval filters in the prevention of pulmonary embolism in patients with proximal deep-vein thrombosis. Prevention du Risque d'Embolie Pulmonaire par Interruption Cave Study Group. *N Engl J Med* 1998;338:409–415.
32a. Ramos R, Salem BI, De Pawlikowski MP, et al. The efficacy of pneumatic compression stockings in the prevention of pulmonary embolism after cardiac surgery. *Chest* 1996;109:82–85.
33. Comerota AJ, Chouhan V, Harada RN, et al. The fibrinolytic effects of intermittent pneumatic compression: mechanism of enhanced fibrinolysis. *Ann Surg* 1997;226:306–313; discussion 313–314.
34. Pulmonary Embolism Prevention (PEP) Trial Collaborative Group. Prevention of pulmonary embolism and deep vein thrombosis with low dose aspirin: Pulmonary Embolism Prevention (PEP) trial. *Lancet* 2000;355:1295–1302.
35. White RH, Romano PS, Zhou H, et al. Incidence and time course of thromboembolic outcomes following total hip or knee arthroplasty. *Arch Intern Med* 1998;158:1525–1531.
36. Goldhaber SZ. Venous thromboembolism prophylaxis in medical patients. *Thromb Haemost* 1999;70:72–74.
37. Hirsh DR, Ingenito EP, Goldhaber SZ. Prevalence of deep venous thrombosis among patients in medical intensive care. *JAMA* 1995;274:335–337.
38. Goldhaber SZ. Venous thromboembolism in the intensive care unit: the last frontier for prophylaxis. *Chest* 1998;113:5–7.
39. Mismetti P, Laporte-Simitsidis S, Tardy B, et al. Prevention of venous thromboembolism in internal medicine with unfractionated or low-molecular-weight heparins: a meta-analysis of randomised clinical trials. *Thromb Haemost* 2000;83:14–19.
40. Samama MM, Cohen AT, Darmon JY, et al. A comparison of enoxaparin with placebo for the prevention of venous thromboembolism in acutely ill medical patients. Prophylaxis in Medical Patients with Enoxaparin Study Group. *N Engl J Med* 1999;341:793–800.

CHAPTER 19

Pulmonary Embolism

Samuel Z. Goldhaber

The cardiologist is often summoned to help diagnose suspected acute pulmonary embolism (PE) because of familiarity with the differential diagnosis of chest pain and dyspnea, the ability to recognize clinical manifestations of acute pulmonary hypertension, and facility with right ventricular (RV) catheterization, pulmonary angiography, and echocardiography. After the diagnosis of PE is established, the cardiologist is often the specialist asked to stratify risk and to manage patients at high risk by utilizing thrombolysis and, if necessary, embolectomy.

DIAGNOSIS

Clinical Presentation

The clinical presentation can often be helpful in raising suspicion for PE. Major predisposing conditions include surgery, trauma, immobilization, cancer, and cancer chemotherapy. For women, additional risks include pregnancy, oral contraceptives, and hormone replacement therapy.

The most common features of PE are dyspnea and chest pain, which is often pleuritic. Most patients present with normal systemic arterial pressure. Although the heart rate often exceeds 100 beats/minute (bpm) and the respiratory rate is often greater than 16 bpm, anatomically large PE can present with neither tachycardia nor tachypnea. In addition, a low-grade fever may point the clinician toward infection as the principal problem.

When clinical suspicion of PE has been aroused, the next challenge is to use wisely the wide array of available diagnostic tests. The specific diagnostic pathway that is chosen depends largely on the expertise available at a specific hospital and the accessibility and turnaround time for specific tests.

Among the most important principles is to pursue the diagnosis, if strongly suspected, even if some of the initial diagnostic tests are negative. To avoid ordering an unnecessarily wide array of tests, a critical pathway for diagnosis of PE (Fig. 19-1A) is especially useful. The process of discussing and ultimately instituting a diagnostic protocol will promote interdisciplinary communication and cooperation.

Electrocardiography

At Brigham and Women's Hospital (BWH), all patients suspected of PE have an electrocardiogram (1). Although focus on new onset atrial fibrillation or flutter is widely cited, along with a new "S1Q3T3" sign, we find most helpful the more subtle manifestation of right heart strain: T-wave inversion in leads V1 through V4.

Chest X-ray

The chest x-ray is useful for establishing alternative diagnoses such as pneumonia, congestive heart failure (CHF), or pneumothorax. However, it is important to realize that because PE can coexist with other cardiopulmonary illness, it is especially difficult to diagnose under these circumstances (2).

Blood Tests

Arterial blood gases were used for a generation to augment suspicion of PE based on hypoxemia and to exclude PE in the presence of a normal alveolar-arterial oxygen gradient. However, these parameters are unreliable and can mislead the physician who must triage patients suspected of PE (3,4). Specifically, patients who are otherwise healthy can present with a large PE and yet maintain a high arterial $Po2$ and a normal alveolar-arterial oxygen gradient.

The only useful blood test is the plasma D-dimer by enzyme-linked immunosorbent assay (ELISA). D-dimers are released in the presence of PE because of endogenous fibrinolysis. Plasmin dissolves some of the fibrin clot from PE and subsequently D-dimers are released into the plasma. The D-dimers can be recognized by commercially available monoclonal antibodies. The D-dimer ELISA has a high negative predictive value for PE. This means that if the D-dimer ELISA is normal, it is extremely unlikely that PE is present (5).

D-dimers are highly sensitive for the diagnosis of PE. This high sensitivity is crucially important in a screening test.

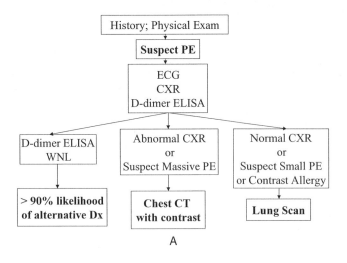

A

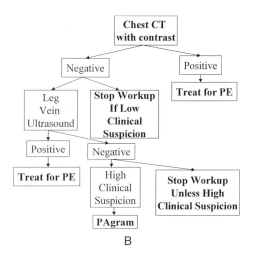

B

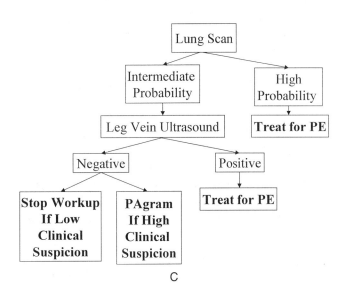

C

FIG. 19-1. A. Global pulmonary embolism diagnostic pathway. B. Chest computed tomography pathway. C. Lung scan pathway.

However, D-dimers are nonspecific and will often be elevated in conditions that mimic PE [e.g., acute myocardial infarction (MI) or pneumonia]. They are also elevated in patients with cancer and in the postoperative state.

Aside from lack of specificity, a more important drawback of D-dimers is that the ELISA has traditionally required highly skilled technological support. Therefore, the availability of this test was usually restricted to the daytime shift on weekdays. Now, however, several assays are commercially available with vastly simplified laboratory procedures and with turnaround times of less than 1 hour. At BWH, we have invested in the VIDAS D-dimer ELISA (6), and this rapid turnaround assay system is pivotal in our Emergency Department's critical pathway for the diagnosis of PE (Fig. 19-1A). Unless we have overwhelmingly high clinical suspicion, we do not pursue the diagnosis of PE further in a patient with a normal D-dimer ELISA. It is important to point out that the commonly available latex agglutination D-dimer (used for screening of suspected disseminated intravascular coagulation) is not sensitive enough

to help "rule out" PE and is not used in our diagnostic protocol.

Imaging Tests

If the D-dimer ELISA is elevated, the next step is to decide between a chest computed tomography (CT) scan with contrast (Fig. 19-1B) and a lung scan (Fig. 19-1C). In the United States, chest CT scanning is quickly becoming the preferred imaging test because it usually provides a satisfying dichotomous "yes" or "no" answer to whether PE is present. The CT scan can also help diagnose pneumonia, cancer, and interstitial lung diseases not apparent on the chest x-ray film. The major limitations of chest CT scanning are the need to administer intravenous contrast and the inability to diagnose small, peripheral PE (7).

Lung scanning has been the standard, noninvasive imaging test for patients suspected of having PE. It is highly specific when the probability for PE is high, but it is not sensitive. Based on the Prospective Investigation of Pulmonary

Embolism Diagnosis (PIOPED) trial, more than half of the patients with PE proved by angiography did not have high probability lung scans (8).

Advantages of the lung scan over chest CT include more extensive validation with pulmonary angiography as well as the ability to detect abnormalities in the periphery of the lung. The principal disadvantage of lung scanning is that most of the scans are of intermediate probability for PE and frustrate the clinician because they do not provide a clear-cut answer to the diagnostic dilemma of whether PE is present.

When the lung scan is equivocal or when the chest CT is negative despite high clinical suspicion, leg vein ultrasonography is often a useful next step. If the venous ultrasound demonstrates deep vein thrombosis (DVT), this usually suffices as a surrogate for PE and the diagnostic workup can stop at this point. However, it is crucial to understand that as many as half of patients with PE will have no evidence of DVT, probably because the clot has already embolized to the lungs (9). Therefore, if clinical suspicion remains high, contrast pulmonary angiography should be obtained at this point (10). Nevertheless, with the diagnostic pathway outlined, only a small proportion of patients will require angiograms (11).

In the future, magnetic resonance will become the preferred imaging test when PE is suspected (12). For now, it should be considered experimental and not sufficiently "mature" to be placed on a diagnosis critical pathway.

MANAGEMENT

Risk Stratification

After the diagnosis of PE is established, other critical pathways are used to streamline, standardize, and optimize therapy. The most important initial step is to stratify risk in PE patients, because the clinical spectrum and severity of PE are wide (Fig. 19-2).

Fortunately, most patients with PE will remain hemodynamically stable and will not suffer recurrent PE or develop chronic pulmonary hypertension as long as they receive adequate anticoagulation. If the PE is anatomically small, involving less than 30% of the lungs, then it is likely that RV function will not be impaired (13), especially if no underlying cardiopulmonary disease is present.

In the United States, intravenous heparin is considered the standard of care for patients presenting with PE. Although low molecular weight heparin has been administered, such patients have been monitored as in-patients for an average of 7 hospital days (14). For those patients who have absolute contraindications to anticoagulation, with active bleeding requiring transfusion, placement of an inferior vena caval filter is worthwhile. Filters are effective in preventing recurrent PE but, paradoxically, are associated with a doubling of the DVT rate.

Further risk stratification should be undertaken for any patient who (a) appears clinically toxic; (b) has evidence of anatomically moderate or large PE; or (c) has small PE anatomically but underlying cardiopulmonary disease. Before the advent of echocardiography, we relied primarily on frequent assessment of systemic arterial pressure and heart rate. When patients became dependent on pressors to maintain adequate systemic arterial pressure, they were labeled as "high risk." At that point, they had obvious cardiogenic shock and often did not respond satisfactorily to aggressive intervention with thrombolysis or embolectomy.

Our approach to risk stratification has changed markedly. We now believe that among normotensive patients, assessment of RV function is pivotal to prognosticate accurately after PE is diagnosed. Patients who develop worsening RV function despite adequate anticoagulation have an ominous prognosis and are at high risk of recurrent PE, including fatal recurrent PE (15).

The International Cooperative Pulmonary Embolism Registry (ICOPER), which enrolled 2,454 patients from 52 hospitals in 7 countries, is the largest prospective registry that has ever been published (16). In ICOPER, age greater than 70 years increased the likelihood of death by 60%. Six other risk factors independently increased the likelihood of mortality by a factor of two- to threefold: cancer, clinical CHF, chronic obstructive pulmonary disease, systemic arterial hypotension with a systolic blood pressure of less than 90 mm Hg, tachypnea (defined as >20 breaths per minute), and RV hypokinesis on echocardiogram, an especially useful sign to identify patients at high risk who might be suitable for aggressive interventions such as thrombolysis (15) or embolectomy.

THROMBOLYSIS

For patients with massive PE (Fig. 19-3) or smaller PE accompanied by moderate or severe RV dysfunction, anticoagulation alone may not yield a clinically successful outcome. When considering thrombolysis, careful screening for potential contraindications is necessary. Pay particular attention to a history of poorly controlled hypertension or presentation with PE and systemic hypertension. Patients should also be questioned about prior head trauma, seizures, or stroke.

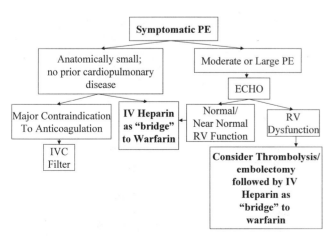

FIG. 19-2. Risk stratification of pulmonary embolism.

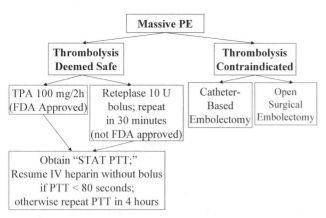

FIG. 19-3. Management of massive pulmonary embolism.

TABLE 19-1. *FDA approved thrombolytic regimens for pulmonary embolism*

Streptokinase:	250,000 IU as a loading dose over 30 min, followed by 100,000 U/h for 24 h—approved in 1977
Urokinase:	4,400 IU/kg as a loading dose over 10 min, followed by 4,400 IU/kg/h for 12–24 h—approved in 1978
rt-PA:	100 mg as a continuous peripheral intravenous infusion administered over 2 h—approved in 1990

Bleeding Complications

The most feared complication is intracranial bleeding. In ICOPER, 3% of the patients suffered intracerebral hemorrhage (16).

In a separate registry of 312 patients receiving thrombolysis for PE in five clinical trials, a 1.9% risk (95% CI, 0.7% to 4.1%) of intracranial bleeding was seen (17). Two of the six patients had preexisting known intracranial disease, but nonetheless received thrombolysis in violation of the exclusion criteria listed in the clinical trial protocols. Two of the six intracranial hemorrhages probably were caused by administration of heparin and not thrombolysis, because they occurred late, 62 and 157 hours after thrombolysis. Diastolic blood pressure on admission was elevated in patients who developed intracranial hemorrhage compared with those who did not (90.3 vs. 77.6 mm Hg; $p = 0.04$).

The mean age of patients with major bleeding was 63 years, whereas that of patients with no hemorrhagic complication was 56 years ($p = 0.005$). A 4% increased risk of bleeding was seen for each additional year of age. Increasing body mass index and pulmonary angiography were also significant predictors of hemorrhage (18).

Predictors of Efficacy

An inverse association is seen between duration of symptoms and improvement on lung scan reperfusion after thrombolysis. We observed 0.8% less reperfusion on lung scanning per additional day of symptoms (95% CI, 0.2% to 1.4%, $p = 0.008$). After controlling for age and initial lung scan defect size, we found 0.7% less reperfusion per additional day of symptoms (95% CI, 0.2% to 1.2%, $p = 0.007$). Thus, delay in administering thrombolysis will attenuate efficacy. Nevertheless, thrombolysis is still useful in patients who have had symptoms for 6 to 14 days (19).

Practical Points

The US Food and Drug Administration (FDA) approved streptokinase (SK) in 1977 and urokinase in 1978 for the treatment of PE; recombinant tissue plasminogen activator (rt-PA) received approval in 1990. None of the regimens (Table 19-1) require laboratory tests during the thrombolytic infusion, and none require dosage adjustments. The low concentration of SK administered over 24 hours is only modestly effective and predisposes to allergic reactions such as fever, chills, and hypotension. Urokinase is unavailable in the United States. Thus, rt-PA is the only contemporary, high-concentration thrombolytic agent that is FDA approved for PE. Recently, the MI dose of reteplase (two intravenous bolus injections of 10 U, 30 minutes apart) was compared with rt-PA. The efficacy of reteplase, as assessed by a decrease in the total pulmonary resistance, appeared to be at least as good as rt-PA (20).

None of the FDA-approved regimens for PE thrombolysis uses concomitant heparin, an important difference when compared with thrombolysis for MI. After administering thrombolysis, a partial thromboplastin time (PTT) should be obtained immediately. Usually, when the PTT is less than 80 seconds, intravenous unfractionated heparin can be initiated (or resumed) as a continuous intravenous infusion, without a loading dose. If the PTT exceeds 80 seconds, heparin should be withheld, and the test should be repeated every 4 hours until the PTT decreases to the recommended target.

EMBOLECTOMY

Catheter-Based Embolectomy

Greenfield demonstrated that transvenous catheter pulmonary embolectomy was feasible. He devised a steerable catheter with a distal radiopaque plastic cup. Syringe suction could be applied to aspirate a portion of the embolus into the cup, and a sustained vacuum by the syringe held the embolus as the catheter was withdrawn (21). This 12 Fr double-lumen, balloon-tipped catheter required femoral or jugular venotomy.

Interventional angiographers favor the "Meyerovitz technique" for aspiration; an 8 Fr or 9 Fr coronary guiding catheter without side holes is placed through a 10 Fr Arrow sheath, and the clot is aspirated with a 60 ml syringe (22). Mechanical fragmentation and pulverization of thrombus can be accomplished with a rotating basket catheter (23), high-pressurized jets of normal saline (24), or with a pigtail rotational catheter

Day #1	Day #2	Days #3-#4	Days #5-#7
Establish PE Dx	Continue IV heparin/warfarin	⟶	⟶
Initiate intensive anticoagulation	Emotional Support	⟶	⟶
Risk Stratify	Educate Patient/Family about PE and warfarin	⟶	⟶
Thrombolysis/ Embolectomy if high risk	Gather additional FH	⟶	⟶
Investigate hypercoagulability; Initiate warfarin	Fit for Vascular Compression Stockings	Make arrangements for outpatient appointments and outpatient F/U of warfarin	Discharge if stable

FIG. 19-4. Length of hospital stay for pulmonary embolism.

embolectomy (25). Mechanical fragmentation can also be combined with thrombolysis (26).

Surgical Embolectomy

Surgical embolectomy is best suited for patients with contraindications to thrombolysis or intracardiac thrombus greater than 1 cm^3 (27), or both. Ideally, patients with massive PE will be referred before the onset of cardiogenic shock. However, if cardiogenic shock has developed preoperatively, mechanical hemodynamic support will be required with an intraaortic balloon pump and, in extreme circumstances, a ventricular assist device. Even at specialized centers, patients having emergency pulmonary embolectomy have a high average mortality rate of approximately 30% to 40% (28–29). Prior cardiac arrest and associated cardiopulmonary disease are associated with an even gloomier prognosis (30–31).

At BWH, we have recently lowered our threshold for embolectomy. All patients had massive PE, but few were pressor dependent before referral for embolectomy. The operation was done on cardiopulmonary bypass with a warm beating heart. Avoidance of intraoperative hypothermia may explain why reperfusion pulmonary edema was rarely problematic.

Pulmonary Thromboendarterectomy

For patients who survive massive PE, failure to establish the diagnosis initially or inadequate therapy at the time of the embolism can lead to chronic thromboembolic pulmonary hypertension. When the quality of life is deteriorating because of this problem, pulmonary thromboendarterectomy can offer improvement in functional capacity. At the University of California at San Diego, an average 3-year follow-up of more than 300 patients who underwent this operation yielded encouraging results (32). More than 75% of patients survived beyond 6 years. Furthermore, more than 90% were in New York Heart Association class I or II.

HOSPITAL LENGTH OF STAY

At BWH, our critical pathway for PE lists a 5- to 7-day hospitalization (Fig. 19-4).

On the first day, the diagnosis is established, blood tests for hypercoagulability are ordered, and intensive anticoagulation is initiated. Risk stratification, usually with echocardiography, is undertaken. Patients at high risk have thrombolysis or embolectomy. Most, however, are managed with intravenous unfractionated heparin as a bridge to full and therapeutic warfarin, target international normalized ratio of 2 to 3. In the absence of thrombolysis or embolectomy,

2 weeks	4 weeks	8 weeks	3 months	6 months
Ensure compliance with warfarin	⟶	⟶	⟶	⟶
Emotional support	⟶	⟶	⟶	⟶
Permit return to work (reduced schedule) if stable	Unrestricted work if stable	Consider ECHO/ cardiopulmonary exercise test if residual dyspnea	Inquire re: residual CP/SOB	⟶
				Consider stopping warfarin

FIG. 19-5. Office visits for pulmonary embolism.

warfarin (usually in a dose of 5 mg) is administered on the first hospital day.

On the second hospital day, anticoagulation continues, and the focus shifts to providing the patient and family with the emotional support and education that they need to begin coping with PE (33). Additional family history is obtained. Patients are fitted for vascular compression stockings to help prevent chronic venous insufficiency.

During the remainder of the hospitalization, anticoagulation, emotional support, and education continue, while the patient is observed for signs or symptoms of recurrence despite adequate anticoagulation. Before hospital discharge, arrangements are made for outpatient office follow-up and for outpatient management of warfarin anticoagulation. At BWH, we have established an anticoagulation service run by a nurse and pharmacist under the supervision of a physician.

OUTPATIENT FOLLOW-UP

Office visits are ordinarily scheduled at 2, 4, 8, and 12 weeks, as well as at 6 months after the PE (Fig. 19-5). At the initial office visit, the focus is on ensuring compliance with warfarin and discussing an optimal schedule for return to work. Generally, patients can return to work at least part-time about 2 weeks after an uncomplicated PE. After the 4-week office visit, patients with uncomplicated courses are permitted to return to work full-time.

At 8 weeks, additional prognostic information can be obtained with echocardiography. Patients with persistent moderate or severe pulmonary hypertension are susceptible to reduction in long-term survival (34).

At the 6-month visit, I usually discontinue warfarin. Data on the optimal duration for anticoagulation are conflicting, especially among patients with PE who do not have associated surgery or trauma. One randomized trial implies that patients should receive indefinite anticoagulation after an initial PE (35). On the other hand, ongoing trials such as the National Heart, Lung, and Blood Institute–sponsored Prevention of Recurrent Venous Thrombolism (PREVENT) trial will provide a definitive answer to this controversy (36). Our critical PE pathway encourages enrollment in clinical trials. At BWH, we have enrolled more than 80 patients in PREVENT.

CONCLUSIONS

Pulmonary embolism remains difficult to diagnose and continues to have a high death rate. The most common cause of mortality is recurrent PE, not cancer. Impending hemodynamic instability caused by massive PE and its attendant ominous prognosis can be detected by rapid identification of moderate or severe RV failure (usually with echocardiography). Among patients with massive PE or impending hemodynamic instability, thrombolysis and embolectomy are being used with increasing skill and improved outcomes. The optimal duration of anticoagulation remains uncertain.

We have found that critical pathways streamline and hasten the diagnosis, risk stratification, and management of patients with PE.

REFERENCES

1. Ferrari E, Imbert A, Chevalier T, et al. The ECG in pulmonary embolism. Predictive value of negative T-waves in precordial leads—80 case reports. *Chest* 1997;111:537–543.
2. Goldhaber SZ, Hennekens CH, Evans DA, et al. Factors associated with correct antemortem diagnosis of major pulmonary embolism. *Am J Med* 1982;73:822–826.
3. Stein PD, Goldhaber SZ, Henry JW. Alveolar-arterial oxygen gradient in the assessment of acute pulmonary embolism. *Chest* 1995;107:139–143.
4. Stein PD, Goldhaber SZ, Henry JW, et al. Arterial blood gas analysis in the assessment of suspected acute pulmonary embolism. *Chest* 1996;109:78–81.
5. de Moerloose P, Michiels JJ, Bounameaux H. The place of D-dimer testing in an integrated approach to patients suspected of pulmonary embolism. *Semin Thromb Hemost* 1998;24:409–412.
6. de Moerloose P, Desmarais S, Bounameaux H, et al. Contribution of a new, rapid, individual and quantitative automated D-dimer ELISA to exclude pulmonary embolism. *Thromb Haemost* 1996;75:11–13.
7. Rathbun SW, Raskob GE, Whitsett TL. Sensitivity and specificity of helical computed tomography in the diagnosis of pulmonary embolism: a systematic review. *Ann Intern Med* 2000;132:227–232.
8. The PIOPED investigators. Value of the ventilation/perfusion scan in acute pulmonary embolism. *JAMA* 1990;263:2753–2759.
9. Turkstra F, Kuijer PMM, van Beek EJR, et al. Diagnostic utility of ultrasonography of leg veins in patients suspected of having pulmonary embolism. *Ann Intern Med* 1997;126:775–781.
10. Stein PD, Athanasoulis C, Alavi A, et al. Complications and validity of pulmonary angiography in acute pulmonary embolism. *Circulation* 1992;85:462–468.
11. Perrier A, Desmarais S, Miron MJ, et al. Non-invasive diagnosis of venous thromboembolism in outpatients. *Lancet* 1999;353:190–195.
12. Meaney JFM, Weg JG, Chenevert TL, et al. Diagnosis of pulmonary embolism with magnetic resonance angiography. *N Engl J Med* 1997;336:1422–1427.
13. Wolfe MW, Lee RT, Feldstein ML, et al. Prognostic significance of right ventricular hypokinesis and perfusion lung scan defects in pulmonary embolism. *Am Heart J* 1994;127:1371–1375.
14. Simonneau G, Sors H, Charbonnier B, et al., for the THÉSÉe Study Group. A comparison of low-molecular-weight heparin with unfractionated heparin for acute pulmonary embolism. *N Engl J Med* 1997;337:663–669.
15. Goldhaber SZ, Haire WD, Feldstein ML, et al. Alteplase versus heparin in acute pulmonary embolism: randomised trial assessing right-ventricular function and pulmonary perfusion. *Lancet* 1993;341:507–511.
16. Goldhaber SZ, Visani L, De Rosa M, for ICOPER. Acute pulmonary embolism: clinical outcomes in the International Cooperative Pulmonary Embolism Registry (ICOPER). *Lancet* 1999;353:1386–1389.
17. Kanter DS, Mikkola KM, Patel SR, et al. Thrombolytic therapy for pulmonary embolism. Frequency of intracranial hemorrhage and associated risk factors. *Chest* 1997;111:1241–1245.
18. Mikkola KM, Patel SR, Parker JA, et al. Increasing age is a major risk factor for hemorrhagic complications following pulmonary embolism thrombolysis. *Am Heart J* 1997;134:69–72.
19. Daniels LB, Parker JA, Patel SR, et al. Relation of duration of symptoms with response to thrombolytic therapy in pulmonary embolism. *Am J Cardiol* 1997;80:184–188.
20. Tebbe U, Graf A, Kamke W, et al. Hemodynamic effects of double bolus reteplase versus alteplase infusion in massive pulmonary embolism. *Am Heart J* 1999;138:39–44.
21. Greenfield LJ, Proctor MC, Williams DM, et al. Long-term experience with transvenous catheter pulmonary embolectomy. *J Vasc Surg* 1993;18:450–458.
22. Goldhaber SZ. Integration of catheter thrombectomy into our armamentarium to treat acute pulmonary embolism. *Chest* 1998;114:1237–1238.
23. Sharafuddin MJA, Hicks ME. Current status of percutaneous mechanical

thrombectomy. II. Devices and mechanisms of action. *J Vasc Interv Radiol* 1998;9:15–31.

24. Koning R, Cribier A, Gerber L, et al. A new treatment for severe pulmonary embolism. Percutaneous rheolytic thrombectomy. *Circulation* 1997;96:2498–2500.

25. Schmitz-Rode T, Janssens U, Schild HH, et al. Fragmentation of massive pulmonary embolism using a pigtail rotation catheter. *Chest* 1998;114:1427–1436.

26. Fava M, Loyola S, Flores P, et al. Mechanical fragmentation and pharmacologic thrombolysis in massive pulmonary embolism. *J Vasc Interv Radiol* 1997;8:261–266.

27. Brodmann M, Stark G, Pabst E, et al. Pulmonary embolism and intracardiac thrombi—individual therapeutic procedures. *Vasc Med* 2000;5:27–31.

28. Meyer G, Tamisier D, Sors H, et al. Pulmonary embolectomy: a 20-year experience at one center. *Ann Thorac Surg* 1991;51:232–236.

29. Gulba DC, Schmid C, Borst HG, et al. Medical compared with surgical treatment for massive pulmonary embolism. *Lancet* 1994;343:576–577.

30. Stulz P, Schläpfer R, Feer R, et al. Decision making in the surgical treatment of massive pulmonary embolism. *Eur J Cardiothorac Surg* 1994;8:188–193.

31. Ullmann M, Hemmer W, Hannekum A. The urgent pulmonary embolectomy: mechanical resuscitation in the operating theatre determines the outcome. *Thorac Cardiovasc Surg* 1999;47:5–8.

32. Archibald CJ, Auger WR, Fedullo PF, et al. Long-term outcome after pulmonary thromboendarterectomy. *Am J Respir Crit Care Med* 1999;160:523–528.

33. Walrath K, Berkovitz P, Morrison R, et al. Frequently asked questions of the Venous Thromboembolism Support Group. Brigham and Women's Hospital, 1999. Available at: http://web.mit.edu.karen/www/faq.html.

34. Ribeiro A, Lindmarker P, Johnsson H, et al. Pulmonary embolism: one year follow-up with echocardiography Doppler and five-year survival analysis. *Circulation* 1999;99:1325–1330.

35. Kearon C, Gent M, Hirsh J, et al. A comparison of three months of anticoagulation with extended anticoagulation for a first episode of idiopathic venous thromboembolism. *N Engl J Med* 1999;340:901–907.

36. Ridker PM, for the PREVENT Investigators. Long-term low-dose warfarin among venous thrombosis patients with and without factor V Leiden mutation: rationale and design for the prevention of recurrent venous thromboembolism (PREVENT) trial. *Vasc Med Rev* 1998;3:67–73.

PART IV

Critical Pathways in the Outpatient Setting

CHAPTER 20

Hypercholesterolemia

Daniel J. Rader

OVERVIEW

Large epidemiologic studies such as the Framingham Heart study (1) and the Multiple Risk Factor Intervention trial (2) suggested a relationship between serum cholesterol and coronary heart disease (CHD). Multiple randomized, controlled clinical trials in both secondary and primary prevention have demonstrated the clinical benefit of cholesterol reduction (see below).

Clinical management of patients with hypercholesterolemia requires a general working knowledge of normal lipoprotein metabolism (3). Lipoproteins transport cholesterol and triglycerides within the blood. They contain a neutral lipid core consisting of triglycerides and cholesteryl esters surrounded by phospholipids and specialized proteins known as apolipoproteins. The five major families of lipoproteins are chylomicrons, very low-density lipoproteins (VLDL), intermediate-density lipoproteins (IDL), low-density lipoproteins (LDL), and high-density lipoproteins (HDL). Chylomicrons are the largest and most lipid-rich lipoproteins, whereas HDL are the smallest lipoproteins and contain the least amount of lipid. Disorders of lipoprotein metabolism involve perturbations that cause elevation or reduction of one or more lipoprotein classes. Many of these disorders have as their most important clinical sequela the increased risk of premature atherosclerotic cardiovascular disease. The remainder of this chapter focuses on the identification, diagnosis, and clinical management of patients with lipid disorders, especially regarding the prevention of atherosclerosis and its associated clinical events.

Apolipoproteins, which are required for the structural integrity of lipoproteins, direct their metabolic interactions with enzymes, lipid transport proteins, and cell surface receptors. Apolipoprotein B (apoB) is the major apolipoprotein in chylomicrons, VLDL, IDL, and LDL. Apolipoprotein A-I (apoA-I) is the major apolipoprotein in HDL. Lipoprotein receptors bind apolipoproteins on the lipoprotein particles. The best understood lipoprotein receptor is the LDL receptor, which is responsible for catabolizing both chylomicron and VLDL remnants as well as LDL (4). The level of LDL receptor expression in the liver plays a major role in regulating the plasma level of cholesterol. The LDL receptor–related protein serves as a second pathway for clearance of apoE-containing chylomicron and VLDL remnants, especially in cases of a deficiency of LDL receptors (5). Lipid-modifying enzymes and lipid transport proteins play a major role in lipoprotein metabolism and, potentially, in atherosclerosis. Lipoprotein lipase (LPL) is an enzyme that hydrolyzes triglycerides in chylomicrons and VLDL. It is bound to the surface of the capillary endothelium, especially in muscle and adipose tissue, and binds to the chylomicrons as they traverse the capillary bed. ApoC-II found on the chylomicrons serves as a required cofactor for LPL. The free fatty acids generated by triglyceride hydrolysis enter the tissue to serve as a source of energy or fat storage and the resulting "chylomicron remnant" is released and eventually taken up by the liver. Hepatic lipase, which is found primarily in the liver, is involved in the metabolism of lipoprotein remnants and HDL. Lecithin:cholesterol acyltransferase (LCAT) converts free cholesterol to cholesteryl ester on lipoproteins (especially HDL) by transferring fatty acids from phospholipids to cholesterol (6). The cholesteryl ester transfer protein (CETP) transfers cholesteryl esters and other lipids among lipoproteins (7). One major role is thought to be the transfer of cholesteryl esters from HDL (formed as a result of LCAT activity) to VLDL and IDL in exchange for triglycerides. This may be a major pathway by which cholesterol obtained from cells by HDL is eventually returned to the liver in a process that has been termed "reverse cholesterol transport." However, some cholesteryl esters are transferred by CETP to VLDL and LDL and, therefore, CETP could promote atherogenesis; the relationship of CETP to atherosclerosis remains unknown. These lipoprotein-modifying enzymes and lipid transport enzymes act in concert to modulate lipoprotein metabolism and probably have important effects on atherosclerosis.

RATIONALE FOR CHOLESTEROL-LOWERING STRATEGIES

Multiple randomized controlled clinical trials in both secondary and primary prevention have demonstrated the clinical benefit of cholesterol reduction.

Secondary prevention trials are those performed in patients who already have documented CHD or other atherosclerotic cardiovascular disease. Secondary prevention clinical trials have confirmed that cholesterol reduction in the setting of established CHD is highly effective in preventing future cardiovascular events and reducing total mortality. The coronary drug project demonstrated a modest benefit of niacin in reducing nonfatal myocardial infarction (MI) after 6 years of treatment (8) and in reducing total mortality after 15 years of follow-up (9). The Program on the Surgical Control of the Hyperlipidemias trial used partial ileal bypass surgery to reduce LDL cholesterol levels and demonstrated a significant 35% relative reduction in fatal CHD and nonfatal MI, although not in total mortality (the primary endpoint of the trial) (10).

Three more recent secondary prevention trials used 3-hydroxy-3-methylglutaryl coenzyme A (HMG-CoA) reductase inhibitors (statins). The Scandinavian Simvastatin Survival Study (4S) (11) was designed to address whether cholesterol reduction with simvastatin in persons with CHD and elevated cholesterol would reduce total mortality (the primary endpoint). Subjects (n = 4,444) with CHD whose total cholesterol levels were between 212 and 310 mg/dl were randomized to placebo or simvastatin and followed for a mean of 5.4 years. A highly significant (30%) relative reduction was seen in total mortality in the simvastatin-treated group ($p < 0.00001$). The relative risk of a major coronary event was reduced by 44% and revascularization procedures were significantly decreased by 34%. Importantly, the quartile with the lowest LDL cholesterol levels at baseline had proportionately as much benefit from treatment as the highest quartile (12). An economic analysis based on the 4S study concluded that in the United States the reduction in hospital costs alone as a result of the treatment would virtually offset the cost of the medication (13).

Most patients with CHD do not have particularly elevated cholesterol levels; in fact, approximately 35% of all persons with CHD have total cholesterol levels less than 200 mg/dl (14). Therefore, another major trial, the Cholesterol and Recurrent Events (CARE) study (15) addressed the previously unanswered question of whether, after MI, patients with "average" cholesterol levels would benefit from further cholesterol reduction with pravastatin. Patients (n = 4,159) 3 to 20 months after MI who had total cholesterol levels less than 240 mg/dl were randomized to placebo or pravastatin (40 mg daily) and followed for an average of 5 years. The mean total cholesterol level was 209 mg/dl in each group and the mean LDL cholesterol level was only 139 mg/dl (range 115–174 mg/dl). After 5 years, 274 subjects in the placebo group had nonfatal MI or CHD death (the primary endpoint), compared with 212 subjects in the pravastatin-treated group,

resulting in a significant 24% reduction in relative risk ($p = 0.003$). Revascularization procedures were reduced by 27%. These results demonstrated that the benefit of cholesterol-lowering therapy extends even to those CHD patients who have average cholesterol levels. The Long-term Intervention with Pravastatin in Ischemic Disease trial (16) was another secondary prevention study in 9,014 patients with CHD who had baseline cholesterol levels of 155 to 271 mg/dl. Subjects were randomized to placebo or pravastatin (40 mg) and followed for an average of 6 years. The CHD mortality rate was reduced by 24% ($p < 0.001$); the overall mortality rate by 22% ($p < 0.001$); and significant reductions in CHD events and strokes were found as well.

The benefit of lipid-modifying therapies aimed at low HDL cholesterol in patients with CHD was recently addressed in the Veterans Affairs High-Density Lipoprotein Cholesterol Intervention Trial (VA-HIT) (17). Treatment with gemfibrozil (1,200 mg daily) in 2,531 patients with CHD, low-levels of HDL (mean 32 mg/dl), and relatively low LDL cholesterol levels (mean 112 mg/dl) resulted in a 22% reduction in the primary endpoint (nonfatal MI and coronary death) compared with placebo ($p = 0.006$) after an average of 5.1 years. Notably, gemfibrozil resulted in a 6% increase in HDL cholesterol and a 31% decrease in triglycerides but no change in LDL cholesterol levels. This important study extends the indication for lipid-modifying drug therapy in patients with CHD to those with well-controlled LDL cholesterol but low HDL cholesterol.

Therefore, the overall body of clinical data strongly supports the use of drug therapy for lipid reduction in virtually all patients with established atherosclerotic vascular disease. Not only is lipid-lowering drug therapy clinically effective in secondary prevention, it is cost-effective as well. Aggressive cholesterol reduction in patients with CHD or other atherosclerotic disease is now the standard of care, as agreed in a joint statement issued by the American Heart Association (AHA) and the American College of Cardiology (18).

Primary prevention of CHD is extremely important, as approximately one fourth to one third of first MIs result in death (19), precluding the opportunity for secondary prevention. Randomized clinical trials support the use of cholesterol-lowering drug therapy in primary prevention as well. The World Health Organization cooperative trial using clofibrate in hypercholesterolemic men (20) found a 25% reduction in relative risk of nonfatal MI (the primary endpoint) after 5 years, although a substantial 47% increase in noncardiovascular deaths. In the lipid research clinics primary prevention trial with cholestyramine in hypercholesterolemic men (21,22), combined fatal CHD and nonfatal MI (the primary endpoint) was reduced by 19%. The Helsinki heart study (23) using gemfibrozil in men with elevated non-HDL cholesterol—more than 200 mg/dl—demonstrated a significant 34% reduction in combined fatal and nonfatal MI.

Two more recent trials with statins have confirmed the efficacy of cholesterol-lowering in primary prevention. The West of Scotland Coronary Prevention study (24) was performed in 6,595 healthy Scottish men aged 45 to 64 years with total cholesterol levels more than 252 mg/dl and LDL cholesterol levels 174–232 mg/dl. Subjects were randomized to pravastatin 40 mg/day versus placebo and followed for an average of 5 years. The primary endpoint of the study was nonfatal MI or CHD death. There were 248 definite events in the placebo group and 174 definite events in the pravastatin group, resulting in a 31% reduction in relative risk of nonfatal MI or CHD death ($p < 0.001$). Findings also showed a significant 32% reduction in cardiovascular mortality and a 37% reduction in revascularization procedures. Importantly, the relative risk of death from any cause (total mortality) was reduced by 22% in the pravastatin-treated group. This trial clearly established that drug therapy for hypercholesterolemia can be an effective method of decreasing risk of cardiovascular events and total mortality, even in persons who do not have prior evidence of CHD.

The Air Force/Texas Coronary Atherosclerosis Prevention Study (AFCAPS/TexCAPS) trials extended these findings to a population with average cholesterol levels (25). A total of 6,608 men and women without clinical cardiovascular disease, with LDL cholesterol level 130–190 mg/dl, and with HDL cholesterol levels less than 45 mg/dl in men and less than 47 mg/dl in women were randomized to lovastatin (20 mg) or placebo and followed for an average of 5.2 years. A 37% relative risk reduction ($p < 0.001$) in the primary endpoint (defined as fatal or nonfatal MI, unstable angina, or sudden cardiac death) was found in the lovastatin-treated group. Revascularizations were also significantly reduced by 33%. Interestingly, only 17% of the subjects in this trial would have met current National Cholesterol Education Program (NCEP) Guidelines for drug therapy. Therefore, the major clinical challenge in the use of drug therapy for cholesterol in primary prevention is the accurate identification of individuals who are likely to develop clinical CHD and who, therefore, are most likely to benefit from drug therapy.

BACKGROUND ON THERAPY FOR LIPID DISORDERS

Nonpharmacologic Therapy

Identify and Treat Secondary Causes of Hyperlipidemia

Secondary causes of hypercholesterolemia should be considered and excluded with appropriate laboratory testing. Hypothyroidism is a relatively common but often occult cause of hypercholesterolemia and the clinician should have a low threshold for obtaining a patient's thyrotropin level to rule out this diagnosis. Many lipid experts recommended the routine screening of thyrotropin in all hyperlipidemic patients to exclude hypothyroidism. Treatment of hypothyroidism usually results in substantial improvement in hypercholesterolemia. Hyperlipidemia often accompanies diabetes mellitus, especially type II diabetes, and usually takes the form of a combined elevation in both triglycerides and cholesterol. A fasting glucose level should always be obtained in the initial

workup of hyperlipidemia, and consideration should be given to obtaining a glycosylated hemoglobin determination in persons with glucose intolerance. Diabetes mellitus should be controlled as effectively as possible, which often results in substantial improvement in hyperlipidemia. Nephrotic syndrome is always associated with hyperlipidemia and should be excluded if clinically suspected. Hypercholesterolemia is a frequent consequence of obstructive liver disease, particularly primary biliary cirrhosis. Regular alcohol intake is a common contributor to moderate hypertriglyceridemia and sometimes hypercholesterolemia, and patients with hyperlipidemia who drink alcohol should be encouraged to decrease their intake. Sedentary lifestyle, obesity, and smoking are all associated with low HDL cholesterol levels. Several medications exacerbate hyperlipidemia or low HDL including immunosuppressive drugs, retinoic acid derivatives for acne therapy, and HIV protease inhibitors.

Counsel Patients on an Appropriate Diet

Dietary modification is an important component of the effective management of patients with lipid disorders. It is important for the physician to make a general assessment of the patient's diet, to provide suggestions for improvement, and to recognize whether a patient will benefit from referral to a dietitian for more intensive counseling. The dietary approach depends on the type of hyperlipidemia. For predominant hypercholesterolemia, the major approach is restriction of saturated fat intake. For moderate hypertriglyceridemia, it is also important to restrict intake of simple sugars. For severe hypertriglyceridemia, total fat intake restriction is critical.

To lower the LDL cholesterol level by diet modification, it is necessary to restrict the intake of saturated fats and cholesterol. The most widely used diet is the "Step I diet" developed by the AHA. If possible, the patient should receive specific instruction in the diet from a dietitian or qualified professional. Responses to this diet vary widely among individuals and it can be difficult to predict which persons are most likely to benefit from dietary intervention. However, most patients have relatively modest (<10%) decreases in LDL cholesterol levels on a Step I diet. If therapeutic goals for LDL cholesterol are not reached after 3 to 6 months on this diet, the patient may be referred to a registered dietitian for more detailed dietary instruction, including a Step II diet, which is further restricted in total and saturated fat. Patients with established atherosclerotic cardiovascular disease should be instructed directly in a Step II diet. Almost all persons experience a decrease in HDL cholesterol when they decrease the amount of total and saturated fat in their diet. Patients should be reassured that a low-fat diet is nevertheless beneficial in terms of overall cardiovascular risk. For patients with hypertriglyceridemia, dietary counseling should also include restriction of simple carbohydrates. Treatment of severe hypertriglyceridemia (triglycerides >1,000 mg/dl) includes restriction of all fat intake, both saturated and unsaturated.

Encourage Regular Aerobic Exercise

Regular aerobic exercise can have a positive effect on lipids. Elevated triglycerides are especially sensitive to aerobic exercise and persons with hypertriglyceridemia can substantially lower their triglycerides by initiating an exercise program. The effect of exercise on LDL cholesterol levels is more modest. Although widely believed to be a method for raising HDL cholesterol, the effects of aerobic exercise on HDL are relatively modest in most individuals. Patients should also be reminded that aerobic exercise has cardiovascular benefits that extend well beyond its effect on lipid levels (26).

Encourage Weight Loss

Obesity is often associated with hyperlipidemia, especially with elevated triglycerides and low HDL cholesterol. In persons who are overweight, weight loss can have a significantly favorable impact on the lipid profile and should be actively encouraged. Along with counseling on other dietary issues, a dietitian should also advise patients on caloric restriction necessary for effective weight loss.

Consider Hormone Replacement in Postmenopausal Women

Hormone replacement therapy decreases LDL cholesterol, raises HDL cholesterol, and decreases lipoprotein(a) levels. However, HRT can raise triglycerides and is relatively contraindicated in women with a triglyceride level above 500 mg/dl. Observational studies suggest that estrogen replacement is associated with reduced cardiovascular risk, mediated both through lipid and nonlipid effects (27). However, in the Heart and Estrogen–Progestin Replacement study (28) of 2,763 postmenopausal women with CHD, HRT for an average of 4.1 years did not reduce the overall rate of nonfatal MI or CHD death. The long-term role and the effect of HRT in primary prevention of cardiovascular disease await the results of ongoing studies, including the women's health initiative study of more than 50,000 asymptomatic postmenopausal women.

Pharmacologic Therapy

Drug therapy for lipid disorders, whenever possible, should be based on clinical trials indicating the benefit of treatment in decreasing the risk of cardiovascular morbidity and mortality. LDL cholesterol levels are associated with increased risk of CHD and abundant data exist that treatment to lower LDL decreases the risk of clinical cardiovascular events in both secondary and primary prevention. Elevated triglycerides are also associated with increased risk of CHD, but this relationship weakens considerably when statistical corrections are made for LDL and HDL cholesterol levels. With the exception of VA-HIT, which targeted patients with low levels of HDL, no trials have been performed specifically to determine whether treatment to decrease triglyceride levels decreases the risk of cardiovascular disease. Only in certain patients should drug therapy be targeted initially toward reducing triglycerides rather than LDL cholesterol. For example, when triglycerides are higher than 1,000 mg/dl, the patient should be treated to prevent the risk of acute pancreatitis. When triglycerides are 400 to 1,000 mg/dl, the decision to use drug therapy depends on the assessment of cardiovascular risk; however, if drug therapy is used, usually, it should be first targeted to reducing the triglycerides, as cholesterol reduction is difficult in the setting of substantially elevated triglycerides. If the triglycerides are less than 400 mg/dl, the initial emphasis in treatment should always be on reducing LDL cholesterol or "non-HDL" cholesterol.

Pharmacologic Therapy for LDL Cholesterol Reduction

HMG-CoA Reductase Inhibitors (Statins)

Inhibitors of HMG-CoA reductase, the rate-limiting step in cholesterol biosynthesis, which are known as "statins," are the first-line therapy for reducing LDL cholesterol levels. Six HMG-CoA reductase inhibitors are currently available: lovastatin (Mevacor), pravastatin (Pravachol), simvastatin (Zocor), fluvastatin (Lescol), atorvastatin (Lipitor), cerivastatin (Baycol). Statins are generally well tolerated, with gastrointestinal and musculoskeletal complaints the most common side effects. Severe myopathy and even rhabdomyolysis have been rarely reported. Liver transaminases should monitored (after 6–8 weeks, then every 6 months thereafter), but significant (more than three times normal) elevation in transaminases is rare. Mild to moderate (less than three times normal) elevation in transaminases in the absence of symptoms need not mandate discontinuing the medication. Other liver function tests (e.g., alkaline phosphatase and gamma GT) are not useful and need not be monitored. Creatine phosphokinase should not be monitored on a routine basis.

Bile Acid Sequestrants

Bile acid sequestrants include cholestyramine (Questran), colestipol (Colestid) and Colesevalam (Welchol). They bind bile acids in the intestine, interrupt their enterohepatic circulation, and accelerate the loss of bile acids in the stool. The decreased intracellular cholesterol content results in up-regulation of the hepatic LDL receptor and enhanced LDL clearance from the plasma. Bile acid sequestrants primarily reduce LDL cholesterol and should not be prescribed for patients with elevated triglyceride levels because they exacerbate hypertriglyceridemia. The bile acid sequestrants are very safe drugs that are not systemically absorbed. However, they are often inconvenient and unpleasant to take. Most side effects are limited to the gastrointestinal tract; bloating and constipation are common and ultimately dose-limiting. In addition, bile acid sequestrants can bind certain other drugs (e.g., digoxin, warfarin) and interfere with their absorption. Bile acid sequestrants are especially effective in combination therapy with statins.

Nicotinic Acid (Niacin)

Nicotinic acid, or niacin, is a B-complex vitamin which, in high doses, is an effective lipid-modifying drug. It reduces LDL cholesterol modestly but can be useful in combination with statins for achieving further LDL cholesterol reductions. The use of nicotinic acid has been traditionally limited because of the cutaneous flushing that it often causes. However, Niaspan (KOS Pharmaceuticals, Inc., Miami, FL), a new controlled-release form of niacin that is administered once daily, is better tolerated than regular crystalline niacin and has greater patient compliance (29). Niacin can exacerbate glucose intolerance, but is not contraindicated in diabetic patients and can often be successfully used. It can cause elevations in uric acid and has been associated with precipitation of acute gout. Niacin has also been associated with exacerbation of peptic ulcer disease. Niacin potentiates the effect of warfarin and should be used cautiously in this setting. Mild elevation in liver transaminases (up to two to three times the upper limit of normal) can occur but does not necessarily mandate discontinuance of the niacin.

Pharmacologic Therapy for Triglyceride Reduction

Triglycerides are now recognized as an independent risk factor for coronary artery disease (CAD). A large number of epidemiologic studies have addressed the potential relationship between elevated serum triglyceride levels and increased cardiovascular risk (30–33). Although triglycerides are increasingly recognized as an independent risk factor, some controversy still exists (34), partly because of the heterogenous metabolic disposition of triglycerides. In addition, triglycerides are transported in a number of different lipoprotein fractions known to have differing atherogenic potential. Elevated triglyceride levels are associated with a number of other proatherogenic metabolic and physiologic changes such as a low HDL level, a procoagulant state, and increased small, dense LDL particles. No clinical trial outcome data are available for drug therapy in patients with a triglyceride level greater than 400 to 500 mg/dl, as all of the clinical trials discussed above excluded persons with triglycerides in this range.

Severe hypertriglyceridemia (fasting triglycerides >1,000 mg/dl) is always an indication of hyperchylomicronemia in the fasting state and points to an underlying genetic predisposition. The most common diagnosis in adults is type V hyperlipoproteinemia (HLP). The label of type V HLP is generally used for an adult with triglyceride levels above 1,000 mg/dl who does not have known familial chylomicronemia syndrome caused by to LPL or apoC-II deficiency (see above). Type V HLP is also associated with risk of acute pancreatitis, which can be the initial presentation of this syndrome, and is the major rationale for aggressive treatment of this condition. Type V HLP can also be associated with increased risk of cardiovascular disease, although some patients with type V do not appear to be at significantly increased risk. Type II diabetes mellitus or glucose intolerance frequently accompanies type V hyperlipidemia, but type V also occurs in people with normal glucose tolerance. Some patients with nephrotic syndrome can develop severe hypertriglyceridemia. Estrogen replacement therapy can exacerbate moderate hypertriglyceridemia and lead to a more severe type V hyperlipidemia, as can heavy alcohol use. Finally, treatment with isotretinoin or etretinate sometimes causes severe hypertriglyceridemia.

The management of severe hypertriglyceridemia is first targeted to decreasing triglycerides to reduce the risk of pancreatitis, followed by further lipid lowering, depending on the presence of CAD or other risk factors for cardiovascular disease. Women taking estrogen and patients taking isotretinoin or etretinate should be encouraged to discontinue them if their triglyceride level is above 1,000 mg/dl. Diabetes mellitus should be controlled as optimally as possible. Patients should be referred to a registered dietitian for dietary counseling. In general, dietary management includes restriction of total fat as well as simple carbohydrates in the diet. Alcohol should be avoided. Regular aerobic exercise can have a significant impact on triglyceride levels and should be actively encouraged. If the patient is overweight, weight loss can help to decrease triglycerides as well.

Fibric Acid Derivatives (Fibrates)

Fibrates are agonists for the nuclear hormone receptor PPAR-α and have multiple effects on lipoprotein metabolism. Fibrates lower triglyceride levels effectively and generally raise HDL cholesterol levels modestly, but they have limited ability to lower LDL cholesterol levels. In the United States, this class includes clofibrate (Atromid-S), gemfibrozil (Lopid), and micronized fenofibrate (TriCor). Fibrates are generally well tolerated; side effects include gastrointestinal upset and muscle pains. Elevated liver function tests can occur and should be monitored during therapy. Fibrates increase the lithogenicity of bile and, therefore, the risk of gallstones. As with niacin, fibrates potentiate the effect of warfarin. The most straightforward clinical roles of fibrates are in the treatment of significant hypertriglyceridemia and in patients with type III HLP. The VA-HIT study has extended the rationale for the use of fibrates to the prevention of cardiovascular events in patients with established CHD and a low HDL cholesterol in the setting of a controlled LDL cholesterol level.

Fish Oils (Omega 3 Fatty Acids)

Fish oils are highly effective triglyceride-lowering agents and are useful for patients with severe hypertriglyceridemia resistant to or intolerant of gemfibrozil and niacin. They should not be used for hypercholesterolemia and have been reported to raise LDL cholesterol levels in some persons. At least 6 g/day is usually required for a substantial effect and many patients require 9 to 12 g/day. Dyspepsia, diarrhea, and a fishy taste and fishy smell to the breath limit the use of fish oils in many patients. However, in patients with refractory hypertriglyceridemia and pancreatitis, fish oils can be exceptionally effective.

Combination Therapy

Once the triglycerides are adequately controlled, patients often remain significantly hypercholesterolemic. This often raises the issue of a second medication to better control the LDL cholesterol level. In patients with CHD or those at high risk for the development of CHD (e.g., diabetics), the NCEP guidelines are useful in guiding the decision to institute further drug therapy. Most specialists recommend consideration of a second drug (usually in addition to the fibrate used to treat the triglycerides) in patients with CHD who continue to have an LDL cholesterol level above 130 mg/dl or patients at high risk with an LDL cholesterol level above 160 mg/dl. The two options are statins and niacin. Although a small increased risk of myopathy may be associated with either of these combinations, this risk can be minimized by advising the patient to call the physician immediately in the event of generalized muscle pain. Overall, in the patient at high risk for future cardiovascular events, the significant benefit of further cholesterol lowering generally outweighs the very small risk of severe myositis associated with combination drug therapy.

APPROACH TO PATIENTS WITH ISOLATED LOW HDL CHOLESTEROL

High-density lipoprotein cholesterol levels are inversely associated with CHD, independent of total and LDL cholesterol levels (35). However, formal guidelines for the approach to the patient with a low HDL cholesterol level (a condition often referred to as "hypoalphalipoproteinemia") have not yet been developed. Many causes of a low HDL cholesterol level are secondary to other factors. Cigarette smoking, obesity, and physical inactivity contribute to a low HDL cholesterol. Type II diabetes mellitus, end-stage renal disease, and hypertriglyceridemia from any cause are all associated with a

low HDL level. Beta-blockers, thiazide diuretics, androgens, progestins, and probucol can all reduce HDL cholesterol levels. Importantly, a low fat diet often results in a low level of HDL cholesterol; for example, most vegetarians have low levels of HDL cholesterol. In this case, the low HDL level is not considered to be associated with an increased risk of CHD, as persons who eat low fat diets are at substantially reduced risk of premature CHD. However, many persons with low HDL cholesterol levels have a genetic cause of hypoalphalipoproteinemia. Some genetic causes of low HDL include mutations in apoA-I, LCAT, and ABC1 (Tangier disease). However, most patients with low HDL do not have a currently identifiable mutation and have what is called "primary or familial hypoalphalipoproteinemia" (36,37). It is defined as an HDL cholesterol level below the 10th percentile in the setting of relatively normal cholesterol and triglyceride levels, no apparent secondary causes of low HDL, and no clinical signs of LCAT deficiency or Tangier disease. This syndrome is often referred to as "isolated low HDL." A family history of low HDL cholesterol facilitates the diagnosis of an inherited condition, which usually follows the pattern of an autosomal dominant trait.

No formal clinical practice guidelines exist for the management of a patient with an isolated low HDL cholesterol level. However, some general guidelines can be proposed. Secondary factors should be sought and corrected, when possible. Smoking should be discontinued, obese persons should be encouraged to lose weight, and sedentary persons should be encouraged to exercise. Estrogen replacement therapy can substantially raise HDL cholesterol and should be considered in postmenopausal women. When possible, medications associated with a reduced HDL cholesterol level should be discontinued. Diabetes mellitus should be optimally controlled. Patients with CHD or at high risk for CHD should be treated very aggressively to reduce their LDL cholesterol level, regardless of the HDL cholesterol. The difficult issue is whether pharmacologic intervention should be used to specifically raise the HDL cholesterol level in healthy persons. Those at high risk should be treated aggressively to reduce LDL cholesterol levels. Regarding treatment to raise the HDL cholesterol level, niacin is the most effective among current drugs. Fibrates can also raise the HDL cholesterol level modestly, but are generally effective only if the triglycerides are elevated.

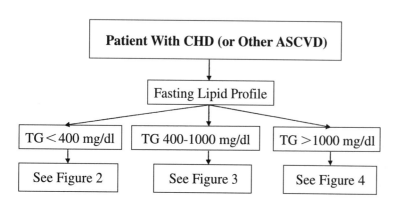

FIG. 20-1. Algorithm for the initial evaluation of lipids in patients with established coronary heart disease or other atherosclerotic cardiovascular disease.

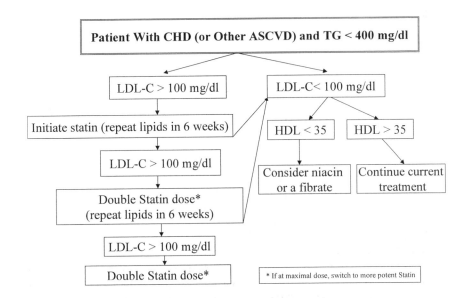

FIG. 20-2. Algorithm for the management of hypercholesterolemia in patients with established coronary heart disease or other atherosclerotic cardiovascular disease who have fasting triglyceride levels less than 400 mg/dl.

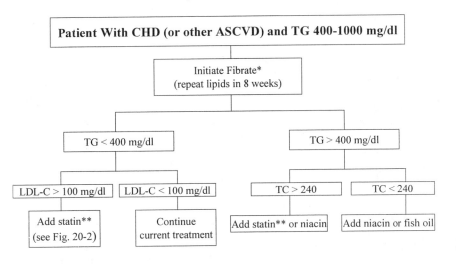

FIG. 20-3. Algorithm for the diagnosis and management of dyslipidemia in patients with established coronary heart disease or other atherosclerotic cardiovascular disease who have fasting triglyceride levels 400 to 1,000 mg/dl.

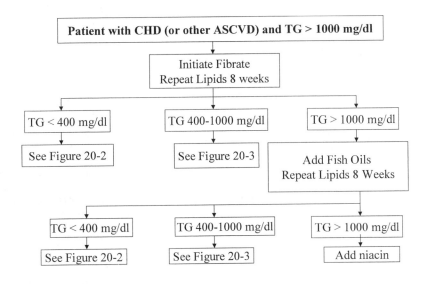

FIG. 20-4. Algorithm for the diagnosis and management of dyslipidemia in patients with established coronary heart disease or other atherosclerotic cardiovascular disease who have fasting triglyceride levels more than 1,000 mg/dl.

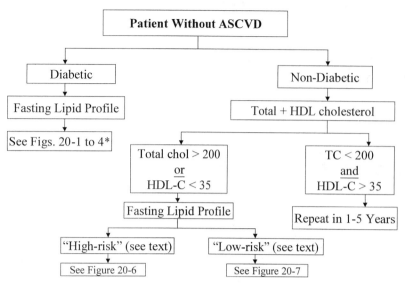

*Diabetics without ASCVD have similar cardiovascular risk as non-diabetics with known ASCVD.

FIG. 20-5. Algorithm for lipid screening in patients without established atherosclerotic cardiovascular disease.

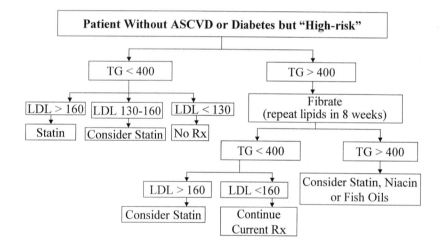

FIG. 20-6. Algorithm for the management of hypercholesterolemia in high-risk primary prevention.

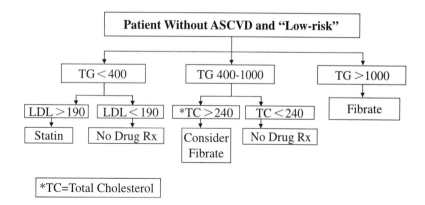

*TC=Total Cholesterol

FIG. 20-7. Algorithm for the management of hypercholesterolemia in low-risk primary prevention.

STRATEGY ALGORITHMS

Strategy algorithms related to the secondary prevention of CHD in patients with known atherosclerotic cardiovascular disease are found in Figs. 20-1 through 20-4.

For primary prevention of CHD in patients without known atherosclerotic cardiovascular, see Figs. 20-5 through 20-7.

REFERENCES

1. Kannel WB, Castelli WP, Gordon T. Cholesterol in the prediction of atherosclerotic disease. New perspectives based on the Framingham study. *Ann Intern Med* 1979;90:85–91.
2. Stamler J, Wentworth D, Neaton JD. Is relationship between serum cholesterol and risk of premature death from coronary heart disease continuous and graded? Findings in 356,222 primary screens of the multiple risk factor intervention trial (MRFIT). *JAMA* 1986;256:2823–2828.
3. Rader DJ, Brewer HB. Lipids, apolipoproteins and lipoproteins. Dordrecht/Boston/London: Kluwer Academic Publishers, 1994;83–103.
4. Brown MS, Goldstein JL. A receptor-mediated pathway for cholesterol homeostasis. *Science* 1986;232:34–47.
5. Beisiegel U. Receptors for triglyceride-rich lipoproteins and their role in lipoprotein metabolism. *Curr Opin Lipidol* 1995;6:117–122.
6. Rader DJ, Ikewaki K. Unraveling high density lipoprotein–apolipoprotein metabolism in human mutants and animal models. *Curr Opin Lipidol* 1996;7:117–123.
7. Tall AR. Plasma high density lipoproteins. Metabolism and relationship to atherogenesis. *J Clin Invest* 1990;86:379–384.
8. The Coronary Drug Project Research Group. Clofibrate and niacin in coronary heart disease. *JAMA* 1975;231:360–381.
9. Canner PL, Berge KG, Wenger NK, et al. Fifteen year mortality in coronary drug project patients: long-term benefit with niacin. *J Am Coll Cardiol* 1986;8:1245–1255.
10. Buchwald H, Varco RL, Matts JP, et al. Effect of partial ileal bypass surgery on mortality and morbidity from coronary heart disease in patients with hypercholesterolemia—report of the program on the surgical control of the hyperlipidemias (POSCH). *N Engl J Med* 1990;323:946–955.
11. Scandinavian Simvastatin Survival Study Group. Randomized trial of cholesterol lowering in 4444 patients with coronary heart disease: the Scandinavian simvastatin survival study (4S). *Lancet* 1994;344:1383–1389.
12. Scandinavian Simvastatin Survival Study Group. Baseline serum cholesterol and treatment effect in the Scandinavian simvastatin survival study (4S). *Lancet* 1995;345:1274–1275.
13. Pederson TR, Kjekshus J, Berg K, et al. Cholesterol lowering and the use of healthcare resources. Results of the Scandinavian simvastatin survival study. *Circulation* 1996;93:1796–1802.
14. Kannel WB. Range of serum cholesterol values in the population developing coronary artery disease. *Am J Cardiol* 1995;76:69C–77C.
15. Sacks FM, Pfeffer MA, Moye L, et al. The effect of pravastatin on coronary events after myocardial infarction in patients with average cholesterol levels. *N Engl J Med* 1996;335:1001–1009.
16. Tonkin AM. Management of the long-term intervention with pravastatin in ischemic disease (LIPID) study after the Scandinavian simvastatin survival study (4S). *Am J Cardiol* 1995;76:107C–112C.
17. Rubins HB, Robins SJ, Collins D, et al. Gemfibrozil for the secondary prevention of coronary heart disease in men with low levels of high-density lipoprotein cholesterol. *N Engl J Med* 1999;341:410–418.
18. Smith J, Blair SN, Criqui MH, et al. Preventing heart attack and death in patients with coronary disease. *Circulation* 1995;92:2–4.
19. Kannel WB, Schatzkin A. Sudden death: lessons from subsets in population studies. *J Am Coll Cardiol* 1985;5:141b–149b.
20. Committee of Principal Investigators. A cooperative trial in the prevention of ischaemic heart disease using clofibrate. *Br Heart J* 1978;40:1069–1118.
21. Lipid Research Clinics Program. The lipid research clinics coronary primary prevention trial results. I. Reduction in incidence of coronary heart disease. *JAMA* 1984;251:351–364.
22. Lipid Research Clinics Program. The lipid research clinics coronary primary prevention trial results. II. The relationship of reduction in incidence of coronary heart disease to cholesterol lowering. *JAMA* 1984;251:365–374.
23. Frick MH, Elo O, Haapa K, et al. Helsinki heart study: primary-prevention trial with gemfibrozil in middle-aged men with dyslipidemia. Safety of treatment, changes in risk factors, and incidence of coronary heart disease. *N Engl J Med* 1987;317:1237–1245.
24. Shepherd J, Cobbe SM, Ford I, et al. Prevention of coronary heart disease with pravastatin in men with hypercholesterolemia. *N Engl J Med* 1995;333:1301–1307.
25. Downs JR, Clearfield M, Weis S, et al. Primary prevention of acute coronary events with lovastatin in men and women with average cholesterol levels. *JAMA* 1998;279:1615–1622.
26. Fletcher GF. The antiatherosclerotic effect of exercise and development of an exercise prescription. *Cardiol Clin* 1996;14:85–95.
27. Kafonek SD. Postmenopausal hormone replacement therapy and cardiovascular risk reduction. A review. *Drugs* 1994;47:16–24.
28. Hulley S, Grady D, Bush T, et al. Randomized trial of estrogen plus progestin for secondary prevention of coronary heart disease in postmenopausal women. Heart and Estrogen/Progestin Replacement Study (HERS) Research group. *JAMA* 1998;280:605–613.
29. Morgan JM, Capuzzi DM, Guyton JR, et al. Treatment effect of Niaspan, a controlled-release niacin, in patients with hypercholesterolemia: a placebo-controlled trial. *J Cardiovasc Pharmacol Ther* 1996;1:195–202.
30. Hokanson JE, Austin MA. Plasma triglyceride level is a risk factor for cardiovascular disease independent of high-density lipoprotein cholesterol level: a meta-analysis of population-based prospective studies. *J Cardiovasc Risk* 1996;3:213–219.
31. Castelli WP. Epidemiology of triglycerides: a view from Framingham. *Am J Cardiol* 1992;70:3H–9H.
32. Jeppesen J, Hein HO, Suadicani P, et al. Triglyceride concentration and ischemic heart disease: an eight-year follow-up in the Copenhagen male study. *Circulation* 1998;97:1029–1036.
33. Miller M, Seidler A, Moalemi A, et al. Normal triglyceride levels and coronary artery disease events: the Baltimore coronary observational long-term study. *J Am Coll Cardiol* 1998;31:1252–1257.
34. Bass KM, Newschaffer CJ, Klag MJ, et al. Plasma lipoprotein levels as predictors of cardiovascular death in women. *Arch Intern Med* 1993;153:2209–2216.
35. Gordon DJ, Rifkind BM. High-density lipoproteins—the clinical implications of recent studies. *N Engl J Med* 1989;321:1311–1316.
36. Third JL, Montag J, Flynn M, et al. Primary and familial hypoalphalipoproteinemia. *Metabolism* 1984;33:136–146.
37. Genest J, Bard JM, Fruchart JC, et al. Familial hypoalphalipoproteinemia in premature coronary artery disease. *Arterioscler Thromb* 1993;13:1728–1737.

CHAPTER 21

Hypertension

Paul R. Conlin

Recommendations for the treatment of hypertension have evolved significantly over the more than 25 years since the establishment of the National High Blood Pressure Education program (NHBPEP) by the National Heart, Lung, and Blood Institute. The purpose of this program is to increase the awareness, prevention, and treatment of hypertension in the United States population. To achieve this goal, the NHBPEP has convened a joint national committee (JNC) approximately every 4 to 5 years. Previous reports of the JNC have reaffirmed national guidelines for the management of high blood pressure and provided recommendations for evaluating and treating hypertension based on the current state of knowledge in the field. The most recent report (1997) represents the sixth report (JNC VI) of this expert panel (1). The World Health Organization (WHO), in conjunction with the International Society of Hypertension (ISH), issued guidelines in 1999 that came to similar conclusions (2).

Since the first report of the JNC in 1972, information has increased on the awareness, treatment, and control of hypertension in the US population, but substantial room remains for further progress. Although many more individuals are aware of the diagnosis and seek treatment for hypertension, the percentage of patients who are adequately controlled is still small (<30%). Accompanying this increased awareness and treatment of hypertensive patients has been a significant decline in age-adjusted mortality in hypertension-related complications, including stroke. An overall decline of 50% in stroke mortality has occurred since 1972, with a similar decline in coronary heart disease (CHD) mortality (53%) during the same period. However, the steep declines in mortality rate seen since the 1970s have given way to a leveling off of these curves since 1990, with a slight increase in stroke mortality rate between 1992 and 1994. These data, coupled with the small percentage of patients with adequately controlled blood pressure, suggest a large portion of the population has yet to achieve the maximal benefit from treatment for high blood pressure.

EVALUATION, STAGING, AND RISK STRATIFICATION

The appropriate classification of blood pressure in adults emphasizes the importance of blood pressure elevation as a continuum of risk, for both systolic and diastolic blood pressure. A concept first developed in earlier guidelines is the definition of normal and high-normal blood pressure (Table 21-1), which applies to both systolic and diastolic blood pressure. This is based on observations from epidemiologic studies showing the relationship between systolic and diastolic blood pressure and cardiovascular risk. Blood pressure is continuous, independent, and predictive for patients with and without cardiovascular disease. Likewise, the concept of stages of hypertension has been applied to define levels of blood pressure. Many clinicians have continued to use more descriptive terms such as "mild," "moderate," or "severe" hypertension. Because most affected individuals fall into the category previously termed "mild," these patients may not fully understand the significance of risk associated with what they perceive is a "mild" disease and receive mixed messages about the importance of adherence to treatment. Therefore, to avoid confusion between physicians and patients regarding the risk associated with hypertension, it is best to describe the degree of blood pressure elevation using a staging system. When systolic and diastolic blood pressure fall into different categories, the higher stage (and therefore the higher risk) should be used to classify the patient's blood pressure because both are independent risk factors for subsequent cardiovascular events.

An important concept in hypertension management is that the risk of cardiovascular disease is determined by both the blood pressure level and the presence or absence of target organ damage. This is quantitated by risk stratification. The major cardiovascular risk factors for patients with hypertension include age, sex, family history of cardiovascular disease, smoking, dyslipidemia, and diabetes mellitus. Each of these factors can independently modify the risk of cardiovascular disease. The greatest risk for subsequent cardiovascular events is within the group of individuals who have already

TABLE 21-1. *Classification of blood pressure in adults*

Category	Systolic (mm Hg)	Diastolic (mm Hg)
Optimal	<120	<80
Normal	<130	<85
High-normal	130–139	85–89
Hypertension		
Stage 1	140–159	90–99
Stage 2	160–179	100–109
Stage 3	≥180	≥110

Adapted from: Joint National Committee on Prevention, Detection, Evaluation and Treatment of High Blood Pressure and the National High Blood Pressure Education Program Coordinating Committee. The sixth report of the Joint National Committee on Prevention, Detection, Evaluation and Treatment of High Blood Pressure. *Arch Intern Med* 1997;157:2413–2446; with permission.

manifested target organ damage, as evidenced by the presence of CHD, stroke, nephropathy, peripheral vascular disease, or retinopathy.

Combining the patient's risk factor profile with the presence or absence of target organ damage can generate an algorithm for the appropriate treatment of those with various stages of hypertension (Table 21-2).

Risk group A includes patients with any level of blood pressure without additional risk factors, target organ damage, or clinical cardiovascular disease. For patients with high-normal blood pressure or stage 1 hypertension it is appropriate to initiate lifestyle modifications for up to 12 months in an attempt to achieve a normal blood pressure level. Those who do not achieve a goal blood pressure level with lifestyle modification alone are candidates for drug treatment. Despite the absence of risk factors or clinical cardiovascular disease, those patients with stage 2 or stage 3 hypertension warrant drug therapy at the time of diagnosis.

Risk group B includes patients who have one or more risk factors (excluding diabetes mellitus), but who do not have target organ damage or clinical cardiovascular disease. This group represents the largest number of patients with hypertension. As for risk group A, it is appropriate to initiate lifestyle modifications for people with high-normal or stage 1 hypertension because of the relatively low short-term risk associated with these blood pressure levels. However, clinicians should also consider the number of risk factors present in their decision-making and consider drug therapy either after a shorter period of lifestyle changes (6 months) or concomitant with the lifestyle modifications.

Risk group C includes patients who have evidence of target organ damage or clinical cardiovascular disease, diabetes mellitus, or both (independent of the presence of other risk factors). These patients are at the greatest risk for future cardiovascular events and are candidates for drug therapy even in the presence of high-normal blood pressure. This is especially true for patients with renal insufficiency, heart failure, or diabetes mellitus. Obviously, lifestyle modifications should be included in the initial treatment plan but should be used as adjunctive as opposed to primary treatment in this group at high risk. Some patients may manifest signs or symptoms suggestive of an identifiable cause of hypertension. Additional diagnostic tests may be appropriate to evaluate individuals in whom age of onset, medical history, examination (including stage of hypertension), or initial laboratory testing suggest that an underlying cause is present. Some secondary causes of hypertension, clinical clues to their presence, and appropriate screening tests are outlined in Table 21-3.

RATIONALE FOR PREVENTION AND TREATMENT OF HYPERTENSION

As noted, a substantial number of individuals are unaware that they have hypertension and an even larger number of individuals with high-normal blood pressure are at risk for developing hypertension (Fig. 21-1). Also, a large portion of cardiovascular disease occurs in individuals whose blood pressure is above optimal levels but not so high as to be diagnosed with hypertension. Whereas the absolute risk for

TABLE 21-2. *Risk stratification and treatment*

Blood pressure stages (mm Hg)	Risk group A[a]	Risk group B[b]	Risk group C[c]
High-normal	Lifestyle modifications	Lifestyle modifications	Drug therapy
Stage 1 (140–159/90–99)	Lifestyle modifications (up to 12 mo)	Lifestyle modifications (up to 6 mo)	Drug therapy
Stage 2 and 3 (≥160/≥100)	Drug therapy	Drug therapy	Drug therapy

[a]No risk factors; no target organ damage (TOD) or clinical cardiovascular disease (CCD).
[b]At least one risk factor, not including diabetes mellitus (DM); no TOD or CCD.
[c]TOD, CCD, and/or DM, with or without other risk factors.
Adapted from Joint National Committee on Prevention, Detection, Evaluation and Treatment of High Blood Pressure and the National High Blood Pressure Education Program Coordinating Committee. The sixth report of the Joint National Committee on Prevention, Detection, Evaluation and Treatment of High Blood Pressure. *Arch Intern Med* 1997;157:2413–2446; with permission.

TABLE 21-3. *Secondary causes of hypertension*

Condition	Clinical clues	Screening test
Cushing's syndrome	Amenorrhea Buffalo hump Diabetes mellitus Edema Hirsutism Moon facies Purple striae Truncal obesity	24-h urine for free cortisol
Hyperparathyroidism	Hypercalcemia Polyuria/polydipsia Renal stones	Serum calcium and parathyroid hormone level
Hyperthyroidism	Anxiety Brisk reflexes Hyperdefecation Heat intolerance Tachycardia Tremor Weight loss Wide pulse pressure	Thyroid-stimulating hormone
Hypothyroidism	Bradycardia Cold intolerance Constipation Fatigue Goiter Weight gain	Thyroid-stimulating hormone
Pheochromocytoma	Labile blood pressure (BP) Most prevalent in young adults Orthostatic hypotension Paroxysms (headaches, palpitations, sweating, pallor) Tachycardia	24-h urine for metanephrines and urinary catecholamines
Primary hyperaldosteronism	$K^+ \leq 3.5$ mEq/L in patients **not** on diuretic therapy; or $K^+ \leq 3.0$ mEq/L in patients **on** diuretic therapy Muscle cramps Polyuria Weakness	Ratio of plasma aldosterone and plasma renin activity
Renal parenchymal disease	Abnormal urine sediment Elevated serum creatinine Hematuria on two occasions or structural renal abnormality Recurrent urinary tract infections Stones	Urinalysis, urine sediment, serum creatinine, 24-h urine for protein and creatinine clearance, or spot urine for albumin/creatinine ratio
Renovascular disease	Bruits over the renal arteries Abrupt onset of severe hypertension Diastolic BP ≥ 110 mm Hg or refractory to multiple medications Initial onset ≥ 50 yr of age Other evidence of vascular disease Worsening BP control when previously stable	Captopril-renogram, magnetic resonance angiogram, renal artery Doppler
Sleep apnea	Chronic obstructive pulmonary disease Daytime somnolence Fatigue Obesity Snoring	Referral for sleep study

Critical Pathway: Hypertension

	Week 0 (Initial Visit)	Week 2-6	Week 6-12	Months 3-6	Months 6-12	Year 1
Goals	○ Determine the Stage of hypertension (see Table 21-1) ○ Evaluate for secondary causes (see Table 3), target organ damage or clinical cardiovascular disease ○ Decide on appropriate treatment (see Table 2) ○ Determine goal BP	○ Re-evaluate effect of treatment ○ Assess compliance and inquire about side-effects of treatment	○ Re-evaluate effect of treatment ○ Assess compliance and inquire about side-effects of treatment	○ Re-evaluate effect of treatment ○ Assess compliance and inquire about side-effects of treatment	○ Re-evaluate effect of treatment ○ Assess compliance and inquire about side-effects of treatment	○ Re-evaluate effect of treatment ○ Assess compliance and inquire about side-effects of treatment ○ Consider step-down of treatment if target BP achieved
Assessment	○ BP measurements- both arms, include orthostatic measures ○ Detailed history- and physical exam	○ BP measurements ○ Review interim history, results of lab tests and effects of treatment and medications	○ BP measurements ○ Review interim history and effects of treatment and medications	○ BP measurements ○ Review interim history and effects of treatment and medications	○ BP measurements ○ Review interim history and effects of treatment and medications	○ BP measurements ○ Review interim history and effects of treatment and medications
Tests	○ Chemistry screen, urinalysis or microalbumin, lipid profile ○ ECG ○ Consider Echocardiogram or other specific tests to evaluate for secondary causes or target organ damage	○ Follow-up tests based on results of initial evaluation or to monitor effect of treatment	○ Follow-up tests based on results of previous evaluation or to monitor effect of treatment	○ Follow-up tests based on results of previous evaluation or to monitor effect of treatment	○ Follow-up tests based on results of previous evaluation or to monitor effect of treatment	○ Follow-up tests based on results of previous evaluation or to monitor effect of treatment
Medications	○ Based on Stage and presence of target organ damage or clinical cardiovascular disease (see Figures 21-2–21-4)	○ Target BP achieved- continue current therapy ○ Not at target BP- consider dose titration or addition of second agent ○ Side-effects limiting use of initial drug- switch to alternative agent	○ Target BP achieved- continue current therapy ○ Not at target BP- consider dose titration or addition of second or third agent ○ Side-effects limiting use of initial drug- switch to alternative agent(s)	○ Target BP achieved- continue current therapy ○ Not at target BP- consider dose titration or addition of second or third agent ○ Side-effects limiting use of initial drug- switch to alternative agent(s)	○ Target BP achieved- continue current therapy ○ Not at target BP- consider dose titration or addition of second or third agent ○ Side-effects limiting use of initial drug- switch to alternative agent(s)	○ Target BP achieved- continue current therapy or consider step-down ○ Not at target BP- Re-evaluate for secondary cause (see Table 21-3) and/or refer to Hypertension Specialist
Other treatments	○ Provide instruction for lifestyle modifications	○ Continue lifestyle modifications	○ Continue lifestyle modifications	○ Continue lifestyle modifications	○ Continue lifestyle modifications	○ Continue lifestyle modifications

FIG. 21-1.

cardiovascular disease as a consequence of hypertension varies in different populations around the world, the relative risk does not—hypertension doubles the risk of a CHD death (3). Efforts to lower blood pressure in a population-wide approach can significantly reduce cardiovascular risk in a large segment of the population.

Lifestyle modifications, which continue to be the cornerstone of prevention and part of the initial treatment of all patients with established hypertension, should certainly be recommended to individuals with high-normal blood pressure. For the first time, the JNC VI report encourages the use of a specific dietary intervention (1). Results of the Dietary Approaches to Stop Hypertension (DASH) study showed that individuals with high-normal blood pressure or stage 1 hypertension had clinically significant declines in both systolic and diastolic blood pressure by adopting a low-fat diet enriched in fruits, vegetables, and low-fat dairy products (4). These favorable effects on blood pressure were independent of weight loss, sodium restriction, or increased physical activity. A recently completed follow-up study evaluated the combined effects of the DASH diet with sodium restriction. In combination, these dietary changes affected blood pressure more so than did either used alone (5). Other independent, well-accepted lifestyle modifications (e.g., weight loss, reduced sodium intake, limited alcohol intake, increased physical activity, and smoking cessation) also form an integral part of the approach to cardiovascular risk reduction.

In some cases, effective lifestyle modifications allow subsequent medication withdrawal once the goal blood pressure level is maintained.

Some of the realities of treating patients with established hypertension are that medication use can pose significant financial burdens and, at times, treatment produces adverse effects that limit the patient's interest in continuing treatment. Additional challenges are that most patients do not make serious attempts to modify their lifestyle; they may not take medications on a regular basis or may not be treated with an appropriate amount of medication to achieve optimal control of blood pressure. Therefore, the goal of prevention and management of hypertension is to "reduce morbidity and mortality by the least intrusive means possible" (1). Target levels of blood pressure are appropriately set at systolic blood pressure less than 140 mm Hg and diastolic blood pressure less than 90 mm Hg—as ceiling levels—to prevent stroke, preserve renal function, or slow the progression of heart failure. Attempts to reduce or eliminate other modifiable cardiovascular risk factors should also be included in this treatment scheme. The results of the Hypertension Optimal Treatment (HOT) study actually confirmed that lower levels of blood pressure (particularly diastolic blood pressure <85 mm Hg) are associated with significantly reduced cardiovascular event rates (6). This underscores the importance and significant benefits of achieving blood pressure levels at or below the targets set by JNC VI and the WHO/ISH guidelines.

Isolated systolic hypertension, as defined by systolic blood pressure more than 140 mm Hg and diastolic blood pressure less than 90 mm Hg, is also firmly associated with an increased risk of stroke and cardiovascular disease, and affects two thirds of the elderly population (>65 years of age) who are hypertensive (7). It has taken a long time to convince clinicians of the benefits of treating this condition, but now unequivocal evidence of those benefits exists. Two large, multicenter trials have assessed the ability of antihypertensive drug treatment to reduce the risk of stroke in patients with isolated systolic hypertension (systolic blood pressure >160 mm Hg).

In the Systolic Hypertension in the Elderly program, nearly 5,000 elderly individuals with isolated systolic hypertension (aged >60 years) were randomized to receive either placebo or active treatment with low-dose chlorthalidone (12.5 mg) followed by atenolol, if required (8). After 5 years, systolic blood pressure was 12 mm Hg lower (143 mm Hg) in the active treatment group than in the control group (155 mm Hg); diastolic blood pressure was 68 and 72 mm Hg, respectively. These findings were associated with a 36% reduction in the incidence of total stroke, a 25% reduction in CHD events, and a 50% reduction in heart failure (8,9). Importantly, most patients achieved target blood pressure, and no excess dementia or depression was seen.

The Systolic Hypertension in Europe (Syst-Eur) trial randomized >4000 patients to placebo or the dihydropyridine calcium-channel blocker, nitrendipine, with addition of enalapril and hydrochlorothiazide, if needed. Substantial reductions in stroke (42%) and all cardiac endpoints (26%) were demonstrated (10). The benefits of treatment were particularly marked in patients with diabetes mellitus (11).

PHARMACOLOGIC TREATMENT

Previous recommendation strongly suggest that initial therapy for individuals with uncomplicated hypertension should begin with a diuretic, beta-blocker, or both because of their proved benefits on mortality in controlled clinical trials. At present, these recommendations continue to be valid. Interim results from the large ongoing clinical study—Antihypertensive and Lipid Lowering to Prevent Heart Attack trial (ALLHAT)—show that the diuretic, chlorthalidone, offers the same benefit as doxazosin in preventing fatal and nonfatal CHD. Indeed, chlorthalidone was significantly better than doxazosin in reducing major cardiovascular events, such as stroke, congestive heart failure (CHF), and myocardial infarction (MI) (12). For this reason, the doxazosin arm of the study was discontinued. Yet to be answered in this ongoing trial is whether the calcium channel blocker, amlodipine, or the angiotensin converting enzyme (ACE) inhibitor, lisinopril, offers further benefits than chlorthalidone. Despite these findings from ALLHAT, compelling indications remain for the use of certain antihypertensive medications in specific circumstances, and for their favorable effects on comorbid conditions with some antihypertensive classes (see below).

Recommendations for initiating drug therapy for patients with diastolic and combined systolic–diastolic hypertension and for those with isolated systolic hypertension are summarized in Figs. 21-2 and 21-3. For most patients, antihypertensive therapy should be initiated with a low dose of the initial drug of choice. The optimal drug formulation should provide 24-hour blood pressure lowering with once-daily dosing and a peak-to-trough ratio of more than 50%.

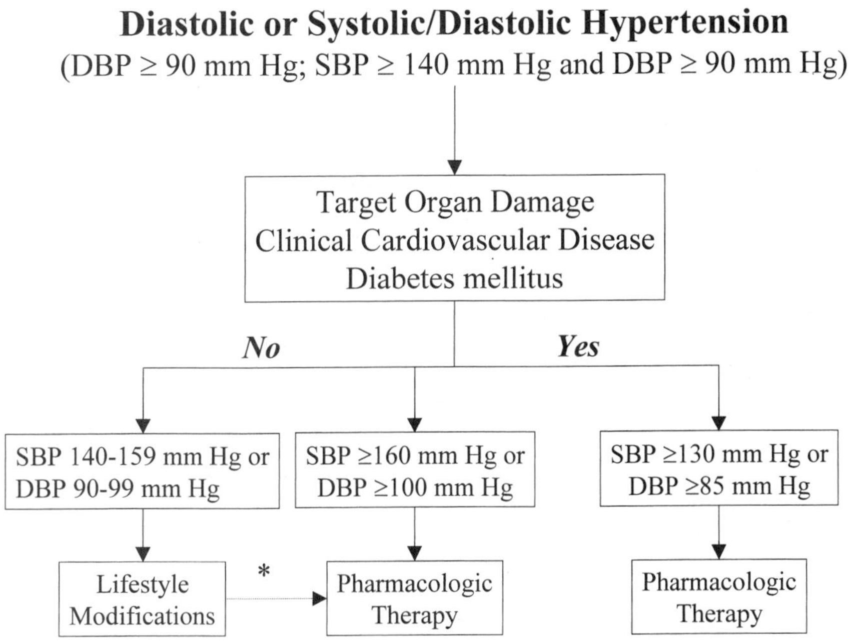

Diastolic or Systolic/Diastolic Hypertension
(DBP ≥ 90 mm Hg; SBP ≥ 140 mm Hg and DBP ≥ 90 mm Hg)

FIG. 21-2. Algorithm for the treatment of patients with diastolic or combined systolic–diastolic hypertension. *Lifestyle modifications should be used as primary therapy for a predetermined time (see Table 21-2), after which the benefits and need for adjunctive pharmacologic therapy should be assessed.

Isolated Systolic Hypertension
(SBP ≥ 140 mm Hg, DBP < 90 mm Hg)

```
              ┌─────────────────────────────────┐
              │    Target Organ Damage          │
              │ Clinical Cardiovascular Disease │
              │    Diabetes mellitus            │
              └─────────────────────────────────┘
              No                           Yes
    ┌──────────────────┬──────────────┐        ┌──────────────────┐
┌────────────────┐ ┌──────────────┐      ┌──────────────────┐
│ SBP 140-159    │ │ SBP >159     │      │ SBP >140 mm Hg   │
│ mm Hg          │ │ mm Hg        │      │                  │
└────────────────┘ └──────────────┘      └──────────────────┘

┌──────────────┐  *  ┌──────────────┐    ┌──────────────┐
│ Lifestyle    │────▶│ Pharmacologic│    │ Pharmacologic│
│ Modifications│     │ Therapy      │    │ Therapy      │
└──────────────┘     └──────────────┘    └──────────────┘
```

FIG. 21-3. Algorithm for the treatment of patients with isolated systolic hypertension. *Lifestyle modifications should be used as primary therapy for a predetermined time (see Table 21-2), after which the benefits and need for adjunctive pharmacologic therapy should be assessed.

Long-acting drug formulations are preferred over short-acting formulations because adherence to therapy is better with once daily dosing; blood pressure control is smooth and persistent; and for some agents, fewer tablets can incur less expense for the patient. Low-dose combinations of medication (with two agents from different classes) may be appropriate for initial therapy. For example, very low doses of a diuretic can potentiate the effects of other agents without producing adverse effects (13,14).

Compelling reasons why agents other than a diuretic or a beta-blocker are chosen as first-line therapy, are based on outcomes from randomized controlled trials. ACE inhibitors have been shown to significantly reduce morbidity and mortality in patients with diabetes mellitus with proteinuria (15,16) and with reduced systolic function and CHF (17). The recently introduced class of angiotensin II receptor antagonists (AIIA) produce similar hemodynamic effects as ACE inhibitors and have none of the most common adverse effects of an ACE inhibitor. However, data are still accumulating on the long-term benefits of this class of agents compared with ACE inhibitors, and their use should not routinely supplant ACE inhibitors in patients with these compelling indications. An example of this is the recent study comparing losartan with captopril in patients with CHF (18). No significant advantage was found to use of losartan, despite an earlier study suggesting benefits, and the mortality rate was similar with the two agents. Several large-scale clinical trials that have enrolled thousands of patients are ongoing to determine whether AIIA offer similar effects in patients at high risk (e.g., after MI, left ventricular hypertrophy, and diabetes mellitus with overt nephropathy).

If blood pressure is not well controlled with a single antihypertensive agent, three alternatives remain: (a) titrate the dose upward, (b) switch to an alternative monotherapy agent, or (c) combine a second agent with the first. Although up-titration of doses may improve blood pressure control in some patients, it also increases the risk of side effects and is subject to diminishing returns. For patients who experience significant adverse affects or have no response to the initial drug selection, an alternative medication from a different class can be substituted. Replacing the ineffective medicine with another or "sequential" monotherapy may ultimately benefit some patients (19), but can be time-consuming for those who do not respond. Several reasons are seen to consider combination drug therapy by prescribing small doses of two drugs with different mechanism of action (13). The goal with combination drug therapy is to maximize efficacy by using agents with additive or synergistic effects on blood pressure, while minimizing side effects. If a diuretic was not chosen as the initial drug, it is appropriate to add one as a second agent because of its ability to enhance the blood pressure–lowering effects of most classes of antihypertensive drugs (14). In some patients, the compliance gained with fixed-dose combination pills is worth the constraints on dosage selection. The most frequently prescribed combinations include a low-dose thiazide diuretic together with a beta-blocker, ACE inhibitor, or AIIA. Combinations of an ACE inhibitor and calcium-channel blocker have also been marketed. All fixed-dose combinations have been shown to be more effective than either agent used alone.

An important point that has escaped the attention of many clinicians is clear from recent studies: to achieve a target blood pressure of less than 140/90 mm Hg (or lower) requires combinations of more than one antihypertensive agent in most patients. This was evident in the HOT study and United Kingdom Prospective Diabetes study where more than two thirds of patients required combinations of antihypertensive agents to achieve a goal diastolic blood pressure level less than 85 mm Hg (6,20).

Hypertension in High-Risk Individuals
(Post-MI, LVH, proteinuria, renal insufficiency, diabetes)

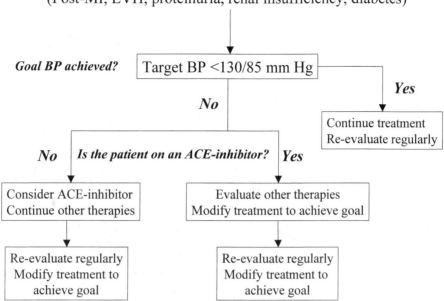

FIG. 21-4. Algorithm for the treatment of patients at high-risk, based on the presence of target organ damage, clinical cardiovascular disease, or diabetes mellitus. Angiotension converting enzyme (ACE) inhibitors have been shown to benefit these individuals. However, an appropriately low target blood pressure level should be sought, through the use of combinations of antihypertensive agents, as necessary.

PROTECTING PATIENTS AT HIGH RISK FOR CARDIOVASCULAR EVENTS

Both the JNC VI and WHO/ISH guidelines for the treatment of hypertension have acknowledged that patients at the highest risk for cardiovascular complications are those who have already manifested target organ damage or clinical cardiovascular disease (1,2). In almost all cases, these patients have been shown to have significant benefit and reduced mortality when treated with an ACE inhibitor. ACE inhibitors significantly prolong survival and prevent recurrent MI in patients with symptomatic CHF or following anterior MI. These findings have now been extended to individuals at high risk based on the presence of diabetes mellitus or other cardiovascular disease risk factors. In the Heart Outcomes Prevention Evaluation study, more than 9,000 patients at high risk for cardiovascular events (including >3,500 patients with diabetes mellitus) were randomly assigned to receive the ACE inhibitor, ramipril, versus placebo, with follow-up for 5 years (21). Underscoring the importance of high-normal blood pressure as a risk factor for progression of cardiovascular complications, the average blood pressure of patients entering the study was 139/79 mm Hg. Those patients receiving ramipril had a significant reduction in subsequent MI, stroke, CHF, or death from any cause. Patients with diabetes mellitus had similar benefits in addition to less progression of microalbuminuria to overt nephropathy (22). Based on these results, recommendations for the treatment of patients at high risk are presented in Fig. 21-4.

SUMMARY

It is through blood pressure lowering that reductions in cardiovascular morbidity and mortality are achieved. Treatment of hypertensive patients should also focus on prevention and management of cardiovascular complications through achieving a target level of blood pressure that is appropriate for the patient's clinical status. In making treatment decisions, it is appropriate to assess patients for the presence or absence of risk factors, target organ damage, and clinical cardiovascular disease. Clinicians should strive to use the least intrusive means possible to achieve goal blood pressure level and the treatment regimen should be individualized for each patient based on the presence or absence of risk factors, concomitant diseases, or comorbid conditions. In many cases, these additional factors can significantly influence what might be an appropriate treatment selection for a given patient with hypertension. Achieving that goal requires selecting the appropriate measures to lower blood pressure, identifying the patients who will benefit the most from treatment, treating to appropriate goals, reducing or eliminating other cardiovascular risk factors, and choosing a treatment plan that is acceptable to the patient.

REFERENCES

1. Joint National Committee on Prevention, Detection, Evaluation and Treatment of High Blood Pressure and the National High Blood Pressure Education Program Coordinating Committee. The Sixth Report of

the Joint National Committee on Prevention, Detection, Evaluation and Treatment of High Blood Pressure. *Arch Intern Med* 1997;157:2413–2446.

2. 1999 World Health Organization. International Society of Hypertension guidelines for the management of hypertension. Guidelines Subcommittee. *J Hypertens* 1999;17:151–183.

3. van den Hoogen PC, Feskens EJ, Nagelkerke NJ, et al. The relation between blood pressure and mortality due to coronary heart disease among men in different parts of the world. Seven Countries Study Research group. *N Engl J Med* 2000;342:1–8.

4. Appel LJ, Moore TJ, Obarzanek E, et al. A clinical trial of the effects of dietary patterns on blood pressure. *N Engl J Med* 1997;336:1117–1124.

5. Sacks FM, Svetkey LP, Vollmer WM, et al. A clinical trial of the effects on blood pressure of reduced dietary sodium and the DASH dietary pattern (The DASH-Sodium Trial). American Society of Hypertension, May 2000(abst).

6. Hansson L, Zanchetti A, Carruthers SG, et al., for the HOT Study group. Effects of intensive blood-pressure lowering and low-dose aspirin in patient with hypertension: principal results of the Hypertension Optimal Treatment (HOT) randomized trial. *Lancet* 1998;351:1755–1762.

7. National High Blood Pressure Education Program Working Group. National High Blood Pressure Education Program Working Group Report on Hypertension in the Elderly. *Hypertension* 1994;23:275–285.

8. SHEP Cooperative Research Group. Prevention of stroke by antihypertensive drug treatment in older persons with isolated systolic hypertension. Final results of the Systolic Hypertension in the Elderly program (SHEP). *JAMA* 1991;265:3255–3264.

9. Kostis JB, Davis BR, Cutler J, et al. Prevention of heart failure by antihypertensive drug treatment in older persons with isolated hypertension. SHEP Cooperative Research Group. *JAMA* 1997;278:212–216.

10. Syst-Eur Trial Investigators. Randomised double-blind comparison of placebo and active treatment for older patients with isolated systolic hypertension. *Lancet* 1997;350:757–764.

11. Tuomilehto J, Rastenyte D, Birkenhager WH, et al. Effects of calcium channel blockade in older patients with diabetes and systolic hypertension. Systolic Hypertension in Europe Trial investigators. *N Engl J Med* 1999;340:677–684.

12. ALLHAT Collaborative Research Group. Major cardiovascular events in hypertensive patients randomized to doxazosin vs chlorthalidone: the antihypertensive and lipid lowering treatment to prevent heart attack trial (ALLHAT). *JAMA* 2000;283:1967–1975.

13. Prisant LM, Doll NC. Hypertension: the rediscovery of combination therapy. *Geriatrics* 1997;52:28–38.

14. Materson BJ, Reda DJ, Cushman WC, et al., for the Department of Veterans Affairs Cooperative Study Group on Anti-Hypertensive Agents. Results of combination anti-hypertensive therapy after failure of each of the components. *J Hum Hypertens* 1995;9:791–796.

15. Lewis EJ, Hunsicker LG, Bain RP, et al. The effect of angiotensin-converting-enzyme inhibition on diabetic nephropathy. The Collaborative Study group. *N Engl J Med* 1993;329:1456–1462.

16. Ravid M, Brosh D, Levi Z, et al. Use of enalapril to attenuate decline in renal function in normotensive, normoalbuminuric patients with type 2 diabetes mellitus. A randomized, controlled trial. *Ann Intern Med* 1998;128:982–988.

17. Garg R, Yusuf S. Overview of randomized trials of angiotensin-converting enzyme inhibitors on mortality and morbidity in patients with heart failure. Collaborative Group on ACE Inhibitor trials. *JAMA* 1995;273:1450–1456.

18. Pitt B, Poole-Wilson PA, Segal R, et al. Effect of losartan compared with captopril on mortality in patients with symptomatic heart failure: randomised trial—the Losartan Heart Failure Survival Study ELITE II. *Lancet* 2000;355:1582–1587.

19. Materson BJ, Reda DJ, Preston RA, et al. Response to a second single antihypertensive agent used as monotherapy for hypertension after failure of the initial drug. Department of Veterans Affairs Cooperative Study Group on Antihypertensive Agents. *Arch Intern Med* 1995;155:1757–1762.

20. UK Prospective Diabetes Study Group. Tight blood pressure control and risk of macrovascular and microvascular complications in type 2 diabetes: UKPDS 38. *BMJ* 1998;317:703–713.

21. Yusuf S, Sleight P, Pogue J, et al. Effects of an angiotensin-converting-enzyme inhibitor, ramipril, on cardiovascular events in high-risk patients. The Heart Outcomes Prevention Evaluation Study Investigators. *N Engl J Med* 2000;342:145–153.

22. Heart Outcomes Prevention Evaluation (HOPE) Study Investigators. Effects of ramipril on cardiovascular and microvascular outcomes in people with diabetes mellitus: results of the HOPE study and MICRO-HOPE substudy. *Lancet* 2000;355:253–259.

CHAPTER 22

Chronic Angina Pectoris

R. Scott Wright and Bernard J. Gersh

BACKGROUND

This chapter presents succinctly our recommendations regarding management of patients with chronic stable angina in the form of critical pathways. It is not intended to be a comprehensive review. A recent consensus statement by the American College of Cardiology, American Heart Association, American College of Physicians, and American Society of Internal Medicine (ACC/AHA/ACP-ASIM) on the guidelines for the management of patients with chronic stable angina, can serve as an excellent reference that provides a comprehensive overview of this topic (1). Unstable angina and acute myocardial infarction (MI) are presented in other chapters.

Chronic stable angina is a medical condition characterized by predictable or intermittent symptoms of chest discomfort (angina pectoris) precipitated by exertion. Most patients with chronic angina pectoris have one or more flow-limiting lesions in the coronary vasculature and suffer angina as a consequence of myocardial ischemia. Some patients with chronic angina pectoris experience symptoms because of microcirculatory impairment or as a consequence of systemic hypertension. The AHA estimates that 6.3 million Americans have chronic angina (2). Almost all patients with chronic angina pectoris are treated with medications to limit symptoms. A great number of patients with chronic angina undergo coronary revascularization because of lifestyle-limiting symptoms. It is estimated that at least 700,000 patients annually have percutaneous or surgical coronary revascularization, mostly for chronic angina pectoris (3). The decision-making process regarding timing and mode of revascularization, which is important in patients with chronic stable angina, is discussed later in this chapter. It is important to use a common classification system for grading angina pectoris. Most clinicians use the Canadian classification system (CCS) as a standardized means for relating symptoms to lifestyle limitation (Fig. 22-1) (4).

EVALUATION OF THE PATIENT WITH ANGINA PECTORIS

Patients with chronic stable angina represent a significant proportion of the ambulatory office visits for evaluation and treatment of coronary artery disease (CAD). Given the recent advances in the successful treatment of acute MI and unstable angina, as well as the advances in preventive adjunctive medical therapies, it is to be expected that the number of patients with chronic stable angina who need periodic evaluation will increase. A patient presenting for the initial evaluation of angina pectoris should be evaluated in a somewhat different manner than that used for an individual with chronic angina who is undergoing routine evaluation as part of a periodic assessment.

Initial Evaluation

Our recommended approach to the evaluation of a patient with new onset angina pectoris is outlined in Fig. 22-2. The evaluation of patient with newly diagnosed angina pectoris should include a comprehensive history and physical examination. A baseline electrocardiogram (ECG) and chest x-ray study should be obtained. Special attention should be given to risk factor assessment. A fasting blood glucose and lipid panel should be obtained. The initial evaluation should attempt to uncover any comorbidities that might have an adverse impact on survival (e.g., peripheral vascular disease, carotid artery disease, or aortic aneurysmal disease). It is imperative to assess left ventricular (LV) systolic function because it is an important determinant of long-term survival and may guide further evaluation. We recommend a functional evaluation to determine the extent of ischemia and to identify individuals at high risk (e.g., those with exercise-induced hypotension, severe ischemia, and ventricular arrhythmias). Pharmacologic stress testing can be used for those individuals who are not able to exercise to a near maximal heart rate response.

Grade	Symptom Descriptions
I	Ordinary physical activity does not cause angina, such as walking, climbing stairs. Angina occurs with strenuous, rapid or prolonged exertion at work or recreation
II	Slight limitation of ordinary activity occurs because of angina symptoms. Angina occurs on walking or climbing stairs rapidly, walking uphill, walking or stair climbing after meals, or in the cold, or in wind, or under emotional stress, or only during the few hours after awakening. Angina occurs on walking **more than 2 blocks** on the level, or climbing more than one flight of ordinary stairs at a normal pace and in normal conditions.
III	There is marked limitation of ordinary activity because of anginal symptoms. Angina occurs on walking **one to two blocks** on the level and climbing one flight of stairs in normal conditions and at a normal pace.
IV	There is an inability to carry on any physical activity without discomfort – anginal symptoms may be present at rest.

FIG. 22-1. An outline of the Canadian Cardiovascular Society classification for angina pectoris.

Follow-Up Evaluation

The most appropriate approach in the periodic evaluation of the patient with chronic angina pectoris is a frequent clinical dilemma. Our suggested approach is shown in Fig. 22-3.

At least annually, the patient with stable angina pectoris should have a focused history and physical examination done by his or her physician. The history should focus on the functional status of the individual patient. The physician should determine whether the patient has experienced any acceleration of symptoms or anything to suggest worsened ischemia, including new dyspnea, fatigue, or any functional limitation. Additionally, the clinician should determine if any signs or symptoms of congestive heart failure (CHF) are present. The examination should focus on whether any clinical indicators of LV dysfunction are present. An annual chest x-ray study can be helpful in this regard because it may reveal early clinical evidence of heart failure or any change in cardiac size. An annual ECG is also essential, as it may reveal intercurrent changes that have not been accompanied by symptoms.

Annual treadmill testing in the asymptomatic patient with chronic stable angina is frequently performed, but only meets class IIB evidence for support according to the ACC/AHA/ACP-ASIM guidelines (1). A common clinical dilemma is that of defining the truly asymptomatic patient, especially in the physically inactive patient or the patient with diabetes mellitus who may not experience angina. Despite the lack of widespread outcome-based evidence to support routine exercise stress testing, we perform annual exercise stress testing on our patients with chronic angina. A normal result is reassuring to the patient, and the results can be used to determine a prescription for exercise. Additionally, annual surveillance provides a basis for demonstrating a pattern of functional decline or uncovering easily provoked silent ischemia and, thus, allows for further evaluation and treatment when clinically indicated. Patients with Wolff-Parkinson-White syndrome, chronic left bundle branch block (LBBB), and any evidence of clinical deterioration meet class I indications for exercise stress testing according to the ACC/AHA/ACP-ASIM guidelines (1). Patients with CCS class III angina, despite maximal medical therapy, should have cardiac catheterization and coronary revascularization instead of functional stress testing.

Periodically, the clinician should determine overall LV systolic and diastolic function. It is important to identify LV dysfunction in patients with CAD (5). A variety of methods

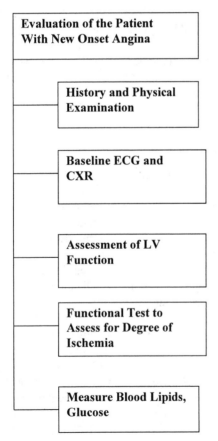

FIG. 22-2. An outline of the suggested approach to the evaluation of the patient with new onset angina pectoris.

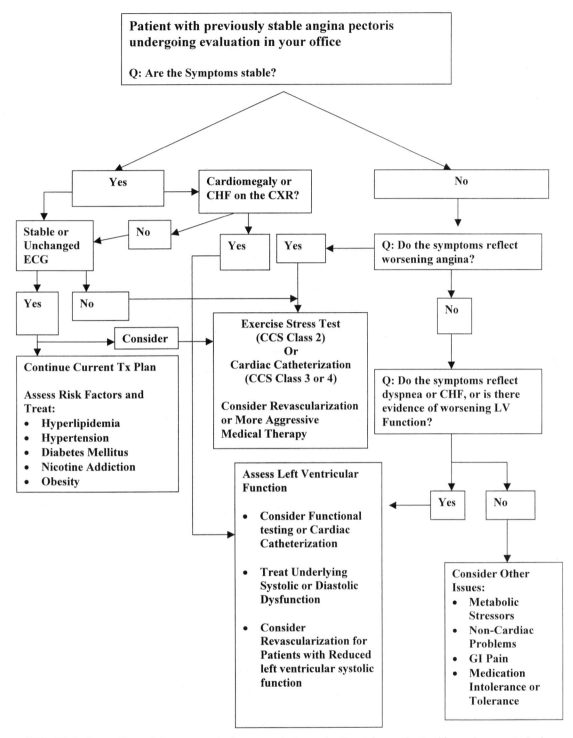

FIG. 22-3. An outline of the suggested approach to evaluation of a patient with angina pectoris for subsequent visits.

are available for determining LV function, including echocardiography, radionuclide angiography, and left ventriculography. It is not necessary to perform annual assessments of LV function (1). The timing of assessment of LV function should be based on a change in symptoms, functional status, or a change on the ECG or chest x-ray study that suggests the development of impaired cardiac performance. It is also important to determine if the patient with CAD has stable blood lipids or any evidence of (a) fasting hyperglycemia or worsening renal insufficiency, (b) uncontrolled hypertension, and (c) peripheral, carotid, or aortic vascular disease. The annual evaluation should include fasting lipids, a fasting glucose measurement, and an assessment of baseline renal function.

MEDICAL MANAGEMENT FOR STABLE ANGINA PECTORIS

The management of the patient with chronic stable angina should be comprehensive and it is imperative to address the following issues: (a) evaluation and intervention of known risk factors; (b) lifestyle modification that promotes regular exercise, cessation of unhealthy behaviors, and proper management of emotional and psychological stresses; (c) use of appropriate adjunctive medications proved to have secondary prevention benefit in patients with CAD (Fig. 22-4); and (d) use of revascularization, when appropriate, for symptom reduction or to enhance long-term survival. Although discussed individually, all of these issues must be addressed concurrently in each patient.

Our recommendations for adjunctive medical therapy are outlined in Fig. 22-4. Aspirin should be used in all patients with CAD who are not allergic to salicylate. Multiple studies have documented the secondary prevention benefit of aspirin therapy (6,7), and it remains the most cost-effective therapy among all adjunctive medications. For patients with an aspirin allergy, clopidogrel can be safely substituted, although it is less well established than aspirin for secondary prevention

(8). Some evidence suggests that the combination of aspirin and clopidogrel is superior to aspirin alone in patients with peripheral vascular disease (8).

All patients should have periodic lipid screening and be treated appropriately for dyslipidemia (Fig. 22-5). Three recent randomized trials have conclusively demonstrated that a statin agent has a profound secondary prevention benefit when used to treat hyperlipidemia in patients with CAD (9–11). The Simvastatin Scandinavian Survival study (4–S), Cholesterol and Recurrent Events (CARE) study, and the Long-Term Intervention with Pravastatin (LIPID) study all demonstrated that aggressive lipid lowering reduced (a) long-term cardiac and noncardiac mortality; (b) recurrence of acute MI and unstable angina; and (c) need for future revascularization with percutaneous coronary intervention (PCI) or coronary artery bypass graft (CABG). Statin agents are well tolerated in patients with CAD and have no long-term adverse consequences. Special attention should also be given to the patient with a low high-density lipoprotein (HDL) cholesterol level. The Veterans Affairs–HDL trial demonstrated that treatment of a low HDL with gemfibrozil significantly reduced future cardiovascular events and improved long-term survival (12). Both fibric acid derivatives and

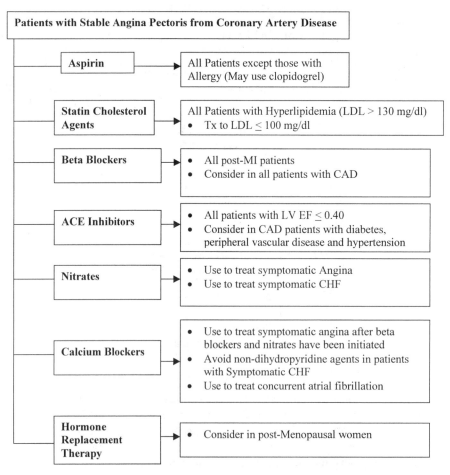

FIG. 22-4. Recommendations for adjunctive medications in patients with stable angina pectoris.

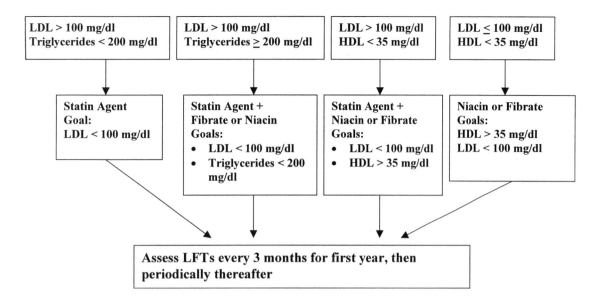

FIG. 22-5. An outline of the suggested treatment of dyslipidemia.

niacin-based compounds raise the HDL cholesterol level; recently, however, several statin agents have also been approved for raising the HDL cholesterol level. It is wise to treat aggressively hypertriglyceridemia, because many believe that elevated triglycerides represent an additional risk factor for CAD progression (13). The fibric acid derivatives and niacin-based agents both reduce triglycerides significantly, and can be used safely in combination with some statin agents.

Among the medical therapies, only two (aspirin and lipid lowering) have been shown convincingly to reduce mortality and morbidity in patients with chronic stable angina and preserved LV function. A large, randomized clinical trial—Heart Outcomes Prevention Evaluation (HOPE)—has provided strong evidence that angiotensin converting enzyme (ACE) inhibitors also reduce mortality and ischemic events in patients at high risk (e.g., those with diabetes mellitus, hypertension, and peripheral vascular disease) (14). Other therapies, including nitrates, beta-blockers, and calcium antagonists, have been shown to improve symptoms, functional status, and exercise performance, but their effect, if any, on survival has not been demonstrated. Nonetheless, a role is seen for ACE inhibitors, beta-blockers, nitrates, and calcium antagonists in patients with CAD as outlined in Fig. 22-4.

Angiotensin converting enzyme inhibitors should be used in all patients with symptomatic or asymptomatic LV dysfunction (15–18). These agents prolong survival and reduce the incidence of hospitalization for CHF. A strong case is proposed for using ACE inhibitors in patients with angina pectoris who are at high risk, namely those with diabetes mellitus, hypertension, and peripheral vascular disease. We cannot recommend widespread use of ACE inhibitors in the patients at less high risk with stable angina who have preserved LV function (14).

Beta-blocking agents, which are potent antianginal agents (19), have established secondary prevention benefit in patients after MI (20–21). Although no widespread evidence supports the routine use of beta-blockers in patients with stable angina pectoris who have not suffered an MI, it is probably best to use them anyway.

Nitrates can be used to treat symptomatic angina pectoris or heart failure, but do not need to be routinely used in patients with stable angina pectoris except for symptomatic relief (22). It is imperative, however, to educate and encourage patients with chronic angina on the prophylactic use of sublingual nitrates in the event of an attack of unstable angina. Calcium blockers are effective antianginal agents and can be safely used in combination with beta-blockers, nitrates, or both (23). Calcium blockers can also be used effectively to treat hypertension.

Vitamin supplements and herbal medicines remain unproved in patients with stable angina pectoris and are not routinely recommended. Chelation therapy is not routinely endorsed for patients with CAD.

SELECTING THE FUNCTIONAL TEST

We practice in an era concerned with cost-effectiveness and clinical value. It is important to consider these issues when selecting a functional test for patients with chronic stable angina (1). It is also critical that the planned functional test should have a direct impact on clinical decision-making, for if the information obtained has no direct impact on how the patient is to be managed, it should not be performed. Fig. 22-6 outlines our suggestions for functional test selection. Some patients with classic symptoms can best be served

with catheterization, especially when the pretest probability of a positive functional tests is high. The ACC/AHA/ACP-ASIM guidelines recommend catheterization for patients with CCS class 3 or greater angina who have symptoms, despite maximal medical therapy (1).

A variety of functional tests can be used in assessing ischemic burden. Most patients are well served with the basic exercise ECG (24). Those with recurrent symptoms and a history of CABG or PCI, those with Wolff-Parkinson-White syndrome, and those with LBBB are best served with an exercise-perfusion or exercise-imaging evaluation because information regarding location and extent of ischemia can have a direct impact on a treatment decision. Patients with a preexisting LBBB may best be served with

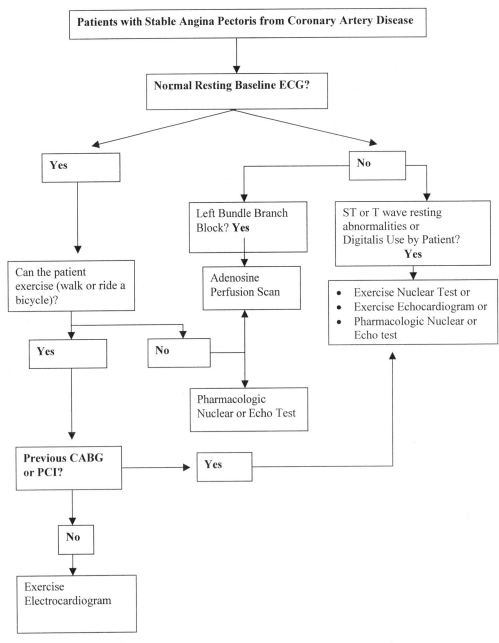

FIG. 22-6. A suggested approach to functional stress testing.

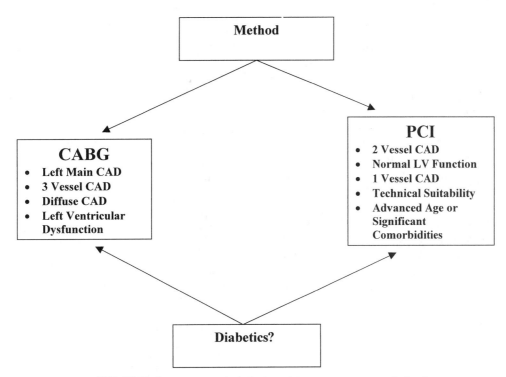

FIG. 22-7. A recommended strategy for coronary revascularization.

an adenosine-imaging test (25). Pharmacologic stress testing should be used for patients who are not able to exercise to a near maximal heart rate response. The major advantages of exercise-perfusion or exercise-imaging functional testing is that of increased sensitivity and the ability to better localize and quantify the degree of ischemia.

Nonetheless, most patients can be fully evaluated without the need for the more expensive functional tests. The results of the stress test can also serve to guide with a prescription for appropriate exercise goals.

INDICATIONS FOR REVASCULARIZATION

It is important to consider coronary revascularization in patients with chronic angina pectoris. Coronary revascularization improves quality of life for patients with limiting angina and prolongs survival in those with LV dysfunction and left main CAD. The decision regarding surgical or percutaneous revascularization (PCI) can be difficult and controversial. The decision should be based on a constellation of factors, including the number and location of diseased vessels, anatomic and technical issues which may have an impact on the success of PCI, the presence of LV dysfunction, the need for complete revascularization, and patient-related issues (e.g., age, occupation, comorbidities, and patient preferences).

The presence of left main coronary disease, three-vessel disease, diffuse coronary disease, and LV dysfunction tilt the decision in favor of surgical revascularization (26–29). The presence of single or double vessel disease, preserved LV function, and anatomic suitability tilt the decision in favor of PCI. The issue of diabetes is more of a controversial one.

The bypass angioplasty revascularization investigation comparing PCI with surgical revascularization suggested that diabetics do best with surgical revascularization (30). Nonetheless, many diabetics in this trial had high risk features such as diffuse disease, three-vessel disease, and LV dysfunction. This may explain why the long-term outcome of diabetics enrolled in the registry did not demonstrate a strong difference in survival between PCI and surgical revascularization (31). Fig. 22-7 is our suggested pathway for decision-making with regard to revascularization.

PATIENTS WITHOUT TRADITIONAL REVASCULARIZATION OPTIONS

Many patients with symptoms of angina pectoris are not considered eligible for traditional revascularization. It is estimated that approximately one million patients in the United States have chronic angina pectoris unrelieved by revascularization or aggressive medical management. A variety of options are now available to these patients. Most of the patients with chronic, persistent angina have had complete revascularization, have reasonably well-preserved LV function, and continue with symptoms, despite triple therapy with a beta-blocker, nitrate, and a calcium antagonist. Two recent options for treatment, which have shown significant promise, are transmyocardial laser revascularization and enhanced external counter-pulsation. Both have been demonstrated to reduce anginal symptoms (32–33). They should be considered when traditional revascularization is not an option, and maximal medical therapy has not alleviated anginal symptoms.

SUMMARY

Patients with stable angina pectoris comprise a large percentage of the patients with CAD. It is important to evaluate these patients carefully on a regular basis, with special emphasis given to issues that have an impact on prognosis and quality of life. It is important to use the appropriate adjunctive therapy in this population as well as to evaluate and treat cardiac risk factors. The treating clinician needs to manage concomitant medical issues (e.g., diabetes mellitus and hypertension) as these conditions can have a negative impact on survival in patients with CAD. Revascularization may need to be considered for certain subpopulations of patients with stable angina pectoris, especially if revascularization can improve quality of life or long-term outcome. One approach to management and decision-making for patients with stable angina pectoris has been suggested in this chapter.

REFERENCES

1. Gibbons RJ, Chatterjee K, Daley J, et al. ACC/AHA/ACP-ASIM guidelines for the management of patients with chronic stable angina pectoris: a report of the American College of Cardiology/American Heart Association Task Force on Practice Guidelines (Committee on the Management of Patients with Chronic Stable Angina). *J Am Coll Cardiol* 1999;33:2092–2197.
2. The American Heart Association. 1999 heart and stroke statistical update. Dallas, TX: American Heart Association, 1999.
3. McGoon MD, Fuster V, Gersh BJ, et al. Coronary revascularization: indications and options. In: Guiliani ER, Gersh BJ, McGoon MD, et al, eds. *Mayo Clinic practice of cardiology*. St. Louis: CV Mosby, 1996:1387.
4. Campeau L. Grading of angina pectoris [Letter]. *Circulation* 1976; 54:522–523.
5. Sanz G, Castaner A, Betriu A, et al. Determinants of prognosis in survivors of myocardial infarction. A prospective clinical angiographic study. *N Engl J Med* 1982;306:1065.
6. Ridker PM, Mafnson JE, Gaziano JM, et al. Low-dose aspirin therapy for chronic stable angina. A randomized, placebo-controlled clinical trial. *Ann Intern Med* 1991;114:835–839.
7. Antiplatelet Trialists Collaboration. Collaborative overview of randomised trials of antiplatelet therapy-I: prevention of death, myocardial infarction and stroke by prolonged antiplatelet therapy in various categories of patients. *BMJ* 1995;308:81–106.
8. CAPRIE Steering Committee. A randomised, blinded, trial of clopidogrel versus aspirin in patients at risk of ischaemic events (CAPRIE). *Lancet* 1996;348:1329–1339.
9. Randomised trial of cholesterol lowering in 4,444 patients with coronary heart disease: the Scandinavian simvastatin survival study (4S). *Lancet* 1994;344:1383–1389.
10. Sacks FM, Pfeffer MA, Moye LA, et al. The effect of pravastatin on coronary events after myocardial infarction in patients with average cholesterol levels. Cholesterol and Recurrent Events trial investigators. *N Engl J Med* 1996;335:1001–1009.
11. The Long-Term Intervention with Pravastatin in Ischaemic Disease (Lipid) Study Group. Prevention of cardiovascular events and death with pravastatin in patients with coronary heart disease and a broad range of initial cholesterol levels. *N Engl J Med* 1998;339:1349–1357.
12. Rubins HB, Robins SJ, Collins D, et al. Gemfibrozil for the secondary prevention of coronary heart disease in men with low levels of high-density lipoprotein cholesterol. Veterans Affairs high-density lipoprotein cholesterol intervention trial study group. *N Engl J Med* 1999;341:410.
13. Carlson LA, Bottiger LE, Ahpeldt PE. Risk factors for myocardial infarction in the Stockholm prospective study: a 14-year follow-up focusing on the role of plasma triglycerides and cholesterol. *Acta Med Scand* 1979;206:351–360.
14. The Heart Outcomes Prevention Evaluation Study Investigators. Effects of an angiotensin-converting-enzyme inhibitor, ramipril, on cardiovascular events in high-risk patients. *N Engl J Med* 2000;342:145–153.
15. Pfeffer MA, Braunwald E, Moye LA, et al. Effect of captopril on mortality and morbidity in patients with left ventricular dysfunction after myocardial infarction. Results of the survival and ventricular enlargement trial. *N Engl J Med* 1992;327:669.
16. The SOLVD Investigators. Effect of enalapril on survival in patients with reduced left ventricular ejection fractions and congestive heart failure. *N Engl J Med* 1991;325:293.
17. The SOLVD Investigators. Effect of enalapril on mortality and the development of heart failure in asymptomatic patients with reduced left ventricular ejection fractions. *N Engl J Med* 1992;327:685.
18. The Acute Infarction Ramipril Efficacy (AIRE) Study Investigators. Effect of ramipril on mortality and morbidity of survivors of acute myocardial infarction with clinical evidence of heart failure. *Lancet* 1993;342:821.
19. Opie LH, Sonnenblick EH, Kaplan NM. Beta-agents. In: Opie LH, Chatterjee K, eds. *Drugs for the heart*, 4th ed. Philadelphia: WB Saunders, 1995:20–23.
20. Gottlieb SS, McCarter RJ, Vogel RA. Effect of beta-blockade on mortality among high risk and low risk patients after myocardial infarction. *N Engl J Med* 1998;339:489.
21. Chem J, Marciniak TA, Radford MJ, et al. Beta-blocker therapy for secondary prevention of myocardial infarction in elderly diabetic patients. Results from the National Cooperative Cardiovascular project. *J Am Coll Cardiol* 1999;34:1388.
22. Parker JD, Parker JO. Nitrate therapy for stable angina pectoris. *N Engl J Med* 1998;338:520.
23. Freher M, Challapalli S, Pinto JV, et al. Current status of calcium channel blockers in patients with cardiovascular disease. *Curr Probl Cardiol* 1999;24:236.
24. Gibbons RJ. Exercise ECG testing with and without radionuclide studies. In: Wenger NK, Speroff L, Packard B, eds. *Cardiovascular health and disease in women*. Greenwich, CT: Le Jacq Communications, 1993: 73–80.
25. Wagdy HM, Hodge D, Christian TF, et al. Prognostic value of vasodilator myocardial perfusion imaging in patients with left bundle branch block. *Circulation* 1998;97:1563–1570.
26. Chaitman BP, Fisher LK, Bourassa MG. Effect of coronary bypass surgery on survival patterns in subsets of patients with left main coronary artery disease. Report of the Collaborative Study in Coronary Artery Surgery (CASS). *Am J Cardiol* 1981;48:765.
27. Passamani E, David KB, Gillespie MJ, et al., and the CASS principal investigators and their associates. A randomized trial of coronary artery bypass surgery. Surgery of patients with a low ejection fraction. *N Engl J Med* 1985;312:1665.
28. Mock MB, Ringqvist I, Fisher LD, et al., and participants in the Coronary Artery Surgery Study. Survival of medically treated patients in the Coronary Artery Surgery Study (CASS) Registry. *Circulation* 1982;66:562.
29. Yusuf S, Zucker D, Peduzzi P, et al. Effect of coronary artery bypass graft surgery on survival: overview of 10-year results from randomised trials by the Coronary Artery Bypass Graft Surgery Trialists Collaboration. *Lancet* 1994;344:563–570 [published erratum appears in *Lancet* 1994;344:1446].
30. The Bypass Angioplasty Revascularization Investigation (BARI) Investigators. Comparison of coronary bypass surgery with angioplasty in patients with multivessel disease. *N Engl J Med* 1996;335:217.
31. Detre KM, Guo P, Holubkov R, et al. Coronary revascularization in diabetic patients: a comparison of the randomized and observational components of the bypass angioplasty revascularization investigation (BARI). *Circulation* 1999;99:633.
32. Horvath KA, Cohn LH, Cooley DA, et al. Transmyocardial laser revascularization: results of a multicenter trial with transmyocardial laser revascularization used as sole therapy for end-stage coronary artery disease. *J Thorac Cardiovasc Surg* 1997;113:645.
33. Lawson WE, Hui JC, Cohn PF. Long-term prognosis of patients with angina treated with enhanced external counterpulsation: five-year follow-up study. *Clin Cardiol* 2000;23:254–258.

CHAPTER 23

Cardiac Rehabilitation in the Post Myocardial Infarction Patient

L. Howard Hartley

OVERVIEW

The management of patients who were recovering from heart attack began to change in the 1950s. In fact, before the 1950s, management could best be described as "convalescence" rather than "rehabilitation," because it was customary to leave patients at bed rest for many weeks. One of the first major breaks from this concept came from Levine and Lown who reported that patients who sat in a bedside chair after myocardial infarction (MI) had better outcomes than those who remained at bed rest (1). Although the report was not an exercise study (patients were lifted to the bedside chair) or randomized (they examined sequential patients), the observation heralded an attitude about activity in the postinfarction period that has led to the cardiac rehabilitation programs of today.

In the 1960s, programs were developed to encourage patients with uncomplicated MI to begin regular exercise for conditioning purposes (2). The programs quickly spread from coast to coast and early review of those experiences indicated that regular physical activity was not harmful (3) and, in fact, resulted in improved physiologic (4) and psychological profiles (5). Also, cardiac rehabilitation began to include major risk factor interventions as a regular part of its agenda.

A number of studies were performed over the ensuing years to examine the efficacy of cardiac rehabilitation programs. Improvement in working capacity was one of the earliest outcomes examined, and an increase was noted in virtually all studies. Data from one such experience is demonstrated in Fig. 23-1 (6). An increase in working capacity, in some cases, resulted from augmentation of maximal cardiac output (7), but in some patients was noted because of a reduction of myocardial oxygen uptake and, hence, less ischemia (8). Reduction in myocardial oxygen demands allowed the achievement of higher work intensities before the onset of ischemia, which is best demonstrated in patients with angina (9). Although specific data are available (8,9), this concept is presented in a idealized figure showing that heart rate

reduction is associated with less ST-segment depression in patients with coronary disease (Fig. 23-2). An increase in coronary blood flow after conditioning was observed in animals with surgically induced coronary stenosis, and the better blood flow seemed to be accounted for by improved collateral circulation (10). Some patients develop angina at a higher double product (heart rate × systolic blood pressure) after conditioning, which also suggests improved blood supply (11), but increased collateral circulation with physical activity has not been convincingly demonstrated. Lessening of the dimensions of coronary arterial lesions has been demonstrated with studies that feature both exercise and low-density lipoprotein cholesterol reductions, but the changes in arterial diameter are small (12). Overall, the evidence that the ischemic myocardium benefits from regular exercise is convincing, but more because of reduced oxygen demands than improved blood supply.

In numerous studies, improvement of other risk factors after participation in cardiac rehabilitation was also reported. Reductions in blood lipids, especially triglycerides, were noted (13). An increase in high-density lipoproteins has been observed, although the amount and duration of activity that is needed to induce that change is greater than is required for most other conditioning effects such as heart rate reduction and increase in working capacity (14). Blood pressure moderation has also been reported with regular conditioning exercise (15). Exercise is also a well-known contributor to successful weight control programs and many reports have pointed out greater success with exercise and diet together than with either alone (16). Hence, an emphasis on risk factors is clearly an appropriate component of cardiac rehabilitation. With the advent of newer pharmacologic agents for the management of blood lipids (17) and blood pressure (18), emphasis was diverted from "self-help" measures of diet and exercise to increasingly frequent reliance on drugs. The antihypertensive and lipid-lowering agents are highly successful, are easily and safely administered, and have been shown by randomized, controlled trials to be efficacious for promoting

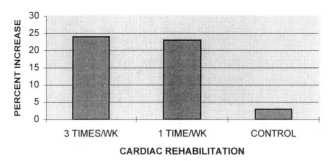

FIG. 23-1. The results of a randomized trial of cardiac rehabilitation in which patients came for either three times per week, once per week, or were in a usual medical care group (controls). Data were collected after 8 weeks in the program and both of the two cardiac rehabilitation groups exercised at least three times per week. The ordinate shows the percent increase in working capacity (measured in watts) over prerehabilitation values. The control group had no significant change.

good risk profiles and for saving lives. However, it is often overlooked that virtually all of the clinical studies of those compounds incorporated diet and exercise in their programs and, hence, the proper recommendation should be that efficacy has been demonstrated if diet, exercise, and pharmacologic agents are used together.

No single study has been performed with sufficient power to address the issue of impact of cardiac rehabilitation on morbidity and mortality. Although studies have been proposed, priorities have never been sufficiently favorable to permit their funding. Pharmacologic studies have been promoted more vigorously because the administration of pills is clearly less labor intensive than cardiac rehabilitation. Also, pharmaceutical companies have encouraged and funded drug studies, but have little enthusiasm for support of other lifestyle studies associated with cardiac rehabilitation.

Because a number of smaller randomized, controlled trials of cardiac rehabilitation have been performed as pilots or with outcomes other than mortality and morbidity, meta-analyses have been performed and reported from two institutions (Fig. 23-3) (19,20). The studies included in these analyses met certain requirements, including exercise as a major component. The results were strikingly consistent. Both showed a clear reduction in mortality for patients in cardiac

rehabilitation programs compared with usual care. However, neither could detect a reduction in rates of reinfarction. The analyses collected data from more than 10 clinical trials with 4,347 patient followed for 3 to 48 months. The reason for the higher total mortality rate with inactivity was not clear, although one of the substudies suggested it might relate to a reduction in sudden cardiac death (21). Of particular interest is the observation that the reduction in mortality is similar to that noted for other major interventions as demonstrated in Table 23-1, derived from the study by Lau et al. (22).

In the era of cost containment, it is also necessary to address cost-effectiveness. One of the early studies showed that attention to ambulation in the hospital resulted in earlier discharge after MI (23). Studies examining costs of medical care, recurrent hospitalizations, and medications concluded that cardiac rehabilitation was certainly very cost-effective per year of quality of life with values that are similar to those observed with pharmacologic agents (24–26). Other studies have reported earlier return to work and greater likelihood of reemployment after participation in cardiac rehabilitation programs (27). Obviously, all cost-effective studies must be viewed with some reservations, but available data do not suggest that formal cardiac rehabilitation carries an unaffordable cost.

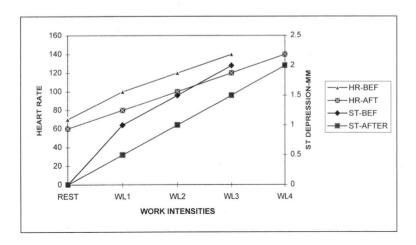

FIG. 23-2. In this idealized figure, the heart rate response to exercise is reduced after exercise conditioning and this reduction is associated with less ST-segment depression. At peak exercise, the heart rate and ischemia are almost the same after conditioning, but occur at a higher work intensity.

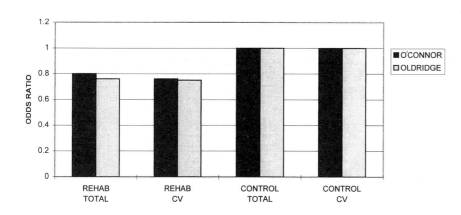

FIG. 23-3. The mean data derived from two meta-analyses of randomized, controlled trials of cardiac rehabilitation. Both show greater than 20% reduction in both total and cardiovascular mortality, which were highly significant. (From O'Connor GT, Buring JE, Yusuf S, et al. An overview of randomized trials of rehabilitation with exercise after myocardial infarction. *Circulation* 1989;80:234–244; and Oldridge NB. Outcome assessment in cardiac rehabilitation health related quality of life and economic evaluation. *J Cardiopulm Rehabil* 1997;17:179–194, with permission.)

However, many people do not have access to cardiac rehabilitation or are unable or unwilling to pay for the service. For this reason, it is important for clinicians to know the requirements for regular physical activity, because the absence of a formal program does not exempt them from the responsibility of promoting the continued good health of the patient who has survived a MI. We recommend referral to a cardiac rehabilitation program, but if that is not available (or not affordable), we provide some guidelines for the clinician to follow.

GUIDELINES FOR GOOD HEALTH

Physical Activity

Two points should be emphasized to patients: First, the amount of activity that is needed and, second, the intensity that is safe. The best safety data come from studies that have examined the experience of large cardiac exercise programs that were conducted in regular classes. This database allows a fairly accurate estimation of the likelihood of adverse events happening in a given time period. Studies of patients with cardiac disease (mostly after MI) who have exercised at higher intensities (jogging and running) report an occurrence of ventricular fibrillation that was approximately 1 in 6 to 12,000 person-hours of exercise in four studies (2,28–30) and 1 in 65,000 for one study (31). The patients who suffered cardiac arrest almost always survived because medical personnel were able to defibrillate them promptly, but they

probably would have died in unsupervised settings. Other reports of accumulated data from patients whose activity was carefully controlled by constant monitoring of the heart rate found the mortality rate was much lower, approximately 1 in 117,000 person-hours of exercise (31). The higher denominator figure is close to the expected random occurrence in patients with coronary heart disease. For this reason, we recommend that patients maintain their activity at a moderate pace, trying to avoid exceeding 80% of maximal oxygen uptake. This translates into a brisk walk (100–110 steps per minute) for most individuals.

The amount of activity that is needed should be expressed in minutes of moderate activity. It should also be emphasized that being on the feet all day (as a salesperson or housekeeper) does not suffice. The activity must be leisure-time activity performed for conditioning. The usual instructions of 5 minutes warm-up, 20 minutes of cardiovascular conditioning, and 5 minutes of cool-down three times per week is probably correct for minimal benefit. However, convincing evidence in the literature indicates that more (quantity, not intensity) is even better. Hence, we recommend that the activity should be carried out for 30 minutes 5 or 6 days per week. Allowing a day off weekly is a good idea because it allows the joints and muscles a brief respite.

Strength training by weight-lifting or resistive exercise does not produce meaningful cardiovascular benefits. However, if such activities are desired for muscle toning purposes, they can be done with low levels of weight. We recommend that weights start at 2 pounds and increase slowly to no more

TABLE 23-1. *Meta-analyses of various secondary prevention approaches*

Agent	Studies	N	Odds ratio	Confidence interval	P
Cardiac rehabilitation	23	5,022	0.8	0.67–0.95	<0.02
Anticoagulants	12	4,975	0.78	0.67–0.90	<0.001
Beta-blockers	17	20,138	0.81	0.73–0.89	<0.001
Cholesterol lowering	8	10,775	0.86	0.79–0.94	<0.001
Antiplatelets	9	13,917	0.83	0.74–0.93	<0.003
Calcium channel blockers	6	13,114	1.01	0.91–1.12	0.91

This table shows the meta-analyses of five common secondary prevention items and permits a comparison with cardiac rehabilitation. The order of magnitude is in the range provided by other interventions.

than 10 pounds of resistance for patients with heart disease. Usually, such exercises are done with weights in the hands while moving the upper extremity carefully through a full range of motion. Careful attention should be paid to joint or muscular pain that might herald problems for the unaccustomed activity. It is important to emphasize to patients that they should do the cardiovascular exercises faithfully and not substitute strength training. Strength training should supplement, not replace the cardiovascular exercise.

Nutrition

If the patient is overweight (a body mass index of $>27\,\mathrm{kg/m^2}$), the nutritional emphasis should be placed on calorie control. Calorie counting can be effective, but it is difficult and very few people will comply with the record-keeping over long periods of time. Our experience has been that qualitative changes in the diet are more likely to be successful over the long run. We recommend that patients follow the guidelines outlined in Table 23-2 (33–36) as a start.

Education

Instructing patients about their disease may seem unnecessary, but experience has shown that misconceptions abound. Many of these misconceptions are harmful, such as the following: "any activity is dangerous," "my heart function is only 50% of normal" (when the ejection fraction is 50%), "my family has heart disease so there is nothing I can do to help myself." Also, a frequent concern in patients after a MI is that any discomfort above the waist is caused by heart problems, angina leads to loss of heart muscle, nitroglycerin is addicting, and many more. It is very important to spend a few minutes discussing with the patients their specific disease, telling them how their outlook is actually good, and that if they adhere to good health measures, they may actually have a life expectancy that is better than it was before their event (most have many reversible risk factors which they have either ignored or not known).

Physician encouragement to the patient to follow a healthy lifestyle is very important. Studies have shown that a physician's recommendation is one of the most powerful

---

TABLE 23-2. *Recommended food habits for calorie control*

- Avoid eating beef, pork, ham, lamb, organ meats (liver, kidney, brain), hot dogs, sausages, hamburgers, duck, or goose. Replace these meats with fish, chicken, turkey, lean veal, or vegetarian substitute for the meat-group contribution to your nonbreakfast meals. These meat group items are lower in fat and calories than red meats (e.g., beef, pork, and lamb).
- Avoid eating ham, bologna, salami, prepared and sliced luncheon meats, liverwurst, hamburgers, hot dogs, or sausages. Luncheon slices of desirable foods such as turkey or chicken are acceptable.
- Avoid eating beef, lamb, or pork (including bacon, ham, and sausages) as breakfast foods.
- Avoid whole eggs for any meal. Egg whites and egg substitutes are healthful, but the yolks contain much cholesterol and should be avoided.
- Avoid whole milk, including buttermilk. Instead, use skimmed milk and products of skimmed milk that are healthy and desirable because the cream that contains the cholesterol and fat has been removed.
- Do not eat ice cream. Even skimmed milk ice cream contains a large amount of refined sugar and therefore is high in calories. Fresh fruits can be prepared as a frozen dessert, but most sherbets contain sugar and should be avoided. Refined sugars are undesirable because they have a tendency to increase blood fats and stimulate the appetite. The sweet taste in fruits is from complex carbohydrates, which are nourishing sources of energy. Hence, fresh fruit rather than refined sugar should be used for sweetening.
- Avoid whipped cream, nondairy whipped cream, cream cheese, sour cream, coffee cream, and nondairy creamer. Plain skim or low fat yogurt, cottage cheese, and fresh fruit purees should be used to minimize the intake of fats.
- Avoid eating cheese that is not low in fat content. Most cheeses have a high fat or oil content. Only those cheeses made with skimmed milk are acceptable.
- Avoid eating butter. Butter contains too much fat and cholesterol. Margarine has little or no cholesterol, but is very high in calories and often contains compounds that the body converts into cholesterol. Low fat cottage cheese can be substituted for butter or margarine.
- Do not eat pie, pastry, sweet rolls, cake, coffee cake, cookies, doughnuts, or candy. Recipes are available for preparing healthful baked foods, but most commercially available baked foods contain whole milk, butter, sugar, or oil (look at the label), which you should avoid. If you are unable to prepare suitable baked foods, please substitute fresh fruits, fruit salads, or ices for desserts or snacks.
- You should not consume more than three caffeine-containing beverages per day. Studies in the medical literature are confusing and often contradictory. Although we admit we are not certain of the exact safe amount, our recommendations are based on studies that have indicated that adverse outcomes increase at a greater rate when consumption of coffee exceeds three cups per day (33), and that serum cholesterol is significantly higher with more coffee consumption than three cups per day (34).
- Three rules about alcohol: If you do not drink alcohol, do not start. If you do drink, limit yourself to one drink per day. If you are trying to lose weight, do not drink any alcoholic beverage (empty calories). Although much has been written about alcohol consumption as a means of lowering the incidence of heart disease, several points need emphasizing. First, many individuals who begin consuming alcohol in moderation become addicted to alcohol and become excessive drinkers, which is clearly harmful. Secondly, alcohol is very caloric, which is a major problem for individuals who are obese. Thirdly, alcohol has some undesirable effects that are especially relevant to heart disease and hypertension: They increase serum triglycerides (35) and raise blood pressure (36).

contributors to smoking cessation (37). This is also undoubtedly true of regular physical activity and good nutrition. Also, attention should be paid to reinforce the need to avoid substance abuses (including alcohol), which carry special risks for the cardiac patient.

CARDIAC REHABILITATION PROGRAMS

If the aforementioned strategies are adequate, why refer to a cardiac rehabilitation program, even if it is available? The added trouble for the patient and the expense would not seem to be warranted. All of the interventions discussed can be done better by trained professionals than by a busy practitioner who had neither the time nor the training to carry them out. More specific physical activity guidelines can be provided because the electrocardiogram and blood pressure can be monitored during the activity. This often enables patients to do much more than is possible with general instructions. Also, it gives patients more confidence because the direct surveillance helps them to feel that all is going well.

Participation in groups enables patients to interact with others who have similar problems, to hear their questions, and to realize that they are not alone. The group dynamic is especially important for assessment of symptoms, and for allaying anxiety about certain activities. Group leaders are adept at encouraging verbalization of problems, both real and imagined.

Surveillance of patients during sessions helps to ensure that all is going well. The discovery of arrhythmias, unsuspected ischemic episodes, or adverse reactions to drugs are additional reasons for repeated surveillance. Many of these outcomes would often either not be noticed by the patient or would be misunderstood.

Finally, the studies that have examined cardiac rehabilitation clearly show that such programs outperform usual medical care. Hence, to deliver optimal care, physicians must either upgrade to cardiac rehabilitation standards (which in most cases is impractical) or refer to established programs.

CRITICAL PATHWAY

A critical pathway for participation in cardiac rehabilitation after MI is shown in Fig. 23-4. As with other secondary prevention tools, it should take its place as a necessary guideline for proper patient follow-up. If cardiac rehabilitation programs are not available, the attending physician must be prepared to ensure that all of the elements of secondary prevention are provided, including physical activity, proper nutrition, and healthy lifestyle.

SUMMARY

Cardiac rehabilitation is an essential part of the management of patients who have survived an MI. Participation has been shown to be efficacious for both quality and quantity

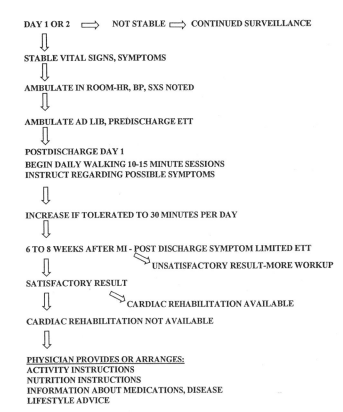

FIG. 23-4. Management pathway for participation in cardiac rehabilitation after myocardial infarction.

of life, and the service is cost-effective. Referral to a cardiac rehabilitation program is preferred; if such services are not available, however, the clinician must be prepared to ensure that they are provided.

REFERENCES

1. Levine SA, Lown B. Armchair treatment of acute coronary thrombosis. *JAMA* 1952;148:1365.
2. Hartley LH. Exercise and cardiac rehabilitation. Proceedings of the New England Cardiovascular Society 1976;28:37–40.
3. Haskell WL. Cardiovascular complications during exercise training of cardiac patients. *Circulation* 1978;57:920–924.
4. Hagberg JM, Ehsani AA, Holloszy JO. Effect of 12 months of intense exercise training on stroke volume in patients with coronary artery disease. *Circulation* 1983;67:1194–1199.
5. Hartley LH. Post myocardial infarction. In: Herd JA, ed. *Behavior and atherosclerosis*. New York: Plenum Press, 1983:II (Pt I):111–116.
6. Sherwood J, Hartley LH. Optimal frequency of follow-up for rehabilitation after myocardial infarction. *Circulation* 1983;68:III-150.
7. Dziekan G, Myers J, Goebbels U, et al. Effects of exercise training on limb blood flow in patients with reduced ventricular function. *Am Heart J* 1998;136:1,22–30.
8. Vanhees L, Fagard R, Lijnen P, et al. Influence of physical training on blood pressure, plasma renin, angiotensin and catecholamines in patients with ischaemic heart. *Eur J Appl Physiol* 1984;53:3,219–224.
9. Detry J-M, Bruce RA. Effect of physical training on exertional ST segment depression in coronary heart disease. *Circulation* 1971;XLIV:390–395.
10. Eckstein RW. Effect of exercise and coronary artery narrowing on coronary collateral circulation. *Circ Res* 1957;5:230–235.
11. Sim DN, Neill WA. Investigation of the physiological basis for increased exercise threshold for angina pectoris after physical conditioning. *J Clin Invest* 1974;54:763–770.

12. Brown G, Albers JJ, Fisher LD, et al. Regression of coronary artery disease as a result of intensive lipid-lowering therapy in men with high levels of apoliproprotein B. *N Engl J Med* 1990;323:1289–1298.
13. Ribeiro J, Hartley LH, Sherwood J, et al. The effectiveness of a low lipid diet and exercise in the management of coronary disease. *Am Heart J* 1984;108:1183–1189.
14. Kokkinos PF, Fernhall B. Physical activity and high density lipoprotein cholesterol levels: what is the relationship? *Sports Med* 1999;28:5,307–314.
15. Halbert JA, Silagy CA, Finucane P, et al. The effectiveness of exercise training in lowering blood pressure: a meta-analysis of randomised controlled trials of 4 weeks or longer. *J Hum Hypertens* 1997;11:641–649.
16. Ribeiro J, Hartley LH, Sherwood J, et al. The effectiveness of a low lipid diet and exercise in the management of coronary disease. *Am Heart J* 1984;108:1183–1189.
17. Knopp RH. Drug treatment of lipid disorders. *N Engl J Med* 1999;341:498–511.
18. The sixth report of the Joint National Committee on prevention, detection, evaluation, and treatment of high blood pressure. *Arch Intern Med* 1997;157:2413–2446.
19. O'Connor GT, Buring JE, Yusuf S, et al. An overview of randomized trials of rehabilitation with exercise after myocardial infarction. *Circulation* 1989;80:234–244.
20. Oldridge NB. Outcome assessment in cardiac rehabilitation health related quality of life and economic evaluation. *J Cardiopulm Rehabil* 1997;17:179–194.
21. Kallio V, Hamalainen H, Hakkila J, et al. Reduction in sudden deaths by a multifactorial intervention programme after acute myocardial infarction. *Lancet* 1979;2:1081–1094.
22. Lau J, Antman EM, Jimenez-Silva J, et al. Cumulative meta-analysis of therapeutic trials for myocardial infarction. *N Engl J Med* 1992;327:248–254.
23. Bloch A, Maeder JP, Haissly JC, et al. Early mobilization after myocardial infarction. A controlled study. *Am J Cardiol* 1974;34:2,152–157.
24. Ades PA, Pashkow FJ, Nestor JR. Cardiac rehabilitation participation predicts lower rehospitalization costs. *Am Heart J* 1992;123:916.
25. Levin L-A, Perk J, Hedback B. Cardiac rehabilitation—a cost analysis. *J Intern Med* 1991:230:427–434.
26. Oldridge N, Furlong W, Feeny D, et al. Economic evaluation of cardiac rehabilitation soon after acute myocardial infarction. *Am J Cardiol* 1993;72:154–161.
27. Dugmore LD, Tipson RJ, Phillips MH, et al. Changes in cardiorespiratory fitness, psychological well-being, quality of life, and vocational status following a 12 month cardiac exercise rehabilitation programme. *Heart* 1999;81:359–366.
28. Fletcher GF, Cantwell JD. Ventricular fibrillation in a medically supervised cardiac exercise program: clinical, angiographic, and surgical correlations. *JAMA* 1977;238:2627–2629.
29. Leach CN Jr, Sands MG Jr, Lachman AS, et al. Cardiac arrest during exercise training after myocardial infarction. *Conn Med* 1982;46:239–243.
30. Mead WF, Pyfer HR, Thrombold JC, et al. Successful resuscitation of two near simultaneous cases of cardiac arrest with a review of fifteen cases occurring during supervised exercise. *Circulation* 1976;53:187–189.
31. Hossack KF, Hartwig R. Cardiac arrest associated with supervised cardiac rehabilitation. *J Cardiac Rehabil* 1982;2:402–408.
32. Van Camp SP, Peterson RA. Cardiovascular complications of outpatient cardiac rehabilitation programs. *JAMA* 1986;256:1160–1164.
33. Lacroix AZ, Mead LA, Liang K, et al. Coffee consumption and the incidence of coronary heart disease. *N Engl J Med* 1986;315:977–982.
34. Bak AA, Grobbee DE. The effect on serum cholesterol levels of coffee brewed by filtering or boiling. *N Engl J Med* 1989;321:1432–1437.
35. Rimm EB, Williams P, Fosher K, et al. Moderate alcohol intake and lower risk of coronary heart disease: meta-analysis of effects on lipids and hemostatic factors. *BMJ* 1999;319:1523–1528.
36. Puddey IB, Beilin LJ, Vandongen R. Regular alcohol use raises blood pressure in treated hypertensive subjects: a randomised controlled trial. *Lancet* 1987;1:647–651.
37. Manley MW, Epps RP, Glynn TJ. The clinician's role in promoting smoking cessation among clinic patients. *Med Clin North Am* 1992;76:2,477–494.

CHAPTER 24

Smoking Cessation

Beth C. Bock and Bruce Becker

EFFECTS OF SMOKING ON HEALTH

Cigarette smoking is the leading cause of preventable morbidity and mortality in the United States today (1). Tobacco use is causally linked to diseases such as cancer, heart disease, stroke, and chronic obstructive pulmonary disease (2), and it is responsible for more than $50 billion in annual healthcare expenditures (3). Each year in the United States, more than 430,000 deaths are linked to cigarette smoking, and one third of deaths among former smokers are directly attributable to tobacco use (4). Moreover, environmental tobacco smoke or "secondhand smoke" has been strongly associated with respiratory illness in children, and with both cancer and heart disease in adults living with smokers. Although the prevalence of smoking decreased in the United States between 1950 and 1980, this trend has not continued (5). Today, one quarter of all adults living in this country smoke (6).

SMOKING CESSATION IN CARDIAC PATIENTS

Coronary heart disease is the leading cause of mortality in the United States, accounting for almost half of all deaths (7). Cigarette smoking greatly increases the risk of death from heart disease and smoking cessation produces marked reductions in cardiovascular risk (2). The experience of hospitalization, particularly for cardiovascular disease, can result in smoking cessation even without intervention (8–10). However, cessation rates vary greatly, depending on the reason for hospitalization, length of stay, and the presence of depressive symptoms (11). For example, Rigotti et al. found high cessation rates (58%) 1 year after hospitalization among patients having coronary bypass, whereas other studies have shown low cessation rates among smokers immediately after hospitalization (13.7%) and at 1-year follow-up (9.2%) (12,13). Most individuals who quit smoking without intervention will relapse within 6 months (14).

PHYSICIAN INTERVENTIONS

Although 70% of smokers visit a physician each year, very few of their doctors use this opportunity to address the patient's smoking (15). Physicians practicing in specialties such as cardiology or emergency medicine are less likely to provide smoking cessation interventions than primary care physicians (16). Possible explanations cited for low physician intervention rates include lack of time, deficient training in counseling skills, and an absence of organizational supports (17–20). This is regrettable because multiple studies have shown that even a brief intervention lasting less than 3 minutes significantly increases the chance that the smoker will quit (21). Formal physician training, the use of cues or reminders, pharmacologic aids, follow-up visits, and supplemental educational materials all increase the effectiveness of physician-delivered interventions (22). Cardiologists seeing smokers with coronary artery disease, hypertension, or histories of recurrent chest pain can be especially effective because the patient's illness can be linked directly to smoking. The clinical encounter is an important opportunity to address smoking cessation, and should not be missed (23). Many physicians, however, do not feel that they have the counseling skills or training to address the issue of smoking cessation effectively. This chapter provides a well-researched, effective, and simple approach that cardiologists can use to counsel their patients who smoke.

TREATMENT APPROACHES

Recent clinical guidelines have been developed through a joint collaboration between the Centers for Disease Control and the Agency for Healthcare Research and Quality (AHRQ) together with the National Cancer Institute, the National Heart, Lung, and Blood Institute, the National Institute on Drug Abuse, the Robert Wood Johnson Foundation, and the University of Wisconsin Medical School Center for Tobacco Research and Intervention (21). The recommendations made as a result of this extensive, systematic review and analysis of the extant peer-reviewed scientific literature form the basis of the approach taken in this chapter.

The key principles underlying these recommendations are:

1. Physicians must identify all of their patients who smoke.
2. Effective treatment is available for tobacco dependence.
3. Physicians must offer treatment to all of their smoking patients who are ready to quit.
4. Physicians should offer treatment even to those smoking patients who are not yet ready or willing to quit because the physician's intervention has been shown to increase the smoker's readiness and motivation to quit.
5. The physician should understand that tobacco dependence is a chronic condition that typically requires repeated intervention before long-term success is achieved.

The best practice model for a brief intervention for smoking cessation is easily summarized by the mnemonic device of the "Five As" (Table 24-1). Each of these As—ask, advise, assess, assist, and arrange follow-up—is summarized below (Fig. 24-1).

Ask

National guidelines recommend that physicians systematically determine the smoking status of all patients at every visit. This can be done by modifying the routine vital sign charting (Fig. 24-2).

Advise

Every tobacco user should be given clear, strong, and personalized advice to quit. Unfortunately, research has repeatedly shown that smoking counseling is not provided at most physician visits (18). Moreover, specialists are less likely to provide smoking counseling than primary care physicians (24).

Counseling does not need to be extensive to be effective. Brief, clear advice from a physician has been shown to **double** quit rates (21). For example, advice to a patient who is currently enrolled in cardiac rehabilitation might sound like this:

- **Clear:** "It is important for you to quit smoking."
- **Strong:** "Because you have already experienced heart disease (or specify condition), the most important thing you can do to avoid repeating this experience is to quit smoking."
- **Personal:** "Your exercise capacity and your ability to be physically active will improve much faster if you quit smoking."
- **Other phrases that work are:** "As your physician, I want you to know that the most important thing you can do to protect or improve your health, is to quit smoking." "Quitting smoking is important for everyone who smokes, but for you its especially important because of (specify current health problem)."

Assess

Assess the patient's readiness to quit smoking and level of nicotine dependence.

TABLE 24-1. *The five As to intervention in smoking cessation*

Ask:	The physician should **ask** all patients if they smoke or have recently quit.
Advise:	The physician should give every tobacco user clear, strong, and personalized **advice** to quit.
Assess:	The physician should **assess** the patient's level of nicotine dependence and readiness to quit.
Assist:	The physician should **assist** the patient in obtaining one or more of the effective treatments that exist for smoking cessation.
Arrange follow-up:	The physician should **arrange follow-up** to reinforce successful efforts and to identify slips early so that barriers can be identified and motivation to try again is renewed.

Readiness to Quit Smoking

Readiness to quit smoking is a key determinant of the treatment approach (Fig. 24-3). Treatment for smokers who are ready to make a serious attempt to quit should be focused on behavioral strategies, including (a) selecting a target quit date; (b) reviewing and arranging appropriate pharmacologic therapies, and (c) referring to self-help or professional programs. Treatment for smokers who are not ready to quit should focus on helping the patient get ready to quit. Treatment for these smokers should focus on the psychological issues surrounding cessation, including reasons for quitting versus reasons for continued smoking, concerns about the cessation process, building the patient's self-confidence, and discussing family or social supports and barriers to quitting.

Motivation, or readiness to quit smoking, has most often been measured using Prochaska and DiClemente's stages of change model (25), which was developed for use in outpatient populations. Because smoking restrictions in the inpatient setting and hospitalization encourage serious thought about smoking habits, this algorithm may tend to misclassify smokers as having more motivation to quit than they actually do. Recent research has shown that asking inpatients a single question regarding how likely it is that they will remain abstinent after hospital discharge may be more predictive of actual motivation (26).

Nicotine Dependence

The most widely used and validated measure of nicotine dependence is the *Fagerstrom Test for Nicotine Dependence* (Table 24-2). Patients scoring 6 or more are highly nicotine dependent. It is important to know the level of nicotine dependence because, although research shows that most smokers benefit from nicotine replacement therapy (NRT), providing NRT is especially important for highly dependent smokers. Overall, smokers who use nicotine replacement show double the success rates as those who do not (21,27). Highly nicotine-dependent smokers are three times

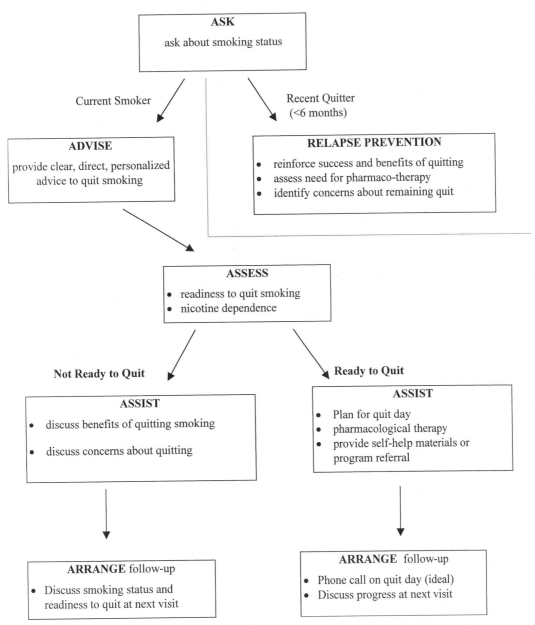

FIG. 24-1. Summary of the "Five As."

more likely to be successful if they use nicotine replacement. Moreover, the physician should choose the initial dose of NRT after considering the patient's level of nicotine dependence.

Assist

Motivational Approach

Many different types of smokers exist. To simplify, however, consider smokers as falling into one of two groups: those who are ready to quit and those who are not yet ready. Research studies have repeatedly shown that physicians who take a motivational approach to addressing smoking with their patients are more successful in helping these smokers to quit. Motivational approaches, including the "transtheoretical" or "stages of change" model and motivational interviewing, are widely used theoretical models of how people change health behaviors (25,28). Developed for use in outpatient populations, the basic tenet of these models is that individuals who are not yet ready to change behavior need to be approached differently than those who are ready to change. In practical terms, this means that treatment goals for smokers who are not yet ready to quit should focus on identifying reasons to quit, enhancing motivation for quitting, and identifying perceived barriers. Treatment for these smokers should avoid immediate behavioral goal-setting (e.g., discussing quit dates or selecting pharmacologic treatments). Conversely, interventions for smokers who are ready to quit should focus on behavioral goals (e.g., choosing a target quit date and pharmacotherapy) and coping strategies.

VITAL SIGNS	Date of visit _____
Blood Pressure_____	Heart rate_____
Weight_____ Temperature____	Respiration_____

Smoking Status: ☐ Current_____ rate (cigarettes/day)

  ☐ Former_____ date last smoked

  ☐ Never

FIG. 24-2. Sample routine vital sign charting.

Concerns About Quitting

Many patients are aware that they should quit smoking, but have concerns about the process of quitting or are discouraged from prior failed attempts. These patients may benefits by exploring their concerns about quitting. The decisional balance worksheet has been used in numerous smoking cessation trials to help smokers identify both their reasons for wanting to quit and perceived barriers to quitting (Fig. 24-4).

Not Ready to Quit

Patients who are not yet ready to quit need help identifying reasons to quit, improving their motivation and confidence in their ability to quit, and identifying barriers to smoking cessation. These patients may lack, or believe they lack, the financial resources to afford NRT or pharmacologic aids to quitting, or information about how smoking is affecting their health. They may have concerns about quitting—possibly related to prior failed attempts (29). The physician can intervene with these patients by providing relevant information that will help them identify barriers to quitting and find the resources necessary to support cessation. Motivational interventions are most successful when the physician is empathic, promotes patient autonomy (provides choices among

ASSESS Readiness to Quit Smoking

Outpatients:

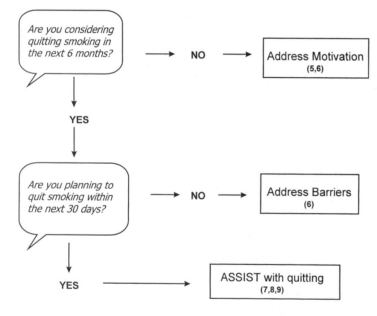

Inpatients:

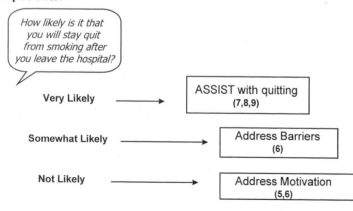

FIG. 24-3.

TABLE 24-2. *Fagerstrom test for nicotine dependence (FTND)*

	Points			
	0	1	2	3
How many cigarettes do you smoke per day?	≤10	11–20	21–30	≥30
Do you smoke more in the morning (or when you first wake up) compared to the rest of the day?	No	Yes		
Do you find it difficult to not smoke in places where smoking is not allowed, like church or the movies?	No	Yes		
How soon after walking do you smoke your first cigarette?	>60 min	31–60 min	6–30 min	<5 min
Do you smoke when you are so ill that you must stay in bed?	No	Yes		
Which cigarette of the day would you most hate to give up?	Any other	The first		

From Heatherton TF, Kozlowski LT, Frecker RC, et al. The Fagerstrom test for nicotine dependence: a revision of the Fagerstom Tolerance Questionnaire. *British Journal of Addiction* 1991;86:1119–1127.

options), supports the patient's sense of self-confidence, and avoids argumentation (30,31).

The "Good Reasons to Stop Smoking Now" and the "Benefits of Quitting Smoking" lists may be helpful (Figs. 24-5A and 24-5B).

Ready to Quit

Effective treatments exist for smoking cessation and should be provided to all smokers who are ready to quit. Effective treatment components include:

- Selecting a target quit day
- Reviewing pharmacologic therapies with the patient and selecting appropriate options
- Anticipating challenges (work schedules, stressors, social supports, and saboteurs)
- Offering referral to self-help materials or specialized programs and resources

Planning to Quit

Guidelines suggested to help those patients planning to quit include the following:

1. Select a target quit date: usually within 2 weeks of the office visit. Total abstinence as of this date is essential.
2. Prepare the environment: If possible, eliminate ashtrays, smoking paraphernalia, and cigarette supply.
3. Past experience: Review what worked, and what caused prior relapses.
4. Plan the day: Patient's need to consider how they will alter their usual routine to avoid smoking. Avoid alcohol. For a few days, the patient may need to avoid people and places associated with smoking. Patients should anticipate triggers and have a coping plan.
5. Recommend pharmacotherapy: Consider using medications if not contraindicated. Explain how these medications can reduce withdrawal symptoms and increase chances of success.
6. Suggest social support: Have the patient identify family, friends, or coworkers who will be helpful. Arrange for other household smokers to restrict their smoking near the patient.
7. Schedule a follow-up visit.

Arrange Follow-up

Follow-up Visits

Ideally, the first follow-up visit should occur within 1 week of the quit date. A phone contact on the quit day is helpful to most smokers. Congratulate and reinforce the patient's success. If the patient has smoked, identify circumstances surrounding slips; reframe slips as learning experiences—not as signs of failure; identify a new target quit day; reassess the need for pharmacotherapy; consider referral to a more intensive program. A second follow-up visit is recommended within 1 month.

Discuss Concerns About Continuing Not to Smoke

Nicotine dependence is a chronic and recurring condition, often requiring several serious quit attempts before permanent success is achieved. Therefore, physicians should be prepared to address relapse prevention with any patient who has recently quit smoking (<6 months abstinence). Physicians should reinforce success, the benefits of quitting smoking, and help patients identify any problems or concerns they may have about staying quit. Even patients who have recently quit smoking may be helped with pharmacotherapy or behavioral therapy and referrals (Table 24-3) (49,50).

Short-Term Coping Strategies

Short-term strategies the clinician can suggest to the patient include (a) remove all smoking-related paraphernalia (e.g., ashtrays, lighters) from the home, office, and car; (b) keep cigarettes out of easy reach (in an out-of-the-way kitchen cupboard, in the garage, in the trunk of the car); (c) be prepared to ask others to modify their behavior for a short while; (d) avoid alcohol; (e) exercise—brief walks during the day reduce stress and get the smoker out of the environment wherein smoking might be triggered; and (f) reward positive change.

PHARMACOLOGIC THERAPIES

All smokers who are ready to make a serious attempt to quit should be strongly encouraged to use pharmacotherapy to aid their quitting efforts, except where contraindicated (Table 24-4). As with other chronic disease conditions,

GOOD REASONS TO STOP SMOKING NOW

Its never too late to quit. The body begins to repair itself within minutes of the last cigarette.

Within 20 minutes of your last cigarette:
- Blood pressure begins to reduce
- Pulse drops to a more normal rate
- The temperature of hands and feet increases to normal

8 Hours:
- Carbon monoxide in the blood returns to normal
- Oxygen level in blood increases

24 Hours:
- Chance of heart attack decreases

48 Hours:
- Nerve endings start re-growing
- Your ability to smell and taste things is improved

72 Hours:
- Bronchial tubes relax, making breathing easier

2 Weeks to 3 Months:
- Circulation improves and walking becomes easier
- Lung function increases up to 30 percent

1 Month to 9 Months:
- Coughing, sinus congestion, fatigue, and shortness of breath all decrease
- Cilia re-grow in the lungs increasing your ability to handle mucus, clean the lungs, and reduce infection
- Your body's overall energy level increases

5 Years:
- The lung cancer death rate for the average smoker is cut in half

10 Years:
- Risk of lung cancer is almost as low as for those who never smoked
- Risk of other cancers (mouth, larynx, kidney, bladder, pancreas) all decrease.

Taken from the American Cancer Society's FreshStart program.

BENEFITS OF QUITTING SMOKING

- ☺ Fresher breath.
- ☺ Cleaner smelling hair and clothes.
- ☺ Whiter teeth.
- $ Saving money (a pack-a-day smoker will save almost $1,000 per year).
- ☺ Freedom from social restrictions and the demands of addiction.
    - → no need to ensure continual cigarette supply.
- ☺ Improved circulation.
- ☺ Improved ability to exercise.
- ☺ Longer and better life.
- ☺ Less chance of having a heart attack, stroke, and cancer.
- ☺ Reduced risk of lung disease, fewer problems with existing respiratory disease.
- ☺ Improved health for the people you live with, especially your children.
- ☺ Better health: ex-smokers have fewer days of illness, fewer health complaints, better self-reported health status.
- ☺ After 10 years the risk of lung cancer for ex-smokers is cut in half.
- ☺ In about 10 years, the risk of stroke for ex-smokers is the same as for people who never smoked.
- ☺ For people with heart disease, quitting smoking reduces the risk of repeat heart attacks and death from heart disease by over 50%

FIG. 24-4. Lists to assist patients who need help identifying reasons to quit.

Concerns about Quitting (decisional balance worksheet)

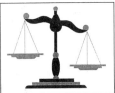

Reasons I'd Like to Quit	Concerns About Quitting Smoking
1. _____	1. _____
2. _____	2. _____
3. _____	3. _____
4. _____	4. _____
5. _____	5. _____
6. _____	6. _____
7. _____	7. _____
8. _____	8. _____

FIG. 24-5. The decisional balance worksheet.

nicotine dependence is best treated using multiple modalities. Physicians are advised to discourage patients from trying a single method and then switching to another single method only if the first approach fails. That strategy is likely to weaken the patient's resolve to quit before achieving success. Two first-line medications are effective for smoking cessation: bupropion and NRT. NRT is currently available in four different delivery formats: transdermal patch, gum, nasal spray, and inhaler. Using either of these pharmacologic options increases the odds of successful cessation by 50% to 150% (32–34). NRT and bupropion can be used simultaneously because they have different mechanisms of action. They are synergistic: using both entities together is more effective than using either alone. Clonidine and nortriptyline have also shown some efficacy for smoking cessation, but they are not recommended as first-line treatment at present (35–37).

Key points related to pharmacologic therapy include:

- Pharmacotherapy doubles quit rates and is safe for most patients.
- Pharmacotherapy is effective for a broad range of patients and should NOT be reserved for "hard core" smokers or heavy smokers.
- Different medication types (e.g., bupropion and NRT) can be combined to enhance chances of success.
- Combining the nicotine patch with self-administered forms of NRT (e.g. gum, inhaler) may be more effective than using a single form of NRT for some smokers.
- Long-term pharmacotherapy can reduce the risk of relapse.

NICOTINE REPLACEMENT IN CARDIAC PATIENTS

When used in medical settings, NRT plus physician advice can produce impressive abstinence rates (38). Soon after the nicotine patch was approved for use, the media reported a possible link between patch use and cardiovascular incidents. The use of NRT in cardiac patients has been of concern because some of the cardiotoxic effects of smoking are attributable to nicotine. Although nicotine does have sympathomimetic effects that increase heart rate and blood pressure, and stimulate vasoconstriction, NRT use generally leads to significantly lower blood nicotine levels compared with smoking, even in patients who smoke during NRT treatment (39–42). NRT use is likely to result in fewer adverse cardiovascular effects than continued smoking. Anecdotal reports of adverse cardiac events have made physicians hesitant to prescribe NRT for cardiac patients (43–45). Systematic research over the past decade finds no reliable association between acute cardiovascular events and the use of the nicotine patch, even among patients who continue to smoke while using the patch (46–48).

Because cigarette smoking in general and nicotine ingestion in particular have cardiovascular effects, some caution is warranted regarding the safety of NRT among certain cardiac patients, such as those with (a) immediate (within 2 weeks) history of myocardial infarction; (b) serious arrhythmias; and (c) severe or worsening angina pectoris. Note that these are cautions, not contraindications. The physician must weigh the benefits of smoking cessation against any possible risk from nicotine replacement. Bupropion is generally well tolerated in cardiac patients, although rare reports have been made of exacerbation of hypertension.

PROGRAM REFERRAL

Most smoking cessation efforts are enhanced by behavioral supports. These can include self-help materials, telephone calls, support groups, and individual therapy for smoking cessation. Intervention intensity is positively associated

TABLE 24-3. *First-line pharmacologic therapies*

Medication	Bupropion (Zyban)	Nicotine patch	Nicotine polacrilex (gum)	Nicotine inhaler	Nicotine nasal spray
Contraindications	Seizure disorder, current bupropion use (e.g., Wellbutrin) or MAO inhibitors, anorexia or bulimia, allergy to bupropion	Severe eczema, allergy to adhesives or other skin disease	Severe temporomandibular joint disease, jaw problems, dentures	None	Presence of asthma, rhinitis, nasal polyps, or sinusitis
Precautions	Usually well tolerated by patients with cardiovascular disease—infrequent reports of hypertension	Recent (2 wk) myocardial infarction, severe arrhythmia, severe angina pectoris	Same as nicotine patch	Same as nicotine patch Use caution with patients who have asthma, wheezing, or other pulmonary disease	Same as nicotine inhaler
Dosage/use instructions	150 mg once a day for 3 d, 150 mg twice per day for 7–12 weeks Start 7–10 days prior to quit date	Available in 7–21 mg doses Treatment usually lasts 4–12 wk with dosage tapering	2 mg and 4 mg One piece every 1–2 h (24/d maximum)	4 mg cartridge (80 inhalations per cartridge); 6–16 cartridges per day; 3–6 months	1–2 doses per hour (5/h and 40/d maximum); 3–6 mo
Availability	Prescription	OTC	OTC	Prescription	Prescription
Adverse reactions (possible remedy)	Dry mouth, insomnia	Skin irritation (hydrocortisone cream/rotate patch sites); vivid dreams (avoid wearing during sleep)	Mouth soreness, hiccups, dyspepsia, jaw ache (review correct chewing technique)	Irritation of mouth, throat, coughing, rhinitis	Irritation in nose and throat, watery eyes, sneezing and cough
Comments	May be used concurrently with nicotine replacement therapy Treatment can be maintained for 6 mo	Vary initial dose with smoking rate (e.g., <15 cigarettes/d should start at lower dosage; >35/d may need higher dose) May work best for regular-interval smokers	May work especially well for light or irregular smokers May help with oral substitution Requires proper chewing technique	May work especially well for light or irregular smokers May help with oral substitution	

MAO, monoamine oxidase; OTC, over the counter.

TABLE 24-4. *Efficacy and estimated abstinence rates for intervention types and intensities*

Level of contact	Number of studies	Estimated odds ratio (range)	Average abstinence rates
No intervention	39	1.0	10.9
Physician advice: (3 min)	10	1.3 (1.1–1.6)	13.4
Self-help	93	1.2 (1.1–1.4)	12.3
Telephone counseling	26	1.2 (1.1–1.4)	13.1
Group counseling	52	1.3 (1.1–1.6)	13.9
Individual counseling	67	1.7 (1.4–2.0)	16.8

Adapted from Fiore MC, Bailey WC, Cohen SJ, et al. Treating tobacco use and dependence. Clinical practice guideline. Rockville, MD: US Dept of Health and Human Services, Public Health Service, June 2000; with permission.

with cessation success: essentially "more is better." Minimal interventions, such as brief (<3 minutes) counseling, from a physician increase the chance of successful cessation by approximately 30%, whereas high-intensity interventions such as individual counseling can more than double quit rates. Therefore, the more intervention resources the physician provides to the patient, the more likely the patient will quit smoking (Table 24-5).

BOOKS AND OTHER SELF-HELP RESOURCES

Numerous books and tapes are available as self-help aids for smokers who are attempting to quit. Most recently, a number of Internet Web sites have sprung up offering assistance to smokers who are trying to quit. Internet sites can be especially helpful to some smokers because chat rooms and other supports are available 24 hours a day. Many helpful books are available to patients who want to quit smoking. A few of these aids are listed below.

Quitting

The Stop Smoking Workbook: Your Guide to Healthy Quitting (Anita Maximin and Lori Stevio-Rust, New Harbinger Publications, 1995).

This stop-smoking guide is outstanding because of its comprehensive content and its interactive workbook format. The practical exercises take smokers through a structured process that enables them to understand the realities of addiction and the different phases of quitting to help them make the changes in their lives that are necessary to quit for good.

No-Nag, No-Guilt: Do-It-Your-Own Way Guide to Quitting Smoking (Tom Ferguson, Random House, Inc. 1998). Dr. Ferguson is an experienced medical writer who avoids antismoking rhetoric. Instead, he offers a reasonable, practical program for smokers who want to quit.

American Cancer Society's "Fresh Start." This is a 21-day gradual smoking reduction program that is helpful for smokers who wish to quit without using NRT. This book addresses coping with cigarette cravings, withdrawal symptoms, and the benefits of quitting smoking.

Quit Smoking for Good: A Supportive Program for Permanent Smoking Cessation (Andrea Baer, Crossing Press, 1998). This book focuses on making emotional and behavioral changes needed to prepare for permanent smoke-free living.

American Lung Association 7 Steps to a Smoke-Free Life (Edwin Fisher, Jr. and C. Everett Koop, John Wiley & Sons, 1998). Based on the American Lung Association's "Freedom from Smoking" program, this book helps smokers identify smoking triggers and develop coping strategies. Contains worksheets, checklists, and quick quit tips.

The Complete Idiot's Guide to Quitting Smoking (Lowell Kleinman, Deborah Messina-Kleinman, and Mitchell Nides, Macmillan Publishing, 2000). A solid, comprehensive guide to smoking cessation and pharmacotherapy.

TABLE 24-5. *Problem solving*

Problem/concern	Possible solution
Strong, continued withdrawal symptoms or cravings	Nicotine replacement therapy If quit >1 wk, start at lower dose (7 mg patch) Consider therapy with bupropion
Depressive symptoms or negative mood	Provide counseling If significant, prescribe medication OR Refer to specialist
Weight gain	Emphasize healthy diet (no strict dieting) Suggest increasing physical activity Most people gain <10 lbs and is self-limiting Consider medications known to delay/reduce weight gain (e.g., nicotine gum, bupropion)
Lack of support for cessation	Schedule follow-up visit Identify social or family supports Refer to organization for support
Low motivation	Assess for cravings/withdrawal symptoms Recommend rewarding activities Emphasize benefits of quitting smoking

When It Hurts Too Much To Quit: Smoking and Depression (Gerald Mayer, Desert City Press, 1997). This book presents information about the special challenges facing smokers who are trying to quit while experiencing clinical depression. It addresses the relationship between smoking and depression, the basics of brain chemistry, the essentials of effective treatment, and making choices about getting help.

Relapse Prevention

Out of the Ashes: Help for People Who have Stopped Smoking. (Peter Holmes & Peggy Holmes, Fairview Press, 1992). This book offers exsmokers new ways to cope with the challenges of remaining smoke-free.

Web Sites

Many patients are familiar with computers and may have access at home or work to the Internet. This form of support can be particularly helpful to smokers who are having difficulty. They can access help and support on a 24-hour basis. The following is a list of smoking cessation support sites with a brief review of their contents. All site addresses (in bold) begin with http://www. except for the Nicotine Anonymous site.

Clever.net/chrisco/nosmoke/cafe.html

A long, convoluted Web address with a high-quality Web site at the other end: the "No Smoke Cafe." The site includes "Counselor Larry": pages containing a wealth of information about making psychological and behavioral changes needed to quit. This site also features chat rooms, message boards, and inspirational information about tobacco use and quitting.

Quitsmoking.about.com

This site is part of the "About.com" network of health-related Web sites. The site contains a lot of information about smoking cessation methods, the "Ash Kickers" discussion forum, and links to many other resources.

Lungusa.com

The American Lung Association Web site featuring "Freedom from Smoking" and "7-Steps to a Smoke-Free Life" programs. This site offers help in English and Spanish.

Nicorette.com

This SmithKline Beecham Web site features Nicorette gum and the "Committed quitters" program—a sound self-help cessation program for NRT gum users. Available in English and Spanish.

Zyban.com

This is the Glaxo Wellcome site is dedicated to providing information about Zyban and the "Zyban Advantage" smoking cessation support program.

Smokehelp.org

The "Smokers Helpline" Web site, this site has general information about quitting smoking, the dangers of tobacco use, and so on. Caution: this site states that quitting cold turkey is the "best way" for most people to quit, and discourages NRT use.

Cancer.org

This, the American Cancer Society Web site, is difficult to navigate and has only generalized informational pages about smoking-related issues, without providing much hands-on help. For example, clicking on their "Fresh Start" program brings up a single page telling you that "Fresh Start" is a program to help people quit smoking—with no content about the program, information, or links to any actual program.

http://nicotine-anonymous.org

The Nicotine Anonymous Web site has contacts for local chapters and instructions on setting up a nicotine anonymous (NA) group. NA follows a traditional 12-step model of addiction recovery. Caution: this site states that "Nicotine Anonymous accepts that nicotine is a toxic, addictive substance that endangers our quality of life," but goes on to say: "We neither endorse nor oppose such devices as nicotine gum or patches." This resource might be helpful to smokers who need group support, but the apparent bias against NRT and confusion between tobacco versus nicotine as toxic substances warrants caution.

SUMMARY AND CONCLUSIONS

Because 75% of all smokers will visit a physician at least once each year (1), smoking cessation interventions delivered in medical settings can reach a wide range of smokers who otherwise might not present for treatment (15). Medical settings can also provide a unique, teachable moment in which to influence patients' perception of risk from smoking-related illness, and to enhance their motivation to quit (51,52).

Tobacco use is unique in that it constitutes a highly significant public health threat, for which clinicians tend not to intervene consistently, despite the presence of effective treatments. Specialists are even less likely to provide smoking counseling than primary care physicians (16,24). This is particularly unfortunate because smokers are more likely to quit when counseling is provided within the context of a sick visit (23). The reluctance of many physicians to provide counseling can be traced to many factors, including lack of counseling skills, inadequate training, time pressures (e.g., patients per hour), and absent organizational support. Large, multilayered hospital systems, third-party insurers, and administrative structures often create barriers to physicians trying to provide preventive health counseling. Physicians should not bear the entire blame for this unfortunate deficit in proactive preventive health intervention. However, physicians can and should always strive to address smoking with their patients with the same vigor with which they address hypertension. The guidelines for physician intervention presented in this chapter reflect recommendations for clinician intervention produced by the AHRQ and US Public Health Service (21). These recommendations should become the standard of care for the millennium and be embraced by physicians, mid-level providers, and healthcare systems as they strive together to free their patients once and for all from the addiction to nicotine and the morbidity and mortality that inevitably surround tobacco use.

REFERENCES

1. US Department of Health and Human Services. Cigarette smoking among adults—United States 1994. *MMWR* 1996;45:588–590.
2. US Department of Health and Human Services. Health benefits of smoking cessation. Report of the US Surgeon General. Washington, DC: US GPO DHHS Pub. No. (CDC) 90–8416, 1990.
3. Miller LS, Zhang X, Rice DP, et al. State estimates of total medical expenditures attributable to cigarette smoking, 1993. *Public Health Rep* 1998;113:447–458.
4. Peto R, Lopez AD, Boreham, et al. *Mortality from smoking in developing countries: 1950–2000.* Oxford: Oxford University Press, 1994.
5. Giovino GA, Henningfield JE, Tomar SL, et al. Epidemiology of tobacco use and dependence. *Epidemiol Rev* 1995;16:48–65.
6. Centers for Disease Control and Prevention. Health objectives for the nation. Cigarette smoking among adults—United States, 1997. *MMWR* 1999a;48:993–996.
7. Centers for Disease Control. Mortality patterns—United States, 1997. *MMWR* 1999b;48:664–668.
8. Houston-Miller N, Smith PM, DeBusk RF, et al. Smoking cessation in hospitalized patients: results of a randomized trial. *Arch Intern Med* 1997;157:409–415.
9. Orleans CT, Ockene JK. Routine hospital-based quit-smoking treatment for the post myocardial infarction patient: an idea whose time has come. *J Am Coll Cariol* 1993;22:1703–1705.
10. Rigotti N, Arnsten JH, McKool KM, et al. Efficacy of a smoking cessation program for hospital patients. *Arch Intern Med* 1997;157: 2653–2660.
11. Glasgow RE, Stevens VJ, Vogt TM, et al. Changes in smoking associated with hospitalization: quit rates, predictive variables, and intervention implications. *American Journal of Health Promotion* 1991;6:24–29.
12. Rigotti N, McKool KM, Shiffman S. Predictors of smoking cessation after coronary artery bypass graft surgery. *Ann Intern Med* 1994;120: 287–293.
13. Stevens VJ, O'Malley MS, Villagra VG, et al. A smoking cessation intervention for hospital patients. *Med Care* 1993;31:65–72.
14. Perkins K. Maintaining smoking abstinence after myocardial infarction. *J Subst Abuse* 1988;1:91–107.
15. Goldstein MG, Niaura R, Willey-Lessne C, et al. Physicians counseling smokers: a population-based survey of patient's perceptions of health care provider delivered smoking cessation interventions. *Arch Intern Med* 1997;157:1313–1319.
16. Thorndike AN, Rigotti NA, Stafford RS, et al. National patterns in the treatment of smokers by physicians. *JAMA* 1998;279:604–608.
17. Cohen SJ, Katz BP, Drook CA, et al. Encouraging primary care physicians to help smokers quit. A randomized controlled trial. *Ann Intern Med* 1989;61:822–830.
18. Cummings SR, Stein MJ, Hansen B, et al. Smoking counseling and preventive medicine. A survey of internists in private practices and health maintenance organizations. *Arch Intern Med* 1989;149:345–349.
19. Lewis CE, Clancy C, Leake B, et al. The counseling practices of internists. *Ann Intern Med* 1991;114:54–58.
20. Strecher VJ, O'Malley MS, Villagra VG, et al. Can residents be trained to counsel patients about quitting smoking? Results from a randomized trial. *J Gen Intern Med* 1991;6:9–17.
21. Fiore MC, Bailey WC, Cohen SJ, et al. Treating tobacco use and dependence. Clinical practice guideline. Rockville, MD: US Department of Health and Human Services, Public Health Service, June 2000.
22. Ockene JK, Kristeller J, Pbert L, et al. The physician-delivered smoking intervention projects: can short-term interventions produce long-term effects for a general outpatient population? *Health Psychol* 1994;13:278–281.
23. Daughton D, Susman J, Sitorius M, et al. Transdermal nicotine therapy and primary care: importance of counseling demographic and participant selection factors on 1-year quit rates. *Arch Fam Med* 1998;7:425–430.
24. Jaen CR, Stange KC, Tumiel LM, et al. Missed opportunities for prevention: smoking cessation counseling and the competing demands of practice. *J Fam Pract* 1997;45:348–354.
25. Prochaska JO, DiClemente CC. Stages and processes of self-change of smoking: toward an integrative model of change. *J Consult Clin Psychol* 1983;51:390–395.
26. Sciamanna CN, Hoch JS, Duke GC, et al. Comparison of five measures of motivation to quit smoking among a sample of hospitalized smokers. *J Gen Intern Med* 2000;15:16–23.
26a. Heatherton TF, Kozlowski LT, Frecker RC, et al. The Fagerstrom test for nicotine dependence: a revision of the Fagerstrom Tolerance Questionnaire. *British Journal of Addiction* 1991;86:1119–1127.
27. Leischow S, Muramoto ML, Cook G, et al. OTC nicotine patches: effectiveness alone and with brief physician intervention. *Am J Health Beh* 1999;23:61–69.
28. Miller W, Rollnick S. *Motivational interviewing: preparing people to change addictive behavior.* New York: Guilford, 1991.
29. Rundmo T, Smedslund G, Gotestam KG. Motivation for smoking cessation among the Norwegian public. *Addict Behav* 1997;22:377–386.
30. Colby SM, Barnett NP, Monti PM, et al. Brief motivational interviewing in a hospital setting for adolescent smoking: a preliminary study. *J Consult Clin Psychol* 1998;66:574–578.
31. Prochaska JO, Goldstein MG. Process of smoking cessation. Implications for clinicians. *Clin Chest Med* 1991;12:727–735.
32. Cepeda-Benito A. Meta-analytical review of the efficacy of nicotine chewing gum in smoking treatment programs. *J Consult Clin Psychol* 1993;61:822–830.
33. Henningfield JE. Nicotine medications for smoking cessation. *N Engl J Med* 1995;333:1196–1203.
34. Jorenby DE, Leischow S, Nides M, et al. A controlled trial of sustained-release bupropion, a nicotine patch or both for smoking cessation. *N Engl J Med* 1999;340:685–691.
35. Hall SM, Reus VI, Munoz RF, et al. Nortriptyline and cognitive-behavioral therapy in the treatment of cigarette smoking. *Arch Gen Psychiatry* 1998;55:683–690.
36. Hughes J, Goldstein MG. Recent advances in the pharmacotherapy of smoking. *JAMA* 1999;281:72–76.
37. Wei H, Young D. Effect of clonidine on cigarette cessation and in the alleviation of withdrawal symptoms. *British Journal of Addiction* 1988;83:1221–1226.
38. Sachs DPL, Sawe U, Leischow SJ. Effectiveness of a 16-hour transdermal nicotine patch in a medical practice setting, without intensive group counseling. *Arch Intern Med* 1993;153:1881–1890.
39. Benowitz NL. Pharmacologic aspects of cigarette smoking and nicotine addiction. *N Engl J Med* 1984;319:1318–1330.
40. Benowitz NL, Fitzgerald GA, Wilson M, et al. Nicotine effects on eicosanoid formation and hemostatic function: comparison of transdermal nicotine and cigarette smoking. *J Am Coll Cardiol* 1993;22:1159–1167.
41. Transdermal Nicotine Study Group. Transdermal nicotine for smoking cessation: six months results from two multi-center controlled clinical trials. *JAMA* 1991;266:3133–3138.
42. Joseph AM, Westman EC. Transdermal nicotine therapy for older medically ill patients: a pilot study. *J Gen Intern Med* 1995;10[Suppl]: 101.
43. Warner JG Jr., Little WC. Myocardial infarction in a patient who smoked while wearing a nicotine patch. *Ann Intern Med* 1994;120: 695.
44. Jackson M. Cerebral arterial narrowing with nicotine patch. *Lancet* 1993;342:236–237.
45. Arnaot MR. Treating heart disease: nicotine patches may not be safe. *BMJ* 1995;310:663–664.
46. Benowitz NL, Gourlay SG. Cardiovascular toxicity of nicotine: implications for nicotine replacement therapy. *J Am Coll Cardiol* 1997;29: 1422–1431.
47. Joseph AM, Norman SM, Ferry LH, et al. The safety of transdermal nicotine as an aid to smoking cessation in patients with cardiac disease. *N Engl J Med* 1996;335:1792–1798.
48. Mahmarian JJ, Moye LA, Nasser GA, et al. Nicotine patch therapy in

smoking cessation reduces the extent of exercise-induced myocardial ischemia. *J Am Coll Cardiol* 1997;30:125–130.

49. Brandon TH, Tiffany ST, Obremski K, et al. Postcessation cigarette use: the process of relapse. *Addict Behav* 1990;15:105–114.

50. Carroll KM. Relapse prevention as a psychosocial treatment: a review of controlled clinical trials. *Exp Clin Psychopharmacol* 1996;4:46–54.

51. Emmons K, Goldstein MG. Smokers who are hospitalized: a window of opportunity for cessation interventions. *Prev Med* 1992;21:262–269.

52. Bock BC, Becker B, Partridge R, et al. Physician intervention and patient attitudes among smokers with acute respiratory illness in the emergency department. *Prev Med* (in press).

Subject Index

Note: Page numbers followed by *f* indicate figures; page numbers followed by *t* indicate tables.

251